The
BACK STAGE®
Handbook for
Performing
Artists

W9-DHO-035

The
BACK STAGE®
Handbook for
Performing
Artists

3

Revised and Enlarged Third Edition

The How-to and Who-to-Contact Reference for Actors, Singers, and Dancers

Compiled and Edited by

Sherry Eaker

BACK STAGE BOOKS
An imprint of Watson-Guptill Publications, New York

Sherry Eaker is the editor of *Back Stage*, the national trade publication geared to the performing artist in both the commercial and nonprofit theatre arenas. As editor since 1977, she has overseen the growth of the paper, which was founded in 1960, to its present form as a national performing arts weekly. She serves on the board of the League of Professional Theatre Women and is both a Tony Award and Drama Desk Award voter. She is a member of the National Theatre Conference and the Manhattan Association of Cabarets and Clubs. She frequently produces and moderates panel discussions focusing on the working actor and issues in the theatre community.

Copyright © 1995 by BPI Communications, Inc.
This edition first published in 1995 in the United States by Back Stage Books, an imprint of Watson-Guptill Publications, a division of BPI Communications, Inc., 1515 Broadway, New York, NY 10036-8986

Library of Congress Cataloging-in-Publication Data:

The Back stage handbook for the performing artist : the how-to and who-to-contact reference for actors, singers, and dancers / compiled and edited by Sherry Eaker. — Rev. and enl. 3rd ed.
     p.   cm.
   Includes index.
   ISBN 0-8230-7599-0 (alk. paper)
   1. Acting—Vocational guidance—United States—Directories.
   2. Performing arts—Vocational guidance—United States—Directories.
   I. Eaker, Sherry.
PN2055.B27 1995   95-39667
791'.023'73—dc20   CIP

Senior Editor: Paul Lukas
Associate Editor: Dale Ramsey
Designer: Jay Anning
Production Manager: Ellen Greene

Manufactured in the United States of America.

2 3 4 5 / 99 98 97 96

*To my father, who raised the curtain for me
and made it all possible, and to my mother,
who's been coaching me along the way.*

I'd like to thank Michèle LaRue and Diane Snyder for their invaluable assistance on this project. Many thanks as well to my assistant Randee Bayer-Spittel; to the editorial staff of *Back Stage*, including Andy Buck, Scott Proudfit, and Emily Kapnek; to Dale Ramsey, the book editor on this project; and to Paul Lucas, who provided editorial assistance. My gratitude to Actors' Equity Association, Screen Actors Guild, the American Federation of TV and Radio Artists, the Casting Society of America, Jill Charles, and *PerformInk* for their cooperation. Finally, a sincere acknowledgment to all the freelance feature writers, columnists, and reviewers who have made valuable contributions to *Back Stage* throughout the years.

Contents

List of Advertisers

Preface

How do you succeed in business without really trying? In show business, you simply don't. Choosing a career in the performing arts goes beyond just having a natural talent. It takes a lot of effort on one's part to climb that ladder of success. It calls for continuous training (in all types of skills), auditioning, making the rounds, periodic mailings, networking—and one hasn't even mentioned the performing aspect yet: That's just a fringe benefit of the job. You'll have to face up to the fact that most of your time will be taken up by looking for and finding the work.

One of the key factors for success in this business is being aware of the range of opportunities that are out there. Another key factor is learning how to take advantage of those opportunities that are right for you.

In essence, that's what this book is all about: helping the artist identify the wide range of jobs that exist in the performing field and learn how to make the necessary contacts in order to pursue them.

This is also the focus of *Back Stage*, the weekly trade paper geared to the performing artist. Each week, aside from carrying audition information for film and stage productions going on in New York and around the country, *Back Stage* features "how-to" articles designed to help actors, singers, dancers, directors, playwrights, and other talents move ahead in their careers.

The idea of putting all these articles together in book form is the result of the countless requests I receive asking for specific back issues. In response to those requests, the first edition of *The Handbook for Performing Artists* was published in 1989. Its success led to a revised and enlarged edition in 1991; the popularity of that book prompted the decision to publish this third edition.

Whereas the first two books focused primarily on those performers first starting out in the business, this newest handbook emphasizes the many outlets awaiting the talented performer in today's market. As in the past, the more than two dozen essays, written by experts in the performing arts, were culled from *Back Stage*. Topics that were covered in previous editions, such as commercial print, cabaret, stand-up comedy, business theatre, theme parks, cruise lines, and TV commercials, have been completely rewritten. In addition, many new subject areas are covered, including summer stock, voice-overs, jingle singing, soap opera, student films, radio drama, museum theatre, and producing and booking a one-person show. As was the case in previous editions, the text is supplemented by lists of agents, casting directors, personal managers, producers, theatres, acting schools, cabaret and comedy clubs, and union offices. However, in this edition it was decided to run all the lists in an appendix at the end of the 25 chapters; some of them are specific to a particular chapter, others provide more general information.

Twenty years ago when I first entered the business, it seemed as if performers were limited to a small segment of the entertainment industry, specializing in just one or two areas. But times have changed, and so has the business. Competition is fierce, money is tight, but there's also new and growing opportunities all over the country. Whether they present themselves on stage, before the camera, or in front of a microphone, in New York, Los Angeles, or any other city, doesn't really matter. These are all outlets for the performance skills you've been working so hard to perfect. Success comes in all sizes.

—SHERRY EAKER

Putting Your Best Face Forward:
The Actor's Headshot
JILL CHARLES

The actor's number-one marketing tool is the picture/résumé. This 8-by-10-inch business card consists of a black-and-white photo stapled back-to-back at all four corners to a clear and concise résumé. It announces to the industry: "Here I am! Don't you want a closer look?"

Putting together your first picture/résumé (or revamping your old one) will take a few weeks of concentrated effort and considerable expense. But it is time and money well spent, if the result is a compelling photo and striking résumé.

Selecting Your Photographer

Begin by looking at other people's pictures, lots of them. Don't just look for good shots; you can learn what to avoid from studying ineffective ones. Ask other actors how they felt at their shoots: Were they made to feel relaxed and not rushed? Did they achieve a real rapport with the photographer? Were they comfortable asking questions? Did they *enjoy* the shoot? Remember that you are not looking for the "best" photographer, but for the photographer with whom you can work well to achieve the best picture of yourself.

After you have made a list of at least six photographers from all your research, call each one to set a time to stop by to see his (or her) book and to meet the photographer in person. Peruse the book carefully. Do the subjects look different from each other? Do they invite you into the frame with their eyes, so that you want to learn more about them as actors?

Notice the technical facility of the photographer. Are skin tones (textures) realistic? Does lighting show features clearly, neither washing out portions of the face nor hiding any area in shadow? Can you tell which actors are blonds? (That's the hardest hair color to light in a black-and-white photo.)

Ask for complete details about the fee—what number of shots does it include, and what guarantees do you have of getting a shot you are happy with? Are the services of a makeup artist included? Is retouching extra? How does the photographer feel about portrait and headshot styles? What poses and clothing does he think would work best for you? How does he run a shoot? Most important, do you feel that this photographer *wants* to photograph you; is he excited by the prospect of capturing your being on film?

Finally, go home and forget about the whole thing for a day or two. The "right" photographer will pop into your head as the obvious choice.

Photo Styles

While the concept of the picture/résumé has remained constant for many years, photography styles have varied. Fifteen years ago, everyone used glossy, black-and-white headshots with white borders. Then the fashion changed to borderless prints with a matte finish. A couple of years ago, more of the body began to show up, in a "portrait" style, with a wide white border set off by a thin black line. Today, most actors have at least one portrait-style photo taken along with a standard headshot. A good theatrical photographer should be comfortable doing both in the same shooting session.

One thing to remember is that, to show more body, the camera will pull back from the subject; the face will become proportionately smaller, making the eyes less effective. Including the torso only as far down as the elbows will keep the face more important than it is in a shot to the waist or lower.

Peter Principato, a commercial talent agent at William Morris in New York City, feels that the wide white border focuses attention on the actor more than the borderless headshot does. Barry Shapiro, a commercial casting director with New York's Herman & Lipson Casting, comments, "If actors are in their 20s or 30s, and they think their body will help sell them, then they should do more of the body, probably a three-quarter. If the actor is 50 or 60, that's not necessary." Shapiro also cautioned women against being overly made-up for their photos.

You will probably be selecting two or three different shots for reproduction, so it makes sense to vary the amount of body shown: perhaps one headshot (which may include shoulders), one "to the table," and one three-quarter or fully frontal view. However much of your body you decide to show, it's wise to consider the purpose of the shots. When you take a photo with "commercial" in mind, always include a warm, full smile. The photo for theatre and film can be more relaxed, with a casual smile. Your third shot might be more glamorous, if you feel that you fit into the soap opera casting world.

Send the shot you feel is most appropriate for a given job; at an audition, it's fine to offer two different shots if you're not sure which is more suitable, and let the casting people keep the one they prefer.

Preparing for the Photo Session

The more carefully you prepare for a photo shoot, the more relaxed you will be, thus ensuring good pictures.

In thinking about a commercial shot, consider whether you fit more into the all-American or the upscale business-executive type. If the first, choose casual clothes in light colors with open collars. Patterns are acceptable if the contrast is not too stark; stay away from white, and from jewelry, hats, and props.

If you're going for the upscale look, you'll want business clothing such as a blazer or jacket with a tie or a bow blouse complemented by a watch and understated earrings. You might use glasses (without lenses), but no other props. For a theatre/film shot, pick clothing to support a more introspective, thoughtful side of yourself. You might choose garments that you are especially fond of in terms of colors, texture, and history.

For a soap shot, women can go with glamorous evening wear, with a low neckline (make up all skin evenly). For men, the same clothing as for the theatre shot will probably work, with a change of expression we'll discuss later.

It is tempting, but generally unwise, to use photographic means to disguise or hide physical traits like crooked teeth, birthmarks, your weight, or the shape of your nose. This can backfire if a busy casting person calls you in on the basis of what she's seen in a photo, and that's not what she sees when you come in the door.

Makeup

An actress who does not feel completely competent and at ease with her own makeup would be advised to spend the extra money to have a professional do it, so that she can be completely relaxed at the actual shoot.

Women should always wear makeup for the photo, even if they wear little or none in everyday life. The amount to use in your photo depends somewhat on your personal appeal (are you a "natural" or a more "glamorous" type?) and the purpose of the photo (theatre, commercial, soap). An actress who is trying to get those three different photos out of her session will want to change hair and makeup accordingly. The most important thing about the makeup for your theatre and film picture is that it be consistent with the way you will look when you go to an audition. Your commercial makeup might be slightly more styled and upscale, while your soap shot would be a more glamorous evening look.

If you have decided to do your own makeup and hair, keep these things in mind: Use a good-quality base that covers without caking the skin, so your natural skin tones show. Don't attempt to cover attractive skin features, like freckles.

When adding color it's essential to remember that you are making up for black-and-white film, for color is seen as shadow. This means cheek color should go lower to accent the cheekbone; if it is applied on the cheekbone (as in normal daytime makeup, to add color) it will take out the contour. Eye shadow works the same way; it will not read as color, but will deepen your eye sockets. Eyeliner should be soft, applied with a brush sparingly, with very little on the lower lid. Use mascara as you would normally. Lipstick is another example of color being meaningless—it is the contrast to your skin, not the color, that will show.

Hairstyling, too, will vary, from casual for theatre and film to more coifed for commercial and glamorously styled for soaps. If you have long, straight hair, you need enough of a set to give it some fullness and body on the sides so that it frames your face attractively.

Men might want to use a little bit of cream base to lighten a very heavy beard, for photos tend to accentuate dark beards. An actor who frequently wears a beard might want to get the most out of a session by doing a full range of facial hair, first shooting with full beard and mustache, then shaving the mustache only, then finally appearing clean-shaven. Shave carefully, and if you have had a beard for a long time be prepared to add makeup to even out the tones of your face.

Finally, schedule your session for the time of day you look and feel your best and most active. You should bring along some of your favorite music, remembering that you want to be alive and "up," not simply relaxed. Don't relax yourself with any alcohol or drugs; even one glass of wine instantly dulls the eyes.

At the Photo Session

It is essential to create an action at the photo shoot, so that the finished photo is a moment captured in active time, not a pose. If during the shoot you're thinking about yourself or what you look like, rather than playing an action, the photo will look posed and frozen. Also, giving yourself an acting task will probably eliminate the tension that some people feel in front of a camera, since you will have something else to concentrate on. To avoid the tension, let the camera eye become a person you care about, and then invite that person into the action.

When setting up your actions, remember: Adjectives freeze, verbs free. Instead of trying to look "happy," you should be thinking something like, "Come here! I really want to show you this!"

Commercial shots need a smile, but it should be an active, natural smile that is integrated—your eyes must smile, as well as your mouth. You want to show your teeth without featuring them and to avoid that wooden, toothy grin. To do this, try creating an active situation for yourself, like sharing a treat with a child, or calling a child to come see something very special. Say a sentence out loud: An enthusiastic "Come with me!" can help present a bright expression, and the word "me" shows teeth. For an upscale commercial shot you want a similar enthusiasm, but at a more adult level, where the stakes are a little higher.

Your theatre and film shot might be more thoughtful or have some mystery to it, but keep it active. Think of planning something or hatching a plot, or think of coiled energy—something is about to happen. Carry this idea into something more provocative for the soap shot, so that there's a sexy, playful secret in your eyes.

After the Shoot

The photographer will give you sheets of the first prints of your pictures. Not yet enlarged to full size, these are called contact prints. Always look at these prints through a magnifying glass and a sheet of white paper with a square the size of one small picture cut out of it. That way you will be looking at each picture individually, which is very different from seeing all of them at once. Trusting your first impressions and following the same criteria you used when you looked at the photographer's portfolio, make rough choices right away. Then take them to a few trusted friends, including a director or casting director if you can. But ultimately you're relying on your own judgment.

In the interest of presenting yourself as you really are, the only retouching that should be done on your full-size photo is to soften lines that normal photography will freeze into an unnatural hardness, and remove blemishes that are not permanent.

Your final step is to have the original print(s), now retouched, reproduced in quantity. It is important that the original print that you get from the photographer be in correct contrast; even black hair should have detail in it, and very light skin have texture. Reproductions generally increase the contrast (light goes lighter, dark goes darker), so these details are important. The reproduction process involves reshooting your original 8 x 10 to produce a larger negative, which then is used to make inexpensive copies. Before the copies are run off from this negative, most labs offer a test print for a little extra cost. When inspecting the test print, look for the closest possible similarity to the original print in terms of contrast and skin tone.

A poor reproduction of your photograph can destroy the uniqueness that you and your photographer worked so hard to achieve.

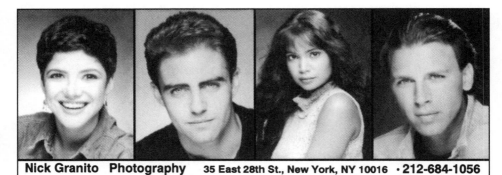

Nick Granito Photography   35 East 28th St., New York, NY 10016 • 212-684-1056

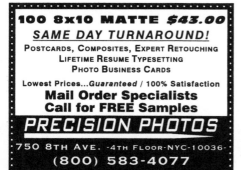
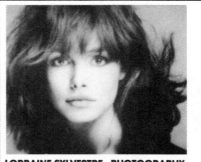

LORRAINE SYLVESTRE - PHOTOGRAPHY

(212) 675-8134-INFO BY APPT

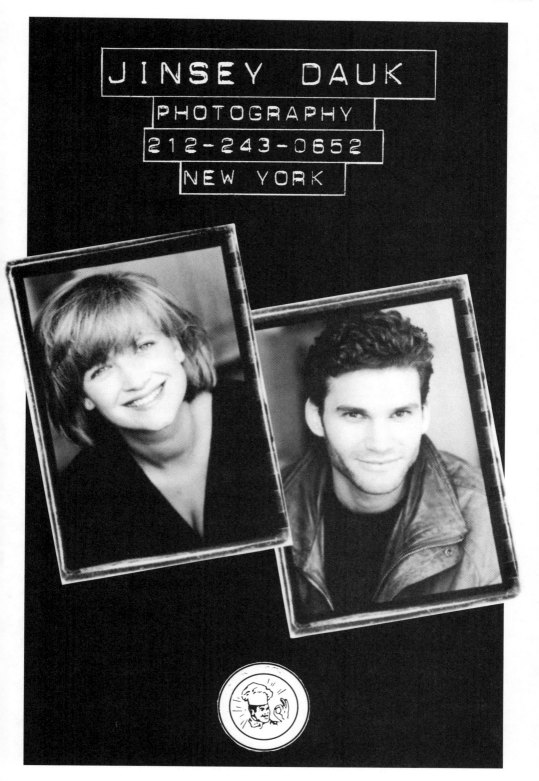

JINSEY DAUK

PHOTOGRAPHY

212-243-0652

NEW YORK

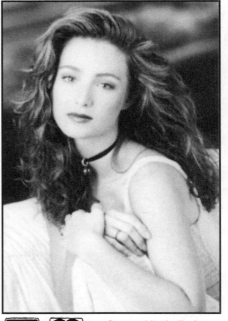

L U K E

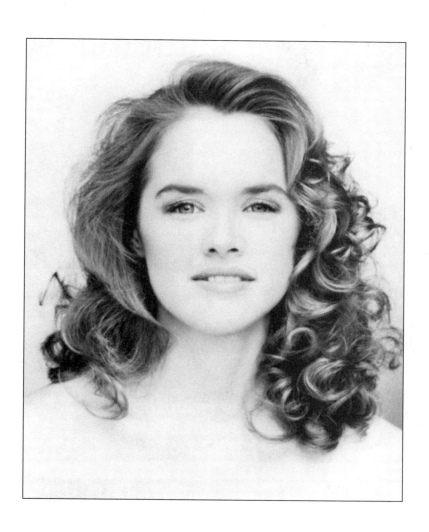

L O I S

594 BROADWAY SUITE 1106 NEW YORK, NY 10012 • (212) 925-4501 FAX (212) 925-4718

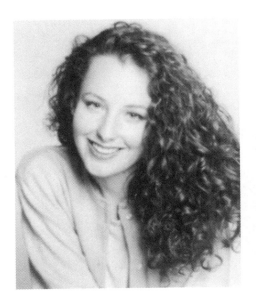

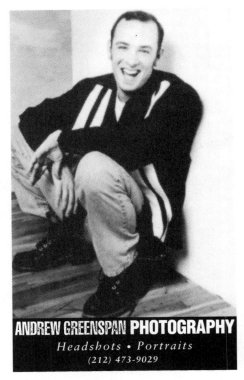

**CHIA MESSINA
PHOTOGRAPHY
212 929 0917**

ANDREW GREENSPAN **PHOTOGRAPHY**

Headshots • Portraits
(212) 473-9029

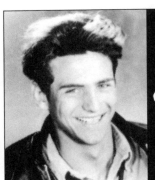

john hart

**The Best Headshots
...naturally
(212) 873-6585**

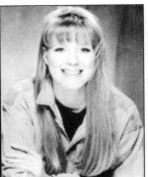

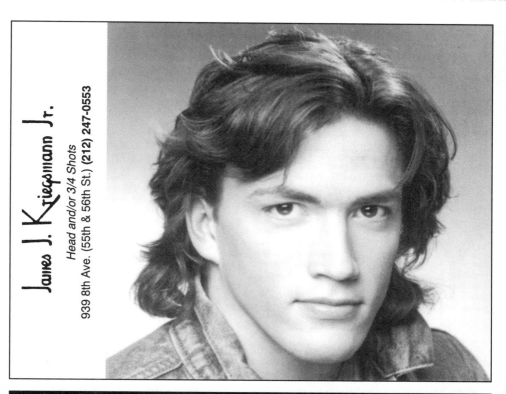

James J. Kriegmann Jr.
Head and/or 3/4 Shots
939 8th Ave. (55th & 56th St.) (212) 247-0553

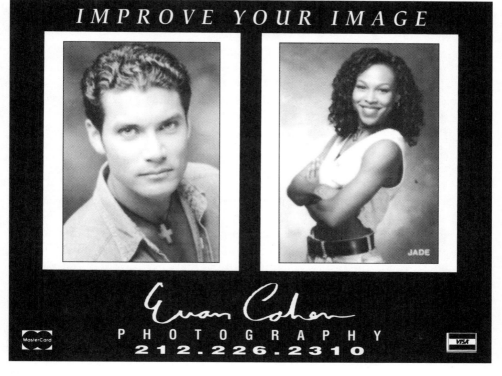

IMPROVE YOUR IMAGE

JADE

Evan Cohen
PHOTOGRAPHY
212.226.2310

MasterCard

VISA

21

2

The Flip Side:
The Actor's Résumé

JILL CHARLES

Your résumé is your chance to represent your experience, training, and skills to the casting person behind the table at an audition. Begin by making a list of your acting credits and training, then think about the best light in which they can be shown. For example, if you're a young actor with few professional credits, you can include the names of highly respected professionals who directed or taught you, or an apprenticeship at a good Equity theatre. No one expects a 20-year-old to have the kind of credits a 35-year-old has accumulated; it is the depth of training and the caliber of the people one has worked with that will stand out on a young actor's résumé.

The best credits in the world won't do any good if they're not read—and they may not be if the résumé is cluttered. Drop all dates, and put credits on a résumé in order of importance, not in chronological order. And *never* lie on a résumé. It's too easy to be found out, and having discovered one lie, the casting person will distrust everything else on your résumé, too.

The professional actor's résumé consists of three sections: vital statistics, credits, and training and special skills.

Vital Statistics
Every résumé should have on it the actor's name, contact phone number, union affiliations, and talent agent, if the actor is represented. Don't list a home address or home phone number unless, instead of a service, you use an answering machine at your home.

Vital statistics are your height, weight, and eye and hair color. The casting person must have immediate reference to these facts. It is not necessary to list your age or age range (let the casting person determine that), nor do you need to list measurements or clothing sizes except in a modeling résumé.

You might include your social security number (some agents prefer that their clients do so), but this is not essential because it's not needed until you're hired for a job. You might want to include "U.S. Citizen" or "Naturalized Citizen."

Some performers note "Singer" or "Actor–Singer" under their names. Such a label can emphasize your strengths, but it can also take you out of consideration for other categories. "Actor" implies one who doesn't sing at all; "Singer" implies that acting skills are secondary or even negligible. However, listing a vocal range is important if you can sing at all; if there is no mention of vocal range and no musical credits, the assumption is that you're tone deaf. If you can carry a tune, put your voice range on the résumé. The extent of your singing ability should be evident through any musical credits listed and by your training.

Credits

The section that lists your credits is usually organized by genre: "Theatre," "Film," "Television," and "Commercials." If you have sufficiently diverse experience, you may want to break "Theatre" down into subsections like "Broadway," "National Tours," "Off-Broadway," "Showcase," "Stock," and "Regional." Or you may want to distinguish simply between "New York" (which can encompass Showcases, Off-, and Off-Off-Broadway) and "Regional and Stock."

Which category comes first on the résumé depends on where your emphasis as a performer is and where your best credits are. If you work a good deal in more than one genre, it is a good idea to have two résumés with different layouts, so that your film résumé lists film and TV credits first and in depth, while your theatrical résumé has the theatre credits first and then a simplified film listing.

As a general rule, your credits are the most important section on your résumé, since casting people tend to look for "sure bets." If they're casting Max in *Lend Me a Tenor,* for instance, a role in a Feydeau farce holds more weight than having played Hamlet at a summer Shakespeare festival. For that reason it's a good idea to cover as many bases as possible on your credit list. Consider your credits carefully as you add and delete them from your résumé. (A role you did years ago might still deserve a place, if it's your best example of classical work.)

"List upon request" may be all you wish to put under the commercial section if you have a significant number of those credits. If you have only a few, you may wish to list them to make it obvious that you have on-camera experience. For smaller film and TV parts you can just cite the show, rather than "under five," "day player," etc., since one assumes that a larger part will have a character name.

Theatre credits should always state where a listed role was played. The phrase "representative roles" is a transparent camouflage for "roles I did in scene study class" or "roles I would like to play." Your résumé should represent your actual experience: the role, the play, and the theatre where you played it. This is important not only to give credence to your résumé, but because directors may pick up on mutual acquaintances, which gives you something to talk about at an audition or interview and makes you more memorable. Whether you list all the directors you've worked under or just the better-known ones is a choice you should make based on the impressiveness of the list and the overall look it will give to the layout. It is not necessary to list playwrights' names, unless you worked on a new play and want to emphasize that fact.

Training and Special Skills

In the "Training" section, if you have trained with well-known teachers, include their names; otherwise, the type and duration of training is sufficient. The purpose of this section, for the casting director, is twofold: to see where (and with whom, if applicable) you trained, and to determine the areas and extent of your training in acting, voice, dance, and related theatre skills.

The "Special Skills" section should show related talents that might be useful in commercial work or that could be an extra attraction to a theatre company. Start with theatre-related skills like stage combat, acrobatics, musical instruments, accents, and dialects. Include athletic abilities and whether you drive a car (standard and/or automatic). You can add to the list almost anything you do well—photography, graphic design, American Sign Language, carpentry, electronics, and so on. Most commercial agencies have a "special skills" file to run to when they're looking for jugglers, equestrians, and so forth. The list of skills that could be useful to a theatre company or in a particular commercial or industrial is almost endless, and these things, too, can generate conversation at an interview or audition.

Printing Your Résumé

You should give the layout and composition of your résumé every bit as much energy as you devoted to your photo. Go to a copy center where there is a display of résumés and step back from a group of them. Which draw your eye? Typefaces, borders and rules, margins and other open space, and arrangement of copy are factors in making a résumé not only striking but easy to read. Remember that the layout of the résumé must fall within an 8 x 10 space so it can be trimmed to match your photo without overlapping edges.

You may be able to do your résumé yourself on a computer with a high-quality (preferably laser) printer. If you can't do your own, be sure you find a service that offers not only high-quality graphics, but a storage service, so that your résumé can be simply—and cheaply—updated as needed. Once you are satisfied with the look of the original, you're ready to reproduce it.

The job is complete when you've securely attached your résumé to your photo, either by staples in all four corners or by rubber cement or another paper glue around the edges. It may seem inconsequential, but résumés that are bigger than their photos or aren't securely attached are a pet peeve of casting people. They're also likely to become separated in casting files, so don't let sloppy assembly ruin your chances for an audition.

The Finished Product

Assembling your picture/résumé is a painstaking procedure. But you'll find it worth the effort when, finally, you march up to those casting people with a package you're proud of. That's the best start to a great audition.

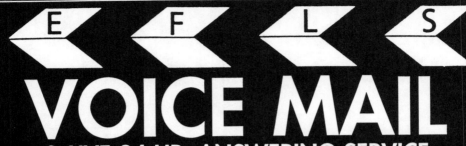

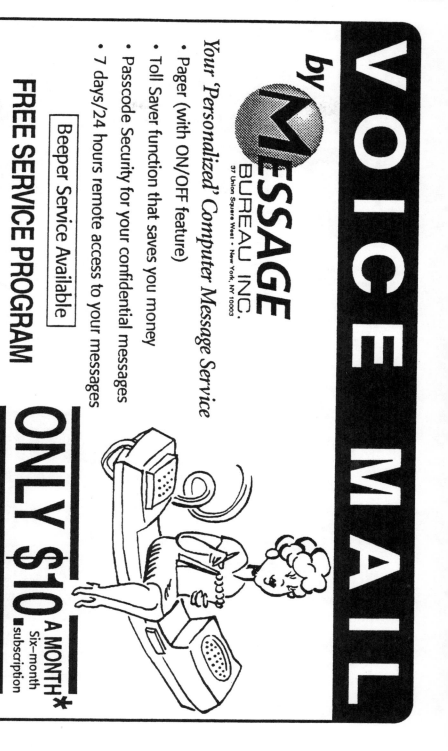

VOICE MAIL

VOICE MAIL by

MESSAGE BUREAU INC.
37 Union Square West · New York, NY 10003

Your 'Personalized' Computer Message Service

- Pager (with ON/OFF feature)
- Toll Saver function that saves you money
- Passcode Security for your confidential messages
- 7 days/24 hours remote access to your messages

Beeper Service Available

FREE SERVICE PROGRAM

ONLY $10 A MONTH*
■ Six-month subscription

Call (212) 255-3155 for immediate service.

Joining the Unions:
The Why, When, and How
MICHÈLE LaRUE

For many performers, "being union" means being professional. But getting your membership card *does not* automatically make you a mature pro, and it certainly doesn't guarantee you work. Like any important career move, joining a performers' union requires careful research and deliberation—and it also helps to be the right person in the right place at the right time. Certainly, "How do you get in the union?" is a critical question. But before you tackle that "how," you should very carefully study the "why" and "when."

We interviewed representatives from the largest of the several performers' unions: Actors' Equity Association (AEA, which protects principals, chorus, and stage managers in live theatre), Screen Actors Guild (SAG, whose jurisdictions are primarily television commercials and film), and the American Federation of Television and Radio Artists (AFTRA, which represents performers on radio and TV, audio and video tape, phono, cable TV, and slide films).

Two other major unions are the American Guild of Musical Artists (AGMA, for musical performers in opera, dance, oratorios, concerts, and recitals), and the American Guild of Variety Artists (AGVA, for singers, dancers, and comedians in revue or variety situations). SAG, AFTRA, and Equity have for many years been discussing a merger, but until that complicated proceeding is negotiated, each of these unions abides by its own rules.

The "Why"
Peter Harris has been an Equity member for 54 years and a staffer in the New York office for nearly 25. As business rep for Theatre for Young Audiences for more than 21 years, he introduced thousands of young actors to the union. Now officially retired but still active on Equity's TYA Committee, he gives several reasons why one would join a union.

The first is professionalism. Equity membership assures your potential employers and co-workers that you are serious about the theatre, that acting or stage-managing is not interim employment; it's your profession. Second, union contracts set salary minimums which are usually higher than those volunteered by nonunion producers. They include benefits almost never offered outside the union, like health insurance coverage and pension points.

As collective bargaining agencies, unions exist to promote and protect their members' welfare. They monitor employers to ensure that agreed-upon monies and benefits are received on time; that performers work in safe, sanitary environments and get ample rest; that they are compensated for extra rehearsal and performance time; and that they are respected by producers, directors, and fellow members.

For the health of the unions and the profession as a whole, Harris explains, unions discipline their members, too. Thereby they guarantee employers that their investment in union performers will secure professional behavior—no unlearned lines, no late arrivals or no-shows for rehearsals or performances, no physical, drug, or alcohol abuse on the job.

Each union has its own membership "perks," as well. Equity, SAG, and AFTRA communicate with their members, via newspapers and magazines, and arrange professional seminars throughout the year. The three jointly manage the Actors' Federal Credit Union, which is sympathetic to performers' needs and provides banking services and some shopper discount plans.

Unions support the welfare of the theatre community by contributing to national organizations like The Actors' Fund of America, the SAG AIDS Task Force, and Broadway Cares/Equity Fights AIDS. Equity, SAG, and AFTRA sponsor the In-School Reading Program in New York, Los Angeles, and Chicago. Several scholarship programs are available to the children of AFTRA members. Equity members frequently are "comped" for live shows, and in New York and Los Angeles, SAG's Film Society offers sizeable discounts on screenings of new features. Additional services may be available in your area's union offices. In New York, for instance, SAG and AFTRA offer equipment and instruction in on-camera and film performance; Equity, SAG, and AFTRA hold periodic lotteries that introduce members to agents.

The "When"

If you're right out of college or conservatory, you may dream of quick validation of your talent through union membership. But even if you're precocious—or lucky—enough to get an immediate offer, think twice before taking it. If you become Equity at too young an age, you can price yourself out of the market. There are far more young performers than there are suitable roles for them, and those roles are generally easy to fill cheaply with young non-Equity actors. Nonunion companies offer a great deal of work, and the more experience you have before you "go union," the better your chances of employment as a union member.

"A student-age person unfamiliar with the business, even if eligible, should not rush in and join," counsels SAG's executive administrator in New York, Bill Weiner. First, he says, "try to get as much exposure in as many ways as possible—in live showcases, in classes, by speaking to as many actors as you can about what it's like trying to make a living in the business. Make sure this is a career choice, not a hobby."

Because joining the unions is an expensive process and a long-term commitment, Weiner advises that you "do your homework before you come to this decision." Be sure acting is what *you*—not your mother or great uncle—want for yourself. Before you join, get high school and college experience, and, urges Equity's Harris, be sure you have another source of income lined up.

The "How"

Each union has its own membership qualifications and procedures. We'll begin with the least complex:

AFTRA

Founded in 1937, AFTRA represents 79,000 members, including actors, newscasters, announcers, disk jockeys, sportscasters, panelists, moderators, and specialty acts. They work in radio, on phonographic recordings, and on live and videotaped television. These performers are served by a national board of 116 members from every geographic area and every category of membership, and by 37 locals across the nation.

AFTRA's initiation fee varies by local office, ranging from $125, in Peoria, Illinois, to $800, in New York City and Los Angeles. Each local also sets its own semiannual dues and caps. In New York, the minimum, $42.50 twice yearly, is based on annual income of $0 to $2,000. An additional 1.5 percent is assessed on earnings, with a $792.50 semiannual cap. Los Angeles' base dues are also $42.50 twice yearly, but its semiannual cap is $1,585.

A performer may join AFTRA, with or without a job offer, by applying to his or her local office.

SAG

Founded in 1933, SAG is a national union representing 73,000 performers working in films (including theatrical, TV, industrial, educational, and experimental) and in music videos. In some cases, TV shows on tape go to SAG, as well. Upon joining, the eligible performer pays SAG's $1,008 initiation fee, plus the union's basic dues, $42.50 twice yearly, which are paid by all members on SAG earnings of $5,000 or less. Additional dues on earnings above this amount are tiered: Members are assessed 1.5 percent of their SAG income over $5,000, to a limit of $150,000. SAG, like Equity and AFTRA, reduces this amount for members who joined through other, "parent" unions.

An actor satisfying any of the following qualifications may join SAG by making an appointment with its New Membership Department.

1. Entering SAG via *Employment as a Principal Performer* requires, within two weeks, proof of employment, or prospective employment, by a SAG signatory company in a principal or speaking role in a SAG film, videotape, TV program, or commercial. You may apply as soon as you have your contract in hand or, if you prefer, after you have completed the work. Your proof of employment will be a signed contract, a payroll check or check stub, or a letter from the company. This document *must* include your name and Social Security number, the name of the production or commercial, the salary, and the date(s) of employment.

2. Entering via *Employment as an Extra* requires proof of employment as a SAG-covered extra player at full SAG rates and conditions for a minimum of three work days. The employer must be signed to a SAG Extra Players Agreement for a SAG film, videotape, TV program, or commercial. Proofs of employment conditions are virtually identical to those listed above for principal performers.

3. If you are already a paid-up member of an affiliated performers' union for a period of at least one year *and* have worked at least once as a principal in that union's jurisdiction, you are eligible for SAG membership. Affiliates are Equity, AFTRA, AGMA, AGVA, the Hebrew Actors' Union (HAU), the Italian Actors' Union (IAU), the former Screen Extras Guild (SEG), and Canada's ACTRA.

Actors' Equity

The oldest of the three major U.S. actors' unions, Equity was founded in 1913. A national organization, it represents 40,000 legitimate principals, chorus members, and stage managers. Equity's initiation fee, $800, is reduced by as much as $400 for those who are already members of AGMA, HAU, IAU, or APATE (Asociacion Puertorriquena de Artistas y Tecnicos del Espectaculo). Annual dues are paid in two $39 installments.

You can "go Equity" in three ways:

1. If you are offered an Equity standard contract, you are eligible to join the union upon its signing. Standard contracts include all Production (primarily Broadway and national tours), LORT (League of Resident Theatres), Stock, and Dinner Theatre contracts. Some tiers of Equity's lesser contracts require you to meet length-of-employment and wage-earning minimums, too. These include LOA (Letter of Agreement), SPT (Small Professional Theatre), TYA (Theatre for Young Audiences), and Mini (a scaled-down Off-Broadway contract). Some contracts allow producers to economize by hiring a small percentage of non-Equity cast members; only in these instances may you as a nonunion member work in an Equity production.

2. Participation in Equity's *Membership Candidate Program* allows nonprofessionals to credit their work toward Equity membership. To become a candidate for this program, you must secure a nonprofessional position at an Equity theatre offering it. Next, you must complete the registration form provided by the theatre and submit it to Equity with a $100 registration fee, which is deducted from your initiation fee when you join. After 50 weeks of work (which may be nonconsecutive) at one or more accredited theatres, a registered candidate may join Equity. Or, after 40 weeks of work, a candidate may take a written exam and join if he or she passes. Upon completing the program, you are eligible for five years to join Equity. During that time, you cannot contract with any Equity theatre except *through* Equity. (A list of theatres and additional information about the Membership Candidate Program are available at your regional Equity office.)

3. Finally, Equity takes membership applications from those who, for at least one year, have been members of AFTRA, SAG, AGMA, AGVA, HAU, IAU, APATE, or SEG. You must prove yourself to be an active member in good standing in one of these unions, and to have worked under union jurisdiction on either one principal, one "under-five," or three days of an extra contract.

Non-Equity actors who qualify as "Eligible Performers" can get priority at union calls. To do so, you must meet certain criteria that Equity has established to guarantee that everyone brings a minimal level of professionalism to interviews and auditions. Eligibility is based primarily on the number of weeks worked within a given period of time and minimum salary earned as a performer, whether on stage or in other media. Your regional Equity office will have details.

Leaving the Unions

If, after all, you decide that professional performance is not for you, there are mechanisms for temporary or permanent withdrawal.

For AFTRA, simply write a letter to your local office stating that you want to retire from active membership, for any reason. You may reactivate your membership at any time. You will not be charged dues during your period of withdrawal, although if you work in AFTRA's jurisdiction, your membership will be reactivated. You may continue to perform under the jurisdiction of any other union of which you are an active member in good standing.

SAG has two means of going on inactive status: Honorable Withdrawal and Suspended Payment. Each must be requested by applying in writing to the Membership Department just prior to either dues period (May 1 or November 1). The applicant must have been a SAG member for at least 18 consecutive months and an active member for at least one year. After becoming inactive, he or she must remain so for at least one year.

Honorable Withdrawal is granted to those whose dues are paid in full at the time of their request. Upon returning to active status, the member pays only the dues owed for the current period.

Suspended Payment permits withdrawal by those whose dues are not paid up at the time they apply. Applicants may be no more than two periods behind in dues payment (excluding the current period). When they return to active membership, they must pay the outstanding dues, plus the current period's.

Members choosing either of these options receive an Honorable With-drawal or Suspended Payment card. Inactive members may *not* seek employment under SAG's jurisdiction and therefore are precluded from attending open calls and auditioning.

Equity's *Temporary Withdrawal* is granted to members who request it in writing. Withdrawal can be for any length of time—although after five years, the member loses first rights to his or her professional name. A return to active status requires a $25 reinstatement fee plus payment of dues for the current period.

Equity has a Suspended Payment status also for members who cannot pay their dues. The balance owed is "frozen" and must be paid upon reinstatement, together with a $25 fee and current dues.

Equity members are forbidden to work in non-Equity productions while on Temporary Withdrawal or Suspended Payment. Full resignation from Equity requires special administrative approval from the main office.

Performers who enter the union as children fall under a special rule: Until they reach age 14, young Equity members may work in nonunion as well as Equity shows. (The membership department should be contacted for specific instructions.) From age 14 on, however, their legitimate theatre work must fall under the protection of the appropriate Equity agreement.

Summing Up

If performing is to be your career—and if you're a capable performer—someday the unions will be an important part of your life. In preparation for that time, you should understand what membership will require of you and do for you.

For a list of the performing artists' unions, see Appendix, page 216.

4

Get It in Writing!
Performers' Guidelines for Contract Negotiation
MICHÈLE LaRUE

As an actor, singer, or dancer, you may work with dozens of employers under a variety of conditions each year. Getting the conditions of your employment in writing is crucial. Even pleasant, well-meaning, ethical people make mistakes, misremember details, keep sloppy accounts, get distracted, and/or fall behind on deadlines. Then there are the not-so-ethical people who honor only those agreements that suit their own needs, and the dedicated idealists who are lost in "Art" and blind to realities like paying the piper.

Of course, "getting it in writing" is easy to endorse in the abstract, but in real life, where personal desires and extenuating circumstances color every decision, it's all too tempting to disregard your own good sense, to avoid making trouble, to *not* get it in writing. In a business in which too many people passionately pursue too few jobs, you can hear only what you want to hear, so mere oral agreements affecting your work and income can be dangerous.

A contract is a tool which should not be feared by either party. Lisa Kaplan Zabel, a New York-based arts and entertainment attorney, advises:

> You should think of entering into a contract as an opportunity to explore the proposed working relationship, rather than as an adversarial process. The drafting of a written agreement allows each party to learn about the expectations of the other. The process of negotiating the contract—particularly a written contract—gives both parties the opportunity to define relationships, goals of the collaboration, rights and responsibilties, and, of course, fundamental terms like pay and working conditions. . . . A person who is affronted by your request for a written contract is probably going to take personally many other issues in your business and artistic relationship.

Kaplan Zabel quickly points out that, yes, "even oral agreements are binding in most cases, and the parties do have some redress if the agreement's not honored. *But the difficulty is a matter of proof."* If it isn't on paper, how does a judge, jury, or arbitrator know who is telling the truth, or—in the case of honest mistakes—whose perception of the truth is more accurate?

Disagreements frequently do result from misperceptions, rather than deliberate deceit. "Conflicts can arise in a collaboration just because no one predicted the problem, or because you're acting in good faith but not on the same wavelength," observes Nancy Adelson, senior legal counsel at Volunteer Lawyers for the Arts in Manhattan. By having a mutually agreed-upon written document to which they can refer at any time, two parties can preserve their valued relationship.

Must You Have a Lawyer?

"A contract is simply an agreement, a meeting of the minds: 'I will give you an apple, and you will give me a dime.' It can be as simple or as complicated as you want," explains Adelson. And while she allows that you can write a contract without a lawyer, she does believe that availing yourself of expert advice is a good idea: "If you're just starting out, you can't anticipate what's coming down the pike. A producer may say that he's giving you a 'standard' contract, but how do you know what 'standard' means?"

Performers often seek help from Volunteer Lawyers for the Arts. Founded in New York City in 1969, the not-for-profit VLA is a network that boasts nearly 50 independent affiliates in the United States and Canada. It offers legal advice and assistance to individual artists and arts groups that have specific questions directly related to the arts.

VLA's free Art Law Line is (212) 319-2910; an initial call brings a response within 48 hours. If VLA can't help you, you'll be referred to some other possibilities. If it can, you'll be asked a few questions about your financial situation. VLA's charter empowers it to provide legal aid *gratis* to whose who qualify; those who don't are directed to other sources. If you do qualify, you'll consult with a staff lawyer and be billed only an administrative fee ranging from $30 to $50. NYC–VLA matches cases requiring additional consultation with one of its 800 volunteers in the area.

The VLA National Directory profiles each of the organizations in the network. It's available from:

Volunteer Lawyers for the Arts
1 E. 53rd Street
New York, NY 10022
Att'n: Publications Department

The cost is $15.00, plus $4.00 for shipping.

What Should a Contract Include?

The performers' unions have evolved a variety of standard contracts and agreements. The performer and producer are required to sign and file completed copies of one of these with the appropriate union before rehearsals begin. The basic guarantees these contracts give can be supplemented by mutually agreed-upon "riders" added during negotiations. If you're a nonunion performer, you'll either have a contract presented to you by your would-be employer, or you'll need to create one yourself.

Kaplan Zabel explains, "Some of the particulars that performers will probably want to focus on are the time at which they're to be paid, the form of payment, what happens if the production is closed during rehearsal or performance, what kind of advertising and billing the actor is going to get, and the actor's right to perform in other things concurrently." A performer going on the road will also need to know whether he or she will be paid a per diem; what type of accommodations will be provided, if any; and who pays for transportation, *each way*.

Additionally, you may want to put in writing any specifics about your rehearsal period (how many hours it will take each day or week, and what happens if you go overtime), who supplies the costumes, what kind of security the building has, what kind of dressing rooms will be provided, and whether the performers will be asked to do anything offstage—like move scenery or wait tables.

You can anticipate the producer's responses to some of these questions by doing your homework. For instance, books like Theatre Communications Group's *Theatre Profiles* and Jill Charles' *Regional Theatre* and *Summer Theatre* directories list each theatre company's union affiliations, as does *Back Stage* in its casting notices. Read the trade papers and collect facts from other performers. Those who have worked with a producer can tell you about the kind of working and housing provisions, production schedule, and compensation you can expect from him or her.

Dancers may want to specify what kind of floor they'll be dancing on and may be particularly concerned about issues of health and casualty insurance. Dancers who choreograph, and actors or singers who are asked to improvise while rehearsing a work in progress, should thoroughly explore the question of ownership: Who holds the copyright?

Consider, too, the context in which you're working. If you're doing a showcase or workshop production, you're going to have a low budget, and you're likely to be dealing with a relatively inexperienced director and/or producer. We all have to start somewhere, and overly enthusiastic novices often make mistakes. Being prepared for these may not require the negotiation of an absurdly detailed contract so much as the adoption of a tolerant attitude towards the process of artistic maturation.

On some projects, "profit-sharing can be a reasonable alternative," says Adelson. "It's often worth taking risks and accepting less money initially, because this work may help you go on to make a name for yourself."

Kaplan Zabel concludes: "It's important to understand that, once there is a written contract, it supercedes any oral understandings. For any matter that is covered in the contract, the court will not be willing to hear about oral representations. It's as if anything that's not written does not exist." So if you discover that your contract requires modifications, make them with a written amendment. A handshake isn't enough.

One Union's View

For some general advice from a union perspective, we went to Gareth May, agency representative, and Chuck Blasius, a former business representative at Actors' Equity Association. Like Adelson and Kaplan Zabel, May endorses doing your own research. Producers, he explains, are required to "post bond" with Equity before rehearsals begin. (Bond is an amount of money held in trust by the union until the production has closed and all salaries and claims have been paid to the contracted Equity members. If the producer proves insolvent, the bond generally ensures that members will receive at least the contractual guarantee.) Producers used to post bond much earlier in the preproduction process than they do today. These days, husbanding their front money, producers tend to bond at the last minute—the Friday before the Monday on which rehearsals begin. But each actor must file his or her copy of the contract before beginning work, leaving him only the weekend between bonding and first rehearsal to study the contract—and to try to negotiate additional terms.

Don't wait till the last minute. If you're on your second or third audition with a producer, pick up a copy of the Equity contract applicable to that job and *read* it. Your first task is to understand what it is you'll be agreeing to if you sign: What are your obligations to the producer? What are the producer's obligations to you? What is the producer not obliged to do for you? The provisions which are not guaranteed by the standard contract are those for which you might want to negotiate before signing. A rider, mutually agreed upon and added to your contract at this stage, will define and ensure those provisions.

Riders provide individual performers with rights beyond those guaranteed by the standard Equity contracts. Producers have dozens of standard riders in their computers. Want a per diem or a private dressing room on the road? Somebody presses a key, and there's your rider—just fill in your name.

By the time a producer has cast a given role several times, according to May, the riders as well as the contracts are *pro forma*. But you can still try to negotiate a unique rider if you think something important is missing. Most likely, if the director wants only you for the role, or if you've been asked to play a principal part, you'll have more clout than a chorus member. Generally, the chorus budget is solidly set before casting, but the line item for principals' salaries and perks is more flexible.

The higher-paying contracts tend to be more flexible overall. Don't ask producers operating under a Small Professional Theatre agreement for perks that you'd request on Broadway—they won't have the budgets for it. In these times, nonprofit theatres especially are often unable to negotiate above Equity's contract minimums and conditions. Then, too, certain riders are simply inappropriate to certain contracts. Per diem payments, housing, and transportation, for instance, are add-ons available almost solely to performers working away from home.

Some Specifics About Riders

When producers generate contracts for a production, they will include all the riders they think necessary and will expect not to have to add amendments later. Usually, copies of one contract with its riders will be issued to all members of the company.

Many Equity contracts carry their own standard riders. The Production Contract, for instance, sets terms for minimum additional payment when performers are asked to record a cast album or to perform a scene from the show on Tony night. Another Equity rider ensures increased salaries for roles requiring "extraordinary risk."

One question that frequently arises—especially in the lower-paying contracts and agreements—involves taking time off to do other professional work. The "More Remunerative Employment" (MRE) clause is a provision of many standard Equity contracts and agreements—among them are the Off-Broadway, Letter of Agreement (LOA), Small Professional Theatre (SPT), and Cabaret contracts. The clause allows a performer who is already contracted for a production to leave that show temporarily or permanently for a better-paying job—provided that he or she gives the producer adequate notice as defined by the clause.

This can become a complicated matter. Not only are there contracts in which the MRE clause is *not* an option, like League of Resident Theatres (LORT) and Theatre for Young Audiences (TYA) contracts, but there are those in which the producer can delete the MRE clause entirely by choosing to use Equity's "Run of Play Provision" (ROP) rider. This rider pays the performer a certain premium above the required weekly salary in order to prevent the MRE clause from being implemented. In other words, the producer is spending more money to keep the selected cast intact. Blasius warns performers to be aware of this provision when negotiating. The ROP rider is not available to LOA and SPT producers; it is available in Production, Off-Broadway, Cabaret, and Business Theatre contracts, among others.

Blasius adds that your options for time off can depend on your producer. Some producers will let you do film and TV, even if they are paying you extra under the ROP. May advises that a producer is more likely to grant you days off for a special family event if you specifically request such a rider up front rather than seek a contractual amendment later. (The standard Production Contract actually allows unpaid leave of up to three performances for "compelling circumstances"—a wedding, a funeral, or a serious illness—involving your immediate family.)

Although Equity endorses contractual riders "as long as they're to the general benefit of the member," says May, the union will hesitate to process them if they are unclear and can be misinterpreted. In such cases, Equity sends a letter to the producer, requesting that a new one be written.

Riders can be added to Equity contracts at any time with the mutual consent of the producer and actor. There should be four signed copies: one for you, one for the producer, and one for each of you to forward to the union's Contracts Department. (Remember that Equity can't enforce any side contract between an actor and a producer unless it is on file as a rider with the union.)

"It's up to you to know what you're signing," May states, "and it is the union's responsibility to give you as much information as possible."

Aural Account:
The Voice-Over Business
THOMAS WALSH

You can call them "voice actors," or "voice artists," or "voices of choice." They call themselves very fortunate. The field is voice-overs, and it's one that can prove both satisfying and lucrative for performing artists—a way of making a living as a true performer, though without ever being seen by an audience. "You're magnifying words with the voice, and through that magnification you're making a great impact on an audience," says Steve Harris, a veteran voice-over teacher and performer who is also a regular voice talent on WQCD 101.9-FM in New York.

"You're creating a visual image for a listener and acting with your voice, not with your body or anything else," adds Alice Whitfield, owner of Real-to-Reel Recording, a New York and Los Angeles company that writes, casts, and produces radio and TV voice-overs. "That's why we call it *theatre of the mind*."

When you hear copy being read to accompany a television picture or to deliver a radio message, you're getting much more than a standard sales pitch or a deadpan announcement by a copy-reader. Every syllable of that copy has been vocally shaped by a highly skilled pro who has fused natural ability with years of training to bring out the best from those words. The objective is to convince listeners to respond to the message in a powerful way. And learning to do that consistently is the first step on the road to becoming a successful professional in the intensely competitive and demanding voice-over industry.

TV and radio advertising is certainly the best known, most glamorous, and most profitable area of voice-over work, but there are other, very diverse areas in which voice-over performers are in constant demand, such as documentary narration, animated cartoons, corporate videos, slide shows, "point of purchase" displays, telephone recording systems, training films, and "talking books." In fact, wherever spoken words are needed to help sell a product, promote a service, or provide information to the public, voice-over artists are being hired regularly at attractive pay rates.

Regardless of which segment of the business you're looking to get into, as a craft it is much more difficult than it seems. "A newcomer to the business can be generally naive about most things, and one is that they think this is one of the easiest areas to become an expert in quickly," says Ruth Franklin, who by her count has booked more than 40,000 voice-over jobs and runs a by-audition-only voice-over master class. "They often think that if they can read a book out loud, they can read copy out loud, as though this business is essentially reading out loud. And there's the idea that voice-overs are something to do while waiting for a real career to start, instead of waiting tables. That is absolutely wrong."

"It always has been and always will be a highly competitive field, and it's extremely difficult to break into," notes Maureen Kelly, owner of Just Voices, a New York casting service that handles voice-over jobs only. "But what we look for are actors first, not just good sound."

Voices in Competition

The voice-over game begins with one basic rule: Competition among performers for the available jobs is intense. In good economic times or bad, industry observers have never been terribly optimistic about the prospects for newcomers to break in.

"It's a relentless pursuit," says Harris. The people who are able to work every day number about two dozen. Most voice-over work is born at an ad agency, which relays to the casting director what an ad campaign is about and what kind of talent is needed. Casting directors then describe to the talent agents the types of performers they want to gather for auditions, and the agents follow up by getting in touch with the talent with whom they have worked before and who fit the bill for the project.

Because certain types of voices are better suited to particular products, it is extremely important for performers to determine what "type" they are: Are they great at "character" voices or "spokesperson" voices? What is their age range? What kind of persona does the voice project? Is a young woman better at playing a youthful mother or a young girl? Is a middle-aged man more adept at sounding like a friendly uncle, a "little brother," or a straight-ahead announcer?

Welcome to Training Camp

When veterans of the voice-over profession ask people why they want to work in voice-overs, the most common answer they hear is something to the effect of, "People tell me I have a nice voice," or "a good sound." While those qualities are helpful, they are not nearly enough by themselves to make it in this field.

Talent is vital, but even more important is proper training. Training can take many forms. In New York City alone, several dozen facilities and individuals offer classes, workshops, and seminars that can range from one-shot deals that are a couple of hours long to full-scale courses lasting several months or longer. The teaching techniques also vary widely. Some instructors recommend that their students tape commercials off of television and radio. They offer several reasons: One is to listen to them over and over again to analyze how the performer uses acting skills in reading copy. Another is to imitate the voices on those tapes repeatedly. Other teachers advise students to use good magazine or newspaper ad copy for their reading homework.

Some voice-over teachers have access to sound facilities, where sophisticated microphone and playback equipment is used. Students are frequently asked to bring their homework assignments to these studios for analysis by their instructors and classmates. Other copy reading and acting assignments are often devised on the spot to strengthen abilities further. The main reason that teachers want to get their students into a studio instead of a classroom is to give aspiring performers as many chances as possible to get comfortable in front of a microphone, where they eventually hope to earn a living.

Franklin, a firm believer in strong training, notes:

> The whole point is flexibility, to be able to read differently when necessary. If all you can do is read vegetables, and someone asks you to read face cream, you're sort of out of luck. You need to be able to change deliveries, instead of voices, to suit the product.

On the flip side, Harris maintains:

> I think training and talent are very important, but I've seen people with absolutely no acting experience step up to the mike, read the copy cold, and do a perfect read in 30 seconds. Who can really figure out why some people are naturals at some things? But if you can take classes, you really should. You've often got only 30 seconds to a minute at the audition to be brilliant.

The Audio Résumé

Apart from training and advice, what formal voice-over instruction produces is the single most important tool that a voice-over performer needs: a demo tape. This is a precisely constructed sampling of a voice actor's identity and of what he or she is capable of. It's basically an aural résumé, but unlike a traditional résumé, it is a living document not only of what you've done but what you can do. There is no more fundamental tool than the demo tape, and being without one is like being a graphic artist without a portfolio.

"You have to have a really brilliant professional tape," Franklin declares. "No matter how talented you are, you can't be in the running without it. It has to be competitive with the top people in the field."

The demo is most often an audiocassette tape containing brief snatches of a performer's work from whatever areas he or she has chosen to specialize in. For example, a voice-over artist will generally include on the demo samplings from eight to ten commercials of different kinds—include, for example, spots for an over-the-counter pharmaceutical product, a household product, a food product, a baby product, a local bank, a cosmetic, and so on. Each sample should not be more than 15 or 20 seconds long. (If you are interested in pursuing work doing voice-overs for corporate films, you will need a separate demo with four or five contrasting companies represented.) Pauses between spots shouldn't be excessive (recommendations vary from 3 to 10 seconds). The recommended length for the whole package is generally two to two-and-a-half-minutes, no more, perhaps less.

Only the performer's best material should be on the tape, and of a variety, too, meaning that a commercial for cars shouldn't be followed by one for motorcycles. Says Alice Whitfield, "If the spots on the demo are not sequenced properly, then you're not being heard properly."

The copy used for the demo material should be absolutely top-notch. If you're a student and your class fee includes production of a demo, then copy will probably be provided for you. Some do-it-yourselfers who haven't had a spot produced before and therefore have nothing to read for a demo might try writing their own copy, but several of our experts recommend against it. Magazine or newspaper ad copy is often suggested for those people who don't have credits to their name, and some sound studios have generic copy available.

Professional packaging is strongly stressed, too. Having your name typeset or typewritten on the tape box, instead of hand-lettered, is more likely to sit well with a producer or casting director. The format for listing the tape's contents is another variable; each excerpt can be summarized by a one-word title and its running time in seconds (for example, "Car: 15"), or the client's actual name could be used instead ("Cadillac: 15"). All of the above should be typeset as well, not scrawled.

There are some long-time professionals who prefer to mark the tape with only their name and the words "voice-over demo," letting the spots speak for themselves.

Franklin remarks that "the demo is not meant to be entertaining":

> Many people go wrong on this. It's not meant to be fun, it's only to show skill, and it's a sales tool. When a talent buyer is listening to it, there's a reason, and it's to find a certain voice for a commercial. If it's entertaining, it diverts from the job, and the job is to find an actor.

And Steve Harris adds this advice:

> You shouldn't try to wear a hat that doesn't fit, as far as your type is concerned, and you need to pick really good copy that flatters you. The number-one pet peeve is listening to a demo in which a performer is reading a spot that doesn't make him sound good. If you don't know what you read well, then you're certainly not ready to make a demo. Copy selection is most critical.

A completed demo has to be produced with technical skill. The experts state emphatically that a professional recording studio must be used. As mentioned earlier, many voice-over instructors have access to these studios. If your instructor does not, ask him or her to recommend a recording house, particularly one that specializes in voice-over demos. In the back pages of any issue of *Back Stage* a number of demo experts are listed in the "Services" section. *Shoot* magazine's nationally distributed *Directory for Commercial Production and Postproduction*, published annually, is another source. (To order a copy, send a check for $58, which includes shipping and handling, to: *Shoot* Directory, 1515 Broadway, 12th fl., New York, NY 10036-8986.) The Yellow Pages are also useful in this area.

One way that the demo should *never* be recorded is by you with your own equipment. Even an above-average tape recorder or other consumer sound system cannot match the hardware at a studio. Any facility that produces demos also has the capability to duplicate them, an absolute necessity for any performer. Depending on how serious the voice-over artist is, the number of copies needed varies. Some top people in the field report that they have put several thousand copies of their tapes into the hands of the people doing the hiring.

The dollar figures vary, but basic costs for taking the classes, making a demo, duping it, and mailing copies can range from $500 to well above $1,000. Without classes, you'd be doing well if you spent less than $500 just for studio time, mixing a master copy, and making copies.

Alternative Routes

Though commercials are the primary focus for many voice-over performers, some alternative venues are becoming more and more attractive. Professionals note that most corporations and many good-sized businesses often produce their own training tapes and promotional videos. Public relations firms and some publishing houses produce them for someone else.

When you call certain retail or commercial telephone numbers and you're put on hold, you may hear a promotional spot for those companies; such pitches are being heard more frequently than ever. Just about every voice you hear on those tapes belongs to a voice-over performer. Among the businesses that should be contacted for this kind of work are department stores, travel agencies, airlines, and moving companies.

In fact, there are voice-over talents who use their voices only in these alternative fields and earn six-figure incomes annually, according to several performers and teachers who are doing this. Other areas where voice-over work is in great demand are recorded instructional tapes for community phone systems that tell callers how to get information about a firm ("To speak with a sales representative, press 2 now"), and voice-mail systems. "Talking books"— books read by voice actors and recorded on audiocassettes and compact discs for use by the blind and visually impaired, or for people who simply enjoy listening—are being widely marketed now. In some areas of the country, radio stations seek volunteer voice-over talents to read current newspapers and magazines on the air for visually impaired listeners. Once an aspiring performer identifies potential companies that may need voice-over talent, he or she should send a demo tape to these firms with a brief cover note and should follow up as often as possible.

For artists whose goal is voice-over work in advertising, a key move is to find a list of talent agents, casting directors, performers' unions, advertising agencies, and other entertainment industry resources. A good place to start is with *Ross Reports Television,* a guide published monthly in its edition for the New York market and quarterly in its edition for the national market. Some agents, casting directors, and ad agencies state in their listing that they specialize in representing voice-over performers. Again, the *Shoot* annual directory is another good resource.

Mailing your tape is the most common method of contact, but performers have noted that since you're trying to sell your voice, a phone call can serve as a sort of mini-audition.

Voice-over professionals acknowledge that the chance of becoming a successful voice-over performer without an agent are slim if you are seeking only union work. However, says one experienced artist, "I've seen it happen that a performer without an agent can be sensational, and he gets the jobs."

Cashing In

There are few arguments about the quality of pay in the voice-over field. The basic minimums for jobs covered by the American Federation of Television and Radio Artists and Screen Actors Guild are high, and the money potential for work in nonunion areas can also be high. In the spring of 1994, AFTRA and SAG jointly negotiated a three-year contract with commercial producers, and its coverage includes voice-over work in many segments of advertising on TV and radio. Under the contract, the producer of a commercial made for broadcast TV use under AFTRA and SAG jurisdiction must pay the voice-over artist a minimum of $333.50 per session, and residual payments vary depending on the number of cities in which the spot is aired and the population of these cities. There are additional contracts for cable TV and Spanish-language commercials.

Radio commercials that fall under AFTRA's jurisdiction now pay a minimum rate of $107.15 to $185.00 per session for an announcer. AFTRA has also negotiated minimum salaries with some producers of "point of purchase" promotional spots, telephone recording systems, and other nonbroadcast areas—even talking toys that feature recorded voices and sounds. Also, certain producers of books on tape have paid AFTRA scale to narrators.

A Bright Future

With the huge growth in the cable and satellite-TV businesses and the development of new technologies, especially the computer-compatible compact discs—CD-ROMs and CDIs—the potential for voice-over work seems almost limitless for the performer who knows where to look. Ruth Franklin encourages young voice-over talent with these words:

> If you consider the number of radio stations and commercial and cable TV stations, all of them on 24 hours a day, just imagine the number of voice-over people needed. Think of how much work that is. People who say there's no work out there—well, they're wrong. You just have to know how to find the work—and know how to do it right.

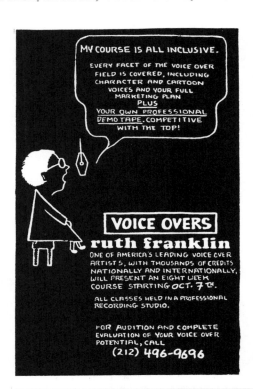
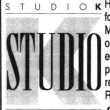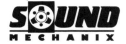

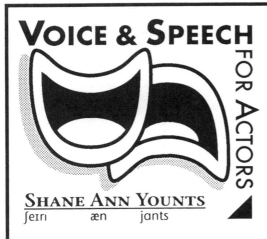

6

Breaking into the Jingle Business

ROBERTA LAWRENCE

Jingles—the brief songs you hear on the radio and TV that tell about the joys of "having it your way" at the fast food chain or note that "This Bud's for you"—represent a way for big business to reach millions of consumers instantaneously. It's a chance to grab them in a minimal amount of time, anywhere from 15 to 60 seconds. Jingles offer an opportunity to sell myriad products, services, and even life-styles to the masses. And the voice you hear singing the tune needs to be one that makes you stop and listen. It must be one that inspires trust, commands attention, and has the ability to persuade. For the lucky few who have vocal cords that are graced with these attributes, entry into the elite world of jingle-singing may be possible.

The rewards can be very lucrative if you get to sing on the right commercials. The highest-paying jobs are usually for national campaigns (ones broadcast across the country) and aired during prime-time shows. A vocalist singing on a national commercial, or "spot," can sometimes make as much as $50,000 in one year, all from a couple of hours in the recording studio.

Payments add up the way they do because of the commercials contracts that were negotiated by the Screen Actors Guild (SAG) and the American Federation of Television and Radio Artists (AFTRA), the two performers' unions whose jurisdictions cover this industry. These contracts include a talent payment scale that is commensurate with how often a spot is being aired, how large a population is being reached, and how much that added exposure benefits the advertiser. That's what residuals, the money periodically paid to singers in addition to the original session fee, actually represent: the mileage that the client is getting from your voice and what that is worth.

Payment for a basic session under SAG and AFTRA contracts varies according to category: whether you're on radio or TV; whether you're on camera or off; and whether you're a group singer or soloist. The highest fee paid is for a solo singer appearing on camera or TV—$333.30 for the session. The other end of the scale is for a group singer or radio spot—$96.30 for the session.

Only AFTRA deals with radio commercials and videotape; SAG deals strictly with film.

The first time you are hired for a union job, you may work even if you are not a member, provided that the producer obtains a Taft-Hartley waiver. This is a written request to hire a nonunion performer and is good for 30 days, after which the singer must join the union before working again under the SAG contract.

Talent and Technique

So how do you become a jingle singer? It takes a combination of talent, luck, skill, and persistence. The reality is, there are not as many spots to go around as there are singers who would like to sing them. That makes it a very competitive field. Novices must keep in mind that they are competing with an elite group of established jingle singers who have already earned their reputations as vocal sharpshooters, and who are probably on every music producer's "A list." This gives you even more reason to do your homework and to be as well prepared as possible before embarking on a campaign to get your foot in the door.

The door is wide open in terms of vocal types that producers and composers are looking for. The spectrum of music written for jingles is wide: easy-listening and show-tune styles, high-energy rock and jazz styles, and whatever style is currently in vogue. Generally, though, the demand for operatic, legitimate, and novelty voices, as compared to pop or rhythm and blues and all the divisions within those genres, is limited to specialized campaigns.

What would be expected of you as far as technique is concerned is another story. One singing coach, the late Ann Countryman, observed, "The better the technique you have, the more responsive you'll be to the demands made upon you in the studio. And the more prepared you are, both musically and technically, the more valuable you will be to a producer."

The requirements for making it as a jingle singer include having good pitch, of course, but also being a quick study; being able to take direction; having the ability to keep reproducing a particular sound (for hours if necessary); and being flexible enough to offer a variety of vocal attitudes.

Group Singers and Soloists

Styles of singing aside, there are two basic categories of singers in the jingle business: group singers and soloists. If you're a group singer, you are usually singing background parts and need to blend with the people you are singing with. The idea is not to have one voice dominate the group, but to mix voices to produce an overall sound with texture and quality. Technical excellence and speed is of paramount importance here, for time and money are critical factors to a music producer. In New York City, for example, the average rate for an hour of recording studio time runs about $275 to $400 for advertising music. So, if you feel you do not have a natural ear for harmonies and rhythms, a course in ear-training and sight-singing are advisable if you want a future in jingle work, especially as a group singer.

For soloists, however, the technical demands are not quite as stringent because other factors are involved. Most people in the business agree that perfection is not what solo singing is about. Drama and magic are the draw here. First of all, music houses are always on the lookout for that great new voice that doesn't sound like anyone else's. "Breaking in as a unique solo talent is always a possibility," according to Jeff Rosner, a producer–rep at JSM Music in New York City. "There's a tremendous demand for someone who has a great voice, and you know it when you hear it. The voice quality just speaks to you. . . . It's a voice that shines."

Jeanne Neary, president of Look, Inc., a New York-based music house, adds, "If singers can 'act' and deliver the message or grab your attention through their belief in the words they are singing, it's more valuable than perfect pitch or a perfect voice." The downside of being a solo singer, as opposed to a group singer, is that because you are always featured as a soloist you run the risk of overexposure—of singing so many commercials that your voice gets too familiar or goes out of fashion. As one producer puts it: "It's a Catch-22 situation, because the more successful you are, the more quickly they get tired of you, and pretty soon they're saying 'Get me somebody *like* him, but not *him.*'" The solution, many agree, is to be able to straddle both categories, solo and group singing.

Your Demo Tape

To be considered for jingle session work, it is necessary to let music houses and advertising agencies with in-house production departments know who you are and what you sound like. This is generally done by sending a demo tape to as many possible sources of musical employment as you can.

The demo tape is your calling card and should be done in as professional an environment as your budget will allow. Call recording studios in your area and compare their hourly rates. Inquire whether they offer any package deals for a finished demo. You don't need a 24-track studio; great things can be done on a 4-track recorder, as well as on 8- and 16-track ones.

The demo tape should contain some musical "sound bites" that demonstrate your singing style and range in a clear and focused way. How you do this depends on how much money you have to spend and how much experience you have. Generally, singers already working in jingles periodically compile a tape that includes the latest spots they have sung. But if you are just starting out, even a well-produced voice-and-piano recording can serve your purpose. Industry insiders suggest that you choose material that complements your voice and is identifiable; the contents don't really matter as long as you sound good and you stand out.

The demo tape should not exceed four minutes. Producers don't always get to listen to your entire tape. Their phones ring, and sessions start, distracting them. You should therefore put your best cuts at the top of the tape. That way, you're assured that they'll be hearing what you really want them to.

Make certain that your tape accurately reflects your *best* voice. If you're a jazz singer, the tape should spell that out. If you're a rocker, there shouldn't be any doubt in any listener's mind as to where to file your tape.

The content should vary. Ideally, it would be great if you had some commercials that you could record as well as excerpts from songs, either well-known ones or good originals. Full backing tracks are good, but many producers also like to hear just a voice-and-piano demo. If you use songs, these should be short segments; a verse and chorus are sufficient. Then move on to the next one.

Don't leave much space in between cuts. Instead, for the listener's sake, aim to cut or fade from one song to the next in as creative and dramatic a fashion as possible. The more exciting an environment you provide for your voice, the better. While still remaining true to your voice, piece your tape together in an interesting way; try varying the tempos and rhythms.

Make sure you get a "DAT" (Digital Audio Tape) demo from the studio. This is a very high-quality tape. You can make more copies as needed and add and delete material as your career grows. Make your copies or "dupes" on high-quality audiocassettes. Label them in a clear way with your name, service phone number, and a listing of contents not only on the insert card but on the cassette itself.

Once you are happy with the sound and contents of your demo tape, try to saturate the market of potential employers with copies. There are industry guides that have listings of music production houses and recording studios, such as *Shoot* magazine's annual *Directory for Commercial Production and Postproduction* (see page 45). Checking your local Yellow Pages may give you leads. You can also call advertising agencies to ask if they handle music for the commercials they produce in-house. In all the above cases, ask if they are amenable to receiving tapes from singers, and to whom you can send yours. Finding out the preferred means of follow-up—by postcard or by phone—is advisable.

Make Yourself Known

Making the demo tape may be the easy part, according to most singers. Getting producers to listen to it and hire you for that first job can prove to be the real challenge. "To get your first chance, you need to be persistent in a nice way," says Sue Cirillo, a New York–based independent music producer:

> You need to call lots of people, and get your tape out to everyone, and let people know who you are and what you do. Be as nice and cordial on the phone as you can. Try to walk that thin line between being a pest and being persistent. Be on the scene where you can meet people who are already involved in the business. I got my education that way, and it was invaluable to me.

Being on the scene may mean going to certain music clubs where other singers, songwriters, and musicians hang out. Jam sessions and open-mike nights can be a good place to be seen and heard. Many music producers and jingle writers frequent these clubs to scout for new talent.

Other singers may also be a possible source of work. If they are not available for a particular jingle session, they can refer you to the client if they know your capabilities and feel you are right for the call.

Once you get the first job, others should more easily follow. Becoming a jingle singer is not usually an overnight process. People in the industry stress the need for patience and perseverance, and for another source of income to support you until your jobs become more frequent. With steady work, you will earn enough money from residuals to cover living expenses.

As Thai Jason, production manager at Crushing Enterprises in New York, puts it:

> This business is not for everybody. You need to have a whole set of factors coincide. You have to have the voice, the pitch, the drive. But I've always maintained that if you want to do this, try to do it. As much as a singer wants to sing in advertising, the people who produce that music need singers to sing. You never know what the next voice will be that catches a producer's ear and sounds new.

That voice could be yours!

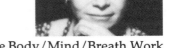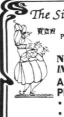
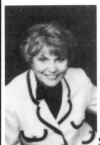

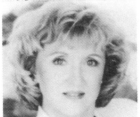

7

The Art and Craft of Auditioning for Film

MAUREEN CLARKE

You're a stage actor, and proud of it. You've got training, experience, and guts. And then one day you get an audition for a fabulous role—in a film. How do you prepare? You've heard all those platitudes about stage versus film—all that stuff about toning it down and making it more real (whatever that means). But the audition's tomorrow, you don't have time to take a class, and the role doesn't sound right for you, and—help! What should you do?

"Stage actors are often mystified by film auditioning. They think it's wildly different, but in reality it's not," says John S. Lyons, an independent casting director in New York City. "The chief difference is that they're generally reading in a smaller space, with just a casting director and a reader. It's just smaller and more intimate." Lyons, whose casting credits include *Housesitter, The Hudsucker Proxy,* and *Lorenzo's Oil,* believes that "anyone who's trained well in the theatre can, with a couple of adjustments in the size of their performance, audition well for film."

But London-based film and theatre director Patrick Tucker disagrees. "Theatre auditions and film auditions are very different," he says. "A stage director, knowing that the actor will rehearse, wants someone who looks like he'll deliver the goods by opening night. In film, since there's no rehearsal, we're not interested in what you can do *someday*—we're interested in what you can do *today.*" Tucker, who is also the author of *Secrets of Screen Acting* (Routledge, 1994), points out that in a theatre audition, "you show us a blank page upon which we can write. In a film audition, we want you to walk in the door already written."

A stage actor's ability to be a "blank page" can be a handicap in a film audition. Glenn Close, in an interview in *New York,* recalled her early film auditions:

> I think a lot of movie directors expect the character to walk in the door. I didn't know how to present myself. If you're auditioning for a play, usually you can read the whole play and you go in and you either sink or swim. But for film, sometimes they will just give

you two pages out of a script you haven't even read. And you go in and you meet with a director and they're looking you up and down, and it's like everybody knows the game and you don't even know the rules. I was at a huge disadvantage to show my abilities.

Finally, at age 35, after ten years of unsuccessful film auditions, Close landed her first film role—Jenny in *The World According to Garp,* for which she received an Academy Award nomination.

Presenting Your Self

When Close said she didn't know how to present herself, she wasn't talking about etiquette or grooming. She meant that she didn't know how to present her *self.*

"There's a story about Robert De Niro and a bunch of guys who used to make the rounds together," recalls casting director Tony Greco of Tony and Maria Greco Casting, in New York:

> They all went to this film audition, and nobody was sure—did the director want a tough guy or a nice guy? They knew they had to make a choice, but what if they chose wrong? Finally, so the story goes, they came up with a solution—they decided to play *charisma.* By playing charisma, no matter which choice they made, at least they were interesting people.

Charisma might be defined as being yourself—only more so. Be confident that your personality is unique. Radiate *yourself,* and don't try to imitate anyone else. "Why try to be Goldie Hawn?" asks Tucker. "She's already a very good Goldie Hawn. Always try to fight on your own battlefield."

If you present your own best self at the audition and you're lucky enough to fit the director's image, you've got a much better chance of being cast. But suppose you took a peek at the script selection and you *know* you're wrong for the part?

The answer is easy: Behave as if you're perfect for the part just the way you are. Play your own charisma. It has happened many times: An actor walks into the audition who's totally wrong but who has such a well-defined personality that the director either changes his or her image of the role or hires the actor for a different part. Diane Tyler, a New York-based actress who has worked at more than a dozen feature film auditions as a reader—the person who reads with auditionees—has seen it happen many times. She recalls:

> One actor who came in for *The Juror* didn't really gel with the director's idea of the character. But there was something so interesting about him, they started thinking about him for other roles. They had him audition for another role, and then another. They finally cast him in the third role—three very different roles from the

one he originally read for. And each time he came in, he made only very subtle changes in his presentation. He was so interesting as himself that they finally found a role he was right for.

It is not unusual for a film director to adapt a role to an actor. In the theatre, a director might say, "She's wonderful, but she's wrong—we can't cast her in the role." In film, he or she can say, "She's wonderful, but she's wrong —we'll change the role."

Presenting your best self has another benefit: It instantly makes auditions easier. You can relax and tell yourself, "Here I am. I'm either right for it, or I'm not." Suddenly it's so much easier to be calm. But be careful that you don't mistake calmness for limpness. Calmness is an alert composure, an energized, focused self-possession that is impossible to fake. The camera loves calmness. Calmness in the audition also signals the director that you'll keep your head during those inevitable moments when lunacy hits the set. As Tyler notes, "Maybe it's because there's so much at stake—so much money, so many reputations—that they're already nervous. They don't want anyone around who's more nervous than they are."

Okay, you're calm. You're bursting with charisma. You and your best self are ready for your film audition. What now?

The Interview and Audition

The interview is often less an audition than a conversation with the director. Does he or she think you have the essence of the character? How will you get along? Making a film means that you're going to be locked together for awhile. If it's a small part, it could be just a day or two, but it could be three months, six months, or longer. There must be compatibility.

Don't forget to use your eyes during the interview—make direct eye contact. Film is all about communication, after all, and the most riveting way to communicate is with your eyes.

In the audition, a video camera may be used. Sometimes it functions simply as a record of the audition, especially if the tapes must be sent to someone (maybe even the director) not present for the actual audition. On the other hand, the director might be present, watching not you but the video monitor during your audition.

Once the camera's running, they'll either "slate" you, or ask you to slate yourself. All you do is say your name pleasantly and directly into the lens. Don't try to impress anyone by suddenly "switching into character" after the slate. Remember, this is film—you don't want them to say, "Wow, what a good actor!" You want them to say, "There, that's the character I envisioned." Slating is a brief and simple moment, but there's a real skill to it, and you should learn to do it well.

Before you get in front of the camera, be sure to ask, "How much of me will be on screen?" This is the only way you'll know how to "size" your performance. In other words, if they're just shooting your head and shoulders, your hand gestures will be wasted—and you will reek of inexperience.

Now's the time to address the biggest complaint most film directors have about stage actors—that they're "too big" for the camera. Often what those directors mean is quite simply that the actor's voice is too loud for the microphone and his gestures are too large for the camera frame.

"I sometimes encounter actors who think they're going to steal a scene by being big and bombastic," says actor Michael Caine in his book *Acting in Film* (Applause, 1990):

> On stage, you have to project your voice, or the words will sink without a trace into the third row of seats. In movies, the microphone can always hear you, no matter how softly you speak. In movies, it is *reaction* that gives every moment its potency. That's why listening in film is so important, as well as the use of the eyes in the close-up. You don't have to shout and scream. You don't ever have to do it big.

Does this mean you should "act less"? Not at all, insists Tucker:

> I've found that many film directors will criticize an actor for being 'too theatrical' when they mean he's simply too loud. Good film actors know how to adjust their vocal levels to the size of the shot. It doesn't mean you do less acting. In a close-up, you sometimes need to do *more* acting than you'd ever do on stage, because the only acting instrument you have is your face. Your face has to do what you'd normally use your whole body to do.

In an interview for the American Film Institute, film director Martin Ritt remarked, "You don't have to tone down anything that is real. You don't want to tone down Babe Ruth. When you have a great thing that is true, then it's pure gold. If it isn't true, then it isn't really great."

Working with "Sides"

When you arrive for the audition, you'll probably be given lines to read from the script—"sides" as they are called. In this snippet of a scene, it's usually impossible to tell what's going on with the story or the characters. Don't panic. "When working with sides, *you* make all the decisions—what the relationship is, what the conflict is, what the game is all about. This is what makes a reading come alive," says Valerie Adami, director of the Weist-Barron School in New York City. "More than anything else, we want to see how you think. There are no wrong choices. The worst thing you can do is make no choice."

There's a delicate balance, however, between making strong choices and overplanning your audition. It's unwise, suggests Diane Tyler, to plan too much. "On film, it's obvious if an actor is being calculating, trying to do something that he practiced at home. It invariably falls flat. It's wiser to stay 'in the moment' and react to what you're given."

Take your time as you do the reading. Look up from the page whenever possible—*especially* when it's not your line. Remember, they want to see your eyes. Keep your face alive at every moment and react instantly to what is said to you. Directors love to cut to listening, reacting actors. Observes Tucker:

> Theatre actors tend to do all their acting on their own lines, and go blank when they're listening. Film actors do exactly the opposite. Concentrate on positively listening to what the other person is saying. React while they're talking. Don't be concerned with your next line. Who cares if you stumble over a word? It's not a reading contest.

Should you try to memorize the script? Adami thinks not. "A lot of actors come into auditions struggling to show that they've memorized their lines, and I think it's unwise. As soon as you put the script down, you're telling me it's a performance, and I'm not asking for a performance; I'm asking for an audition. The last thing I'm worried about is memorization."

Tyler, on the other hand, suggests that "it's helpful to be as off-book as possible. If you have to futz with the script, the sound of the paper is terribly distracting. And when you look down, they lose your face. Nobody minds if you look down in a stage audition, because they've got the rest of your body to look at. But if you look down too much in a film audition, you're just gone."

Finally, don't worry too much about losing your place in the script. A casual attitude towards the text points up the essential difference between film and stage—a screenplay commands nowhere near the same respect that a playscript does. A film script might undergo thousands of rewrites by dozens of people; characters might change age, color, sex, or occupation. "It's not carved in stone, like *The Glass Menagerie,* muses Tyler. "It's virgin territory, and it helps if you're the sort of actor who can roll with the changes and stay in the moment."

Just remember that, at least in the audition, the script is not as important as your image on the screen. Those words might change, but your face will not.

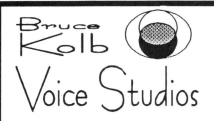

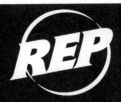

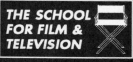

AUDITIONS

SCHOLARSHIPS
FOR
THEATRE TRAINING
IN
NEW YORK CITY

- CHOICE OF PROGRAMS OFFERING THE STUDY OF ACTING FOR THE THEATRE, FILM AND TELEVISION, MUSIC THEATRE AND DANCE
- FACULTY COMPRISED OF PROFESSIONAL ARTISTS
- INTERNATIONAL STUDENT BODY/STUDENT HOUSING PROVIDED

AUDITION LOCATIONS:

ATLANTA	NEW YORK CITY
CHICAGO	ORLANDO
DALLAS	PHOENIX
FORT LAUDERDALE	SAN DIEGO
HOUSTON	SAN FRANCISCO
LOS ANGELES	ST. LOUIS
MIAMI	SEATTLE
MINNEAPOLIS	TAMPA
NASHVILLE	TORONTO
NEW ORLEANS	VANCOUVER

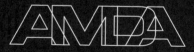

THE AMERICAN MUSICAL AND DRAMATIC ACADEMY
2109 Broadway, New York, New York 10023
1-800-367-7908 OR 212-787-5300
AMDA is an equal opportunity institution.

69

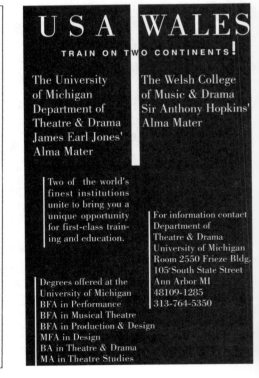

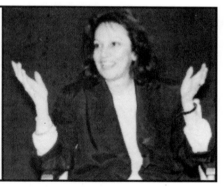

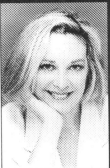

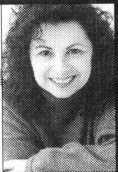

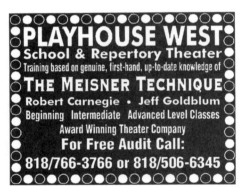

73

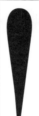
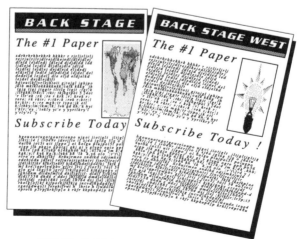

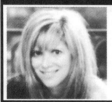

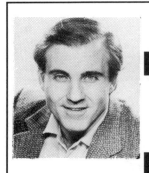

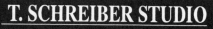

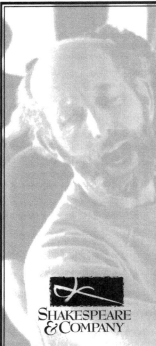
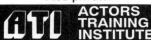

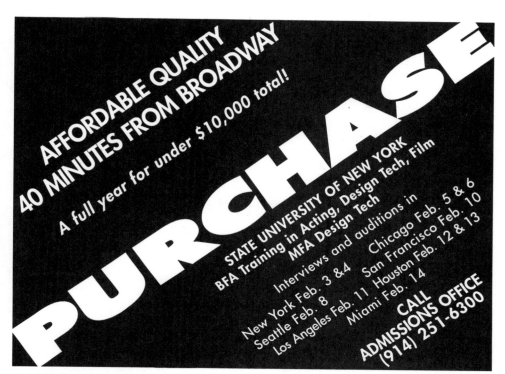

AFFORDABLE QUALITY
40 MINUTES FROM BROADWAY
A full year for under $10,000 total!

PURCHASE

STATE UNIVERSITY OF NEW YORK
BFA Training in Acting, Design Tech, Film
MFA Design Tech

Interviews and auditions in
New York Feb. 3 &4   Chicago Feb. 5 & 6
Seattle Feb. 8   San Francisco Feb. 10
Los Angeles Feb. 11   Houston Feb. 12 &13
Miami Feb. 14

CALL
ADMISSIONS OFFICE
(914) 251-6300

STELLADLER
CONSERVATORY OF ACTING
Two-Year Conservatory Program
Summer Program•Summer Shakespeare Workshop
Part-Time Evening Program•Individual Workshops
Programs for Young Adults

419 Lafayette St., New York, NY 10003•Tel. (212) 260-0525•Fax (212)260-8944

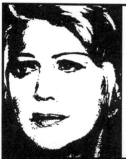

The Birmingham School of Speech & Drama
BSSD

A leading
Drama School
since 1936

3 YEAR PROFESSIONAL
DRAMA DIPLOMA &
1 YEAR POST GRADUATE
DIPLOMA

3 Year Course Accredited by NCDT
Member of The Conference
of Drama Schools

Prospectus from Administration,
45 Church Road, Edgbaston,
Birmingham, England B15 3SW.
Tel: (44) 121 454 3424
Fax: (44) 121 456 4496

"One of the Best Acting Teachers."
Mel Gordon, N.Y.U., author, Stanislavski's Tech.
"She's my Voiceover Guru."
Bill Jumey, CNN, A.T.&T., Disney

MIMI GINA
PRIVATE COACH

Acting Technique • Monologues
Relaxation • Cold Readings
On-Mike Voiceover Training

15th YEAR • Brochure (212) 874-4639
FRM FAC MEM: Lee Strasberg Inst., Berkley Prod. (v.o.)

See: "Choosing Audition Monologues"

8

All the Dish on Soaps:
Getting Work on Daytime Drama
AMY HERSH

Working in daytime drama looks like an almost perfect situation. Soap opera programs offer steady employment, constant acting challenges, and lots of exposure, and they have a following of millions of dedicated fans.

As in all aspects of show business, the acting is not as easy as it looks, and the opportunities aren't easy to come by. Yet breaking in isn't impossible. In fact, casting directors will audition hundreds of actors every year for a whole range of roles. But training and luck are crucial in soap opera, which is becoming more and more competitive.

Soaps may seem omnipresent, but, in fact, only 10 network series were being made at this writing. CBS has *The Young and the Restless, As the World Turns,* and *Guiding Light*—each of them one hour long—and the half-hour series *The Bold and the Beautiful.* ABC also airs four shows: *All My Children, One Life to Live,* and *General Hospital* (one hour each), plus *Loving* (a half hour). NBC has only two: *Another World* and *Days of Our Lives,* both of which are an hour in length.

In the early days of television, New York was the home base of all the soaps. That changed in the mid-1960s, when Los Angeles began to draw the productions westward. Today, four are taped in L.A. studios: *The Bold and the Beautiful, Days of Our Lives, General Hospital,* and *The Young and the Restless.*

Unlike any single television show on prime time, each daytime drama is broadcast five days a week, with a new episode every day. There are no reruns on soaps, so that means many story lines and many characters must be created all year.

Soaps are made under the American Federation of Television and Radio Artists (AFTRA) Network Code contract, which has distinct categories for performers on these shows. Performers with no dialogue fall into the extras' or background players' category. Nonprincipal players who have five lines or fewer are called "under-five" performers. Principals are the most coveted parts, and fall into three categories: Dayplayers who speak more than five lines of dialogue; recurring dayplayers who return in subsequent episodes; and contract roles, the starring roles, which may involve multiyear contracts for their performers.

Fewer Soaps, More Competition

Hiring in soaps has become "more competitive than ever," says Mark Teschner, casting director for *General Hospital*. There were 13 daytime dramas less than a decade ago. As the number of soaps on the air dwindles, so do opportunities for actors.

Yet the appeal of being in a soap is increasing, and many more actors seem to want to do them. "In the past, people looked down their noses a little bit," comments Betty Rea, casting director at *Guiding Light* since 1970. "Now they've discovered it can be a terrific learning experience, it can be very lucrative, and it doesn't stop them from doing films or theatre." Because there are fewer shows and because they're so attractive to performers, "It's not easy to leave one soap and go to another, as it might have been 10 or 15 years ago," Teschner observes.

In addition to being more competitive, soaps have changed in other ways, observes Judy Blye Wilson, casting director at *All My Children*: "There's more freedom in the use of character actors, and more emphasis on minorities and ethnic stories." The typical "hunk" or "beauty queen" type isn't always sought anymore, although good looks help for certain roles.

On the positive side, soaps hire more actors than prime-time shows do. Soap casting directors are busy looking for actors and holding auditions all year round. Teschner estimates that he casts between 8 and 10 contract roles and between 15 and 25 major recurring parts each year. For dayplayers, he adds, *General Hospital* casts "well into the hundreds" annually. "Don't forget—we have approximately 250 episodes a year that last one hour a day. That's the equivalent of casting 10 full seasons of a prime-time show. So it's important that I see as many actors as possible."

The same is true for other casting directors; their job is to find exciting performers, and they have many ways of doing so. One place they look is in large and small theatre productions in New York or Los Angeles. Showcases by leading acting schools, including Yale, Juilliard, and New York University, are another "must," according to Rea. Of course, casting directors also watch for actors on other TV shows and in film.

Making Contacts

When it comes to hearing from actors, casting directors who work in soaps have a no-phone-calls-and-don't-drop-by-either doctrine. You've heard it before, but if you don't have an agent who'll submit your name, a productive way to contact casting directors is to send your headshot. "We get tons of pictures—300 or 400 pictures per week—and the staff and myself go through all of them," reports Blye Wilson. One headshot per actor should do it, though. "I don't recommend sending one picture after another," says Teschner. "If someone's interested, they'll keep you on file. But you can't make somebody see you."

It isn't absolutely necessary to have an agent to get a job on a soap—in fact, Teschner says he's cast major roles with actors who were not signed with representatives. But having an agent certainly helps. "For contract parts, we send out a breakdown to agents," Rea recounts. "Otherwise, agents will call and say, 'We've got somebody new we'd like you to meet.' So we meet them, and file away their headshots." Also, Blye Wilson notes, you don't have to be an AFTRA member for your first soap job, but you'll have to join by the time you're hired the second time.

Even if they're not seeking anyone specific, casting directors hold what they refer to as general auditions. But, unlike general auditions in the theatre, these aren't open calls. "We hold general auditions for people we call in, either because of the picture they've sent to us, or because of recommendations from agents or other actors on the show," says Blye Wilson.

Casting, Coast-to-Coast

New York casting directors go to Los Angeles and L.A. casting directors go to New York to find the right talent for the bigger roles. When they're visiting cities outside their home bases, they will audition as many as 30 or 40 performers a day. If you don't live in New York or Los Angeles, it's still possible to be cast. "We also receive submissions from agents in Chicago, Atlanta, Texas, and Florida," says Rea. "If those people look right, we send them a script and they put themselves on videotape. We may also bring in people from Chicago to put them on tape in New York."

To some extent, the casting on soaps is about types. For example, if a blonde actress who's been on the show for several years decides to leave and the producers want the character to continue, then in recasting the role they'll probably look for an actress who's the same physical type. But type isn't everything; some casting is done against type.

"First and foremost, I look for their strengths as actors or actresses," says Blye Wilson, "and I always look for an inner confidence and focus, as well as education and training." Teschner says, "I'm looking for somebody who takes the page and makes it come alive."

Getting the part is also about luck, when all the pieces fall into place, Rea adds, "Sometimes you see somebody you think is very, very good, and you happen to have just the right part."

There's something about daytime dramas that seems to engender totally unrealistic fantasies among wanna-be performers. Maybe it's the fact that soap actors make their job look so easy. "If you're untrained, the possibility of getting work is practically nil," stresses Rea. "You can't just arrive and look pretty and get a job. You have to know how to approach a part, and you can only do that through studying."

Landing an audition for a soap is a big step. If you are asked to audition, it will certainly help to know at least a little about the show for which you're auditioning. You'll be able, also, to get a copy of the material a few days ahead of time. Having choices ready when you get there is very helpful because it shows more of what you can do, and that you can be creative. As you've no doubt read and heard before, doing your homework is essential.

Ignoring the Speed Limit

Suppose you are cast in a small role. It doesn't mean that you'll have to stay in it your whole life. Blye Wilson says she's had performers move on from smaller roles, and Teschner remarks that he's had major stars who started in roles as waiters. "Having done smaller work on the way up is not going to be a detriment. Every actor has. It's not going to matter, if somebody is special. It's about working, getting better at your craft, and learning," he says. Don't forget, even under-fives aren't easy parts, notes Rea. "You come from nowhere, and go nowhere, and still need to be in character."

You can create your own opportunities on a daytime drama, and a good example of this is James Kiberd's job on *All My Children*. Kiberd was hired to play detective Trevor Dillon on the show in 1989. It was written as a role for eight episodes that would be aired over a period of a month. But thanks to talent, inventiveness, drive, and preparation, Kiberd turned the part into a full-time job, and he's been working on *All My Children* ever since. Along the way, Trevor was "promoted" from a mercenary to a detective to a lawyer. Kiberd's career is also proof that there's room for more than just the "Barbie and Ken" types that are associated with soaps.

When Kiberd first went in to do his role, he already had a whole history and analysis of his character ready to go. He even wrote an eight-page background description of Trevor, which he gave to the producer. The producer ultimately passed the description on to the writers to use. Kiberd also has input into the way Trevor dresses.

That's part of the beauty of soaps. "You can contribute an incredible amount and not be censored, and the positive ideas you have for things will be taken positively," Kiberd reports. "Everybody's creative juices are flowing constantly because there's so little time." Keeping in touch with the show's fans also helps him, and he sometimes incorporates their suggestions.

It takes a lot of special qualities to be successful. Among them is self-discipline and endurance in handling the long, difficult days. "It's not fair to the others if you come in and have only bothered to learn half of what you're supposed to do that day," states Rea. "It throws the whole show off kilter."

Being a fast study is extremely important, because when you're working on a soap, "It's like a train that's moving about 99 miles an hour," says Blye Wilson. Many performers, as they deal more and more with the need to learn quickly, develop speed. "The actor that can learn fast is well ahead of the game," says Teschner.

On *All My Children*, performers get their scripts at least a week ahead of shooting. A typical day on the show starts with "dry blocking" from 7:30 AM to 10 AM, when the actors learn the blocking the director wants for that day's shooting; this is also when final adjustments are made in the script. Dry blocking takes place in a bare rehearsal studio in the same building where the series is shot. From 10 AM to 12 PM, the actors go to the set and do the camera blocking; this teaches the camera and boom operators what to do for each scene.

During a lunch break, actors put on makeup and have their hair fixed, get into their costumes, and go over their lines one last time. Following that, the cast and crew "dress" the show—have a dress rehearsal. After the director's notes are given, the scenes are shot. The day may not end until well into the evening hours. "I'm lucky if I'm out by 8 or 9 o'clock," says Kiberd.

Taping a soap is "almost like doing live theatre," he reports. Doing more than one take is rare, unless an actor stumbles with his or her lines, or there's a technical problem. Kiberd once shot 90 pages in one day. Despite this, learning lines "is the least important thing," he says. "It's not about memorizing—it's about *acting*. What you really need is a strong process in terms of breaking down the script."

If you get cast, Kiberd advises that you stay in acting school or in a class:

> Develop yourself and work at your craft. I've seen hundreds of young actresses and actors—myself included—get into soaps, get some press, and then move on in a few years thinking they're going to be stars in other parts of the industry. But they're eaten alive, and you never hear from them again because they didn't develop their craft.

Working in this medium can be an actor's dream, Kiberd declares. "Where else do you get new material every day to perform in front of millions of people? Only on daytime drama."

Radio Theatre Gives Audiences an Earful
AMY HERSH

The basic elements are so simple: dialogue, sound effects, and music. Even though it doesn't have sets, costumes, lighting, makeup, or any physical movement, radio theatre at its best is a powerful and enjoyable form of entertainment, requiring its audience members to actively participate through their imaginations. It's also a genre that is drawing more and more listeners in the United States and offering opportunities, experience, and exposure for performers.

"Radio theatre can be live or taped, lasting from a few minutes to a few hours," explains Skip Pizzi, who is a technical and radio editor for *Broadcast Engineering* magazine and a consultant to the National Endowment for the Arts and to public broadcasters. A whole range of styles is being produced in radio theatre. Pizzi notes that it runs the gamut, from comedy and political satire to full-length novels and plays—Shakespeare to Noël Coward—experimental and performance art, mystery, science fiction, and short stories. "The interest in radio theatre does seem to be growing, but not at a huge, fad-like rate—it's growing on a consistent, if small, level," Pizzi says. "It's amazing how you can develop an audience for the oddest things, if it's done well."

All Markets, Great and Small
Radio theatre is being produced all over America, in big cities as well as in smaller towns, for a wide market. The variety of producers includes theatre companies, independent production companies formed for the sole purpose of doing radio theatre, and radio stations. Some radio theatre is broadcast only in the city where it's produced. Other programs are bought from local stations and producers and are then distributed via satellite by, primarily, National Public Radio (based in Washington, D.C.) and Public Radio International (based in Minneapolis).

In fact, you don't even have to turn on the radio to hear this genre. Radio theatre productions are becoming available on audiocassettes and compact discs and can be bought in bookstores and from mail-order companies. For example, the Rivertown Trading Company, a for-profit direct-mail company, produces the "Wireless" audio collection catalog and *Garrison Keillor's A Prairie Home Companion Catalog* for Minnesota Public Radio. (Some libraries and museums are becoming good resources for audiotapes, including archival material—for instance, the Museum of Television and Radio, in New York City, which will also open a facility in Los Angeles in 1996; its holdings will duplicate the programs and resources in the New York collection.)

Still, for the most part, public radio stations are the home of this genre. Radio theatre is rarely heard on commercial stations today; in that regard, the genre has changed tremendously over the years. Once a staple of programming, it was first heard in this country on commercial radio networks in the 1920s, and it continued to be popular until television supplanted radio as the favored entertainment medium. Playwrights Arthur Miller and David Mamet worked in the genre early in their careers. Radio drama is still an important part of radio programming in Britain and Canada.

Unfortunately, radio theatre is not an especially lucrative field for actors in the United States. It is covered by the American Federation of Television and Radio Artists' National Public Radio Agreement and its National Code of Fair Practice for Commercial Radio Broadcasting. Under the National Public Radio Agreement in effect at this writing, actors receive $11.30 for each hour of rehearsal time and $87.30 for performing a one-hour show. Scale is $100 under the Network Radio Code for a one-hour drama and $29 for each additional half-hour. There is also a $10-per-hour rehearsal fee. At this writing, AFTRA is renegotiating the previous three-year Network Radio contract, which was extended as of November 15, 1994.

While you probably won't get rich doing radio theatre, it offers a wealth of experience. Radio theatre can help you develop your skills as a voice-over performer in commercials as well as in animation, says Steve Donofrio, director of the Midwest Radio Theatre Workshop. Based at a public radio station in Missouri, MRTW offers two workshops a year and is one of the rare sources of training in this genre. Its week-long fall workshop covers acting, directing, writing, producing, and creating sound effects and culminates in live performances. (For more information, contact: Midwest Radio Theatre Workshop, KOPN-FM, 915 East Broadway, Columbia, MO 65201.)

If you're interested in getting involved in radio theatre, Donofrio recommends that you listen to it to become acquainted with its technique and find out who is producing it where you live. You may want to create your own audiotape demo, which would highlight your range and abilities, and then send it to a local radio theatre producer.

"Everything Is in the Voice"

It takes special skills to be a successful radio drama performer, states Valerie Henderson, executive producer of the Public Media Foundation. Based in Boston, this nonprofit organization was founded in 1979 and began producing radio theatre in 1991. Its mission is to stimulate new American writing and to present contemporary and classic American literature in this form. Since 1992, the Foundation's work has been broadcast on National Public Radio's *NPR Playhouse,* a two-hour weekly series.

The Public Media Foundation has also co-produced broadcasts with the BBC that are heard in the United States and the United Kingdom. Some of the organization's works are also sold on audiocassettes. The Foundation has produced dramatizations of works that include Mark Twain's "The Thirty Thousand Dollar Bequest," Harriet Jacobs' "Incidents in the Life of a Slave Girl," and Edith Wharton's "A Journey."

"In developing a character, everything is in the voice," Henderson says. "An actor can be any size and any age. You're not dependent on physical appearance. You can play virtually any role on radio, which is intriguing to a lot of actors. They love it; there's no question."

On radio, actors don't have to project their voices to the back row of a theatre. "A whisper in radio drama is so much more important than perhaps it would be on the stage," Henderson continues. "You can convey so much quietly through the use of the microphone. There's a great deal of subtlety involved."

NPR estimates that more than 250,000 people listen to its radio theatre programming each week. Henderson notes, "We've got a finished product that goes out to a far bigger audience than actors would have even for an extended run in a theatre."

Performing comedy on radio is similar to performing drama, comments Christine Tschida. Since 1989, Tschida has been the producer of *A Prairie Home Companion,* which has an audience of approximately two million people each week via Public Radio International's satellite service. If there is a "superstar" of radio theatre today, it is Garrison Keillor, who created and hosts the show.

"We look for actors who have a facility for using the voice in all different ways—not only singing, but in developing characters and being able to convey age, background, geographic location, the mood, and what they're feeling," Tschida states.

Sometimes stage performers have a difficult time adapting, because *A Prairie Home Companion* is performed in front of an audience as it's being broadcast live, and stage performers, Tschida explains, tend to play to the audience in the theatre.

> But the real audience is the two million people listening to the radio at home. You reach each one of them individually and on a person-

al level, which is very different from reaching a group of people in an auditorium. Radio is like whispering into one person's ear or talking to someone on the telephone. In radio, smaller is bigger. If actors focus their energy into the microphone, it's a better performance.

Perhaps radio theatre will never return to its Golden Age, when the airwaves were populated with performers such as Jack Benny, the comedian, and Orson Welles, the dramatic actor whose Mercury Theatre production *The War of the Worlds* made headlines. Yet it's still a vibrant medium attracting dedicated actors, directors, writers, and technical experts.

"People who produce radio drama care about it so much," says Andy Trudeau, director of the production and acquisitions unit for NPR Cultural Programming. "I can't think of anywhere else on the radio waves that you hear such creativity."

The Practical Art of Commercial Print

MAUREEN CLARKE

The asthmatic on the subway ads, the young mom on the bank poster, the concerned surgeon in the pharmaceutical magazine—they look like real people, but they're actually models. Not fashion models—print models. In other words, they're actors.

And they must be *good* actors, because they must project fully rounded characters without voice or movement. "When clients call us for print models, they always insist on actors—trained performers who can bring a sense of character to the job," says Scott Powers, president of Powers Productions, Inc., in New York. Actors who can master the skills of print work are exceptionally well-rewarded. According to Powers (who is also a model), "We make about $250 an hour—sometimes more, sometimes less, depending on the client. If you go into overtime, which is generally over eight hours, including lunch—you can make maybe $325 an hour."

And luckily for most of us, you don't have to be young and gorgeous. Fat or thin, young or old, blue-collar or lace-collar, the print world needs all kinds of people. "If a person has a strong look of any particular type, we're interested, as long as the model has very good energy," says Jane Blum of Funnyface Today, one of New York's largest print agencies. "That's what the photographer wants to capture."

The Initial Photo

"All you need is a good, clean, energetic headshot," explains Gary Bertalovitz of Funnyface. "A lot of beginners feel they need a portfolio, but it's just not necessary. We book people from headshots all the time."

Your photo should look like you at your friendliest best. Don't glamorize yourself, and go easy on the retouching. Keep in mind that this isn't fashion modeling; it's print, and the print market wants real people.

You may hear print models talk about "comp cards"—composite photos showing the model in different costumes and poses—but you won't need these until you've got much more experience.

Finding an Agent

So you've got your nice, clean, honest headshot and you mail it to all the print agencies—whoa, not so fast! *All* the print agencies? The pool of print agencies in New York is vast and ever-changing. Every day, one agency opens with a grand flourish while another scurries furtively into the night. And since the quality of print agencies varies wildly, you'll save yourself a lot of time, money, and angst if you do a little homework first.

How do you know where to start? In the Appendix is a list of agents who specialize in commercial print. This list is the best place to begin when you're doing your first mailing. Don't forget to enclose a friendly, businesslike cover letter with your photo, and if you have one, attach your acting résumé to the back of your photo. This will tell them a little more about you.

The Agency Interview

If an agency likes your headshot, you'll be called in for an interview. Be on time, be energetic, be calm, be pleasant, and most of all, arrive looking as much like your photo as possible. Nothing turns an agent off faster than an untruthful headshot.

During the interview, be friendly, but be businesslike. Without being pushy, ask lots of questions. If you don't know anything about this agency, ask how long it has been in business. Ask what kind of clients book its models. Ask to see some photos of the top models, ask how long these models have worked for the agency, and ask to see photos from jobs that have been recently booked.

Should You Sign a Contract?

In short, no. "A long time ago, when there was a lot more work," recalls Powers, "models signed exclusive contracts because an agency could get them a significant amount of work. These days, with the sagging economy, signing a contract is economic folly." Instead, successful print models will have a "verbal alliance" with one agent as their "parent agent," but will also be kept on file with several other agencies. It is understood that the model takes all calls from the parent agency. If a call comes in from another agency, the model can go out for it, so long as the parent agency hasn't called the model for the same job.

If you're just beginning, you might be tempted to open the Yellow Pages and let your fingers do the walking to one of the lesser-known modeling agencies. Don't do it. Until you learn the ropes, it's wiser to start with the larger, well-established, well-respected firms. Unlike theatrical agencies, print agencies are bound by no legal qualifications, licenses, or union requirements. Anyone can hang out a sign and call him- or herself a print agent. Such an ill-regulated system is flypaper for scam artists; most experienced print models can tell hair-raising stories about ending up in the wrong office at the wrong time and being asked to do something fairly unpleasant. (Remember, porn is print too.)

If you find yourself in an agent's office being pressured to sign a contract right away, remember: Legitimate print agencies hardly ever offer contracts anymore, and they *never* offer contracts to beginning models. Never sign anything without letting a lawyer look at it first. (For more about scams, see Chapter 25.)

Commissions

When you book your first print modeling job, look carefully at the paperwork. Notice something interesting? The word "agent" never actually appears. This is because print agents are not really agents. Yes, everyone calls them agents, but legally, they are *managers*.

The difference is crucial. A true talent *agent*, such as a union-franchised agent who books actors for plays or films, cannot legally take a commission of more than 10 percent of a performer's pay. Print *managers*, however, are not bound by these laws, and can take as much of your pay as you agree to give them. Usually, this will be 20 percent of your total pay; then, on top of that, they will take a 20-percent service charge from the client.

Not only is this legal, it is typical. "Some print agents," says Scott Powers, "will take even more than that. Some will take a 35-percent commission from the model, and a 20-percent service charge from the client, and so, in reality, the agency nets 55 cents for every dollar the model nets." This hurts less, of course, when you consider you're making $200–300 an hour, but you should still know what to expect up front.

Because print work isn't governed by a union, nothing is standardized. Working conditions and wages will differ from agency to agency and from job to job. There are some sleazy agencies and some great ones, and you've got no way to protect yourself except by experience and education. If possible, take a print modeling class. Talk to other print models. Ask who's good and who's bad; listen to the stories and remember the names.

The Go-See

The print model's audition is called a go-see. Your agent will call and tell you about it. Again, don't be shy, but ask lots of questions. Ask about the client, the product, and the role; ask what you should wear, where you should go, whom you should see, and what you should expect when you get there. Ask any relevant question you can think of.

Plan to arrive early. It will help you relax and focus, and you can learn a lot from other models who are also waiting. When your name is called, you'll go in and meet the photographer, who will usually take a few quick photos.

How can you prepare for this? Veteran New York print model Bill Bowdren suggests a bit of on-the-spot character work:

> Zero in on the photographer's eyes, and ask a couple of quick questions. I usually ask whether I'm supposed to be happy or sad, rich

or poor, young or old, active or passive. I toss these out very fast, without taking too much time or burdening anyone. Then I try to absorb what I've been told and really talk into the lens. I treat it like a mirror and try to have a good time, because in my 35 years in this business, I've found that when I am who I am, warts and all, I'm at my best.

You Got the Job! Now What?

A couple of days after the go-see, your agent calls and says, "Congratulations, you booked the job!" Now the real work begins.

Squeeze as much information as you can from your agent. Take notes. Ask who, where, what, when, and don't forget the important question: *how much.* Again, since there are no unions in commercial print, every job pays differently. Politely but firmly, find out now exactly how much you'll be paid. It's considered very poor etiquette to talk about pay during the shoot.

Because pay rates aren't standardized, what determines how much you'll get paid? Instead of a contract, you will have a *voucher,* which indicates the pay rate, overtime rate, commission percentages, service charges, hours of work, whether you're entitled to travel time, and any other information pertinent to payment. All this is negotiated between you, your print agent, and the client *before* the shoot. You can't dispute it later—everything is agreed upon in advance and must be stated in the voucher. With a good agent or manager negotiating for you, you'll get everything you deserve, but it helps if you know your stuff. For example, you should know that if they break for lunch, you still get paid. "I've worked on shoots where I'm making $350 an hour, and they take a two-hour lunch break," marvels Scott Powers. "Basically, they buy me my lunch, and then pay me $700 to eat it."

Ask your agent if a makeup artist or hairstylist will be at the shoot. Don't take anything for granted. Will you supply your own wardrobe? If you do, it's a good idea to bring more than they ask for. "If they ask for a couple of shirts and ties, bring four shirts and eight ties," recommends Bill Bowdren. "Photographers absolutely love that."

What else can you do to prepare? Get plenty of sleep the night before. The camera picks up everything.

On the Shoot

Like lack of sleep, discontent reads big on camera. If you're having a bad day, leave it at the door.

Be on time. Lateness is everyone's pet peeve, and chronic lateness is one of the fastest ways to ruin your career. Remember, if you're late, you cost them money.

Focus on the mood the client wants to create. "Try to learn the objective of the shoot," suggests Bowdren. "During a recent job for Vista Hotels, I asked what they were trying to accomplish. They said they were trying to get new weekend business. On weekdays they get lots of corporate travelers, but hotel bookings go way down on weekends. Instantly I knew what they wanted—a relaxed, casual guy having fun on the weekend. Knowing their objective made all the difference."

Pay close attention to every little direction they give you. A seemingly unimportant detail might be crucial to the client, who has spent much time and many dollars on the shoot before you got there. Treat the client's ideas with respect.

And don't forget to have fun. Commercial print work is not only lucrative, it can be artistically satisfying if you see it for what it is, an acting job. The camera is on you—you're the star of the show!

Finally, it's a good idea to keep a notebook and write down the names of everyone connected with the shoot. Send thank-you notes a few days later to tell them how much fun you had, and how much you enjoyed working with them.

There's no better feeling than that moment at the end of the shoot when the client shakes your hand and says that you've done a great job. You can be sure they'll remember you, and if you've done your job well, they'll hire you again.

For a list of commercial print agencies and management firms, see the Appendix, page 266.

Serious Business Theatre:
The Hows and Whys of Doing "Live Industrials"

MAUREEN CLARKE

C an an actor make a good living without doing television, film, or Broadway? Absolutely—by doing corporate stage shows. Usually called "live industrials" or "business theatre," these shows are produced by corporations for conventions or trade shows, usually to highlight a new product or service. Many of these shows use lavish sets, costumes, music, and Broadway-caliber performers. Others require little more than an actor and a slide projector. At either extreme, this kind of work can be lots of fun—and very lucrative.

How does an industrial happen? Buck Heller, executive producer of Heller Creative, Inc., in Putnam Valley, New York, describes the process:

> A corporation has a need—usually in a specific area like marketing, motivation, or sales. They want a theatrical way to illuminate this new product or service at a big meeting or a conference. The corporation—the client—calls several producers and asks each one to develop a proposal. After all the proposals are presented to the client, the project is awarded to one of the producers, who then must bring the proposal to life. If my proposal calls for a lot of audiovisual effects and eight singer–dancers, for example, I begin to put all that together.

The producer assembles a creative team. Depending on the show, there might be a writer, a composer, a choreographer, a director, set and costume designer, and, of course, agents and casting directors.

The Essential Skills

There are agents and casting directors who specialize in industrials. Karen Garber, an agent with the Sanders Agency in New York, describes how she knows whether a performer is right for industrial work:

Because we're dealing with corporate America, we're also dealing with a cross-section of middle America—so we're looking for very middle-American individuals, including members of ethnic groups—as long as it's a very middle-of-the-road look. Our clients want stereotypical business people.

They also want talent and training. If it's a big musical industrial, the performers will be of Broadway quality. John Leavey, senior production coordinator at New York's Caribiner Group, a major industrial producer, notes:

Obviously, a triple-threat is the best possible person: a first-rate actor, singer, and dancer. On top of that, you should be able to handle different styles. When I'm setting up a musical audition, I'm often told that they don't want to hear any Broadway show tunes. The actors are asked to bring in something contemporary, rock 'n' roll, or upbeat. A lot of actors can only belt. On the other hand, I've done shows that relied solely on a show-tune style. You really have to excel at everything.

Including life, according to Karen Garber. "Life skills are a very important part of industrial acting," she asserts.

You must be able to comprehend life on a level other than show business. If you're doing a show for John Deere, for example, be ready to talk about farming equipment. Be able to say, 'Gee, it's interesting—this compactor, or that manure-spreader.' It sounds silly, but this is middle America. You have to be able to talk, not just sing and dance.

Garber acknowledges that such well-rounded performers are rare. "Very few agencies specialize in industrial talent, just for that reason. You can represent excellent actors—but an excellent actor isn't necessarily an excellent industrial actor."

The skill that really makes an industrial performer unique is the ability to make sense of technical copy. "You must have a facility for the English language," says Garber, who auditions actors for copy-reading skills even before she asks them to sing or dance. "Whether you're doing farm equipment or pharmaceuticals, there will be some very technical words. Even if you don't understand what you're saying, you have to come across with authority and enthusiasm."

Industrial producer Ivy Naistadt, president of Ivy Naistadt Creative Communications, in New York, offers some valuable tips for making technical copy come alive:

The key is rehearsing. Get a computer magazine and practice reading it out loud. Find ways to personalize it—learn how to be professional and natural at the same time. Really good performers are actively interested, they want to know how things work, so if you don't understand something in the script, ask. There are always people from the company who are happy to explain things.

If you get called for an industrial audition, ask who the client is. This will help you focus. Naistadt advises:

> Keep the clients in mind. Who are they? What would you wear if you worked for them? They want to cast people who represent themselves, and they're generally a little more conservative. If you're auditioning for a car show, you can wear a sexier outfit, something like you might wear for a regular singing audition. But if you're auditioning for a computer or a pharmaceutical show, it's a good idea to be conservatively well-groomed. And if you're considering working extensively in industrials, it pays to invest in a couple of conservative, quality items of clothing.

While trying to stretch your brain around technical scripts, don't neglect your body. Stay healthy. You'll need a lot of stamina, because rehearsal time is very limited and the hours are long and hectic. When the curtain comes up, it's often at 8:00 in the morning. It's not easy by any means.

Spokesperson Work
Some firms may spend big bucks for fancy sets and costumes, but some just want a spokesperson—an attractive, credible person to stand up at a conference or trade show and talk enthusiastically about a product or service. Companies sometimes start out by asking their own employees to do this—until they discover how hard it is to give the same spiel twice an hour all day long and still be fresh and convincing at the end of the day. "Next time," they groan, "let's hire an actor."

The actor they hire will be both corporate and personable, authoritative and friendly. Even if they don't want you to sing and dance, they'll want you to be facile and spontaneous with multisyllabic, high-tech copy.

Experienced spokespeople handle this in various ways, but a fair number would be lost without their ear prompters. An ear prompter works like this: First, you record your lines on a tape recorder. When it's time to perform, you play the lines back through a hidden earphone, reciting the words as you hear them. The advantages are obvious—no need to memorize difficult material, and last-minute changes are easy. On the other hand, ear prompters aren't easy to use; they're useless for dialogue, and unless you're very skilled, when using one you'll look about as spontaneous as R2D2.

Ear prompters are relatively new in New York. First used in Chicago in the 1980s, they caught on quickly in Boston's booming high-tech industrial market. "People in New York who use them are usually the very experienced industrial actors," cautions Karen Garber. "Novices should be very careful that it doesn't get in the way of the presentation itself."

A professional-quality ear prompter consists of a small tape recorder, a wireless neck loop (worn under your clothes), an earpiece with a volume control, and sometimes a hand-held pause button. [You'll find a more de-tailed description in *Acting in Industrials,* by William Paul Steele, a book about corporate videos (Portsmouth, N.H.: Heinemann, 1994).] Because the earpiece is custom-made to fit entirely within your particular ear, the ear prompter is considered personal equipment. If you're hired to give a presen-tation using one, you'll be expected to supply your own.

Before you spend your money on a professional setup, test yourself. Go into any electronics store and buy a simple earphone on a jack. (Think cheap—this should cost less than $5.) Record a few minutes of technical copy, play it back through the earphone, and recite the words as you hear them.

At first you'll feel like a passenger on a runaway train, but remember, this takes lots of practice. As you improve, challenge yourself with more difficult material. Try a faster pace. Walk and gesture as you speak. Novices tend to sound robotic, so work hard on your spontaneity. Eventually, you should be able to deliver the lines as naturally as if you were improvising.

"Some of the best actors in the business use ear prompters, but you've got to be really good at it or it looks fake," Naistadt acknowledges. She recalls au-ditioning an actor recently:

> There was something a little odd about him. He looked great, but he wasn't connecting with anyone. I asked if he was using an ear prompter, and he said he was. When I asked him to read without it, he refused. I told him we needed him to read the copy off the page so we could see him interact, just for the audition, and he got very defensive. He was using the ear prompter as a crutch; he did-n't want to interact. The key is to learn how to use it without los-ing that spontaneity, that spark of personality, that interaction with your audience—especially the audience at a trade show, where they're standing right in front of you.

Dollars and Sense

Whether you're hired for a big musical extravaganza or a one-person trade show, the pay can be very rewarding. If an industrial producing company wants to use Equity talent (and most of the big ones do), it hires the actors under a Business Theatre contract. A principal performer earns $931 a week under a two-week contract and $1,166 under a one-week contract. Daily rates begin at $388 the first day and are $194 per day thereafter. Under the current contract (which expires June 29, 1997), per diem rates are $65, and the actor is given a single-occupancy hotel room free of charge. These Equity minimums can be negotiated upward by a performer's agent.

Equity's business representative Louise Foisy explains a few rules:

> Industrial producers, like Broadway producers, can employ anyone they want. But if they want to use Equity actors, they must hire them under an Equity contract. If one actor is under contract, they must all be under contract. If they cast a non-Equity actor, that actor will be invited to join the union.

Most actors are happy for the opportunity to join Equity, but in the case of industrials, they aren't required to, because industrial employment usually lasts less than thirty days. "Under state law," Foisy says, "union membership is not required until after thirty days."

Business Theatre contracts are used primarily for large-cast musical industrials. For individual spokesperson work at trade shows, Foisy explains, Equity has long taken the position that contracts are optional:

> If the actor desires it, and the producer is willing, Equity is happy to draw up a contract. Some actors prefer having the contract, because they want the health coverage, and we've made the paperwork very simple to encourage that option. The Business Theatre contract is very painless—only one page, written in plain English.

Breaking into the Biz

There are trade publications (*Ross Reports* in New York, for instance) that specify which agents and casting directors specialize in industrials. In lieu of such a list, you can try calling agents or casting directors to ask if they work in this area. When you send them your picture and résumé, make sure you enclose a typed, businesslike letter telling them you're especially interested in live industrials. Your photo should show you at your most clean-cut, and your résumé should emphasize your most corporate credits.

If you wish to specialize in corporate performing, it wouldn't hurt to have a special résumé which lists your corporate and commercial credits right on top. Mention whether you have or use an ear prompter, and don't forget to indicate all your special skills. Can you juggle? Make sure you juggle well, for even here the competition is fierce. As Carol Nadell, owner of Selective Casting in Manhattan, points out: "An actor who juggles might come to an audition with three lemons and be fine. But real jugglers—who might also be fine actors—will come to an audition with pins, hoops, and costumes, and their own music. There's no contest."

Can you imitate anyone famous? At the 1994 Unix computer show, in New York City, there were *two* David Letterman impersonators. (Two different companies had the same idea, spent tons of money duplicating the Letterman sets, and by sheer coincidence, the shows were set up directly opposite each other. It was a challenging three days for the Dueling Davids.)

If you've never been to a trade show, you have some pleasant homework in store. Call your nearest convention center (such as the Jacob Javits Center in New York City), and get a ticket for the next big trade show. Spend the day there, walk around, see the exhibits and the shows, get a feel for this special world. Watch for well-groomed, friendly presenters who look like corporate executives but are actually actors. (You might check their ears for telltale "buttons.") Ask how they got started, who their agents are. They're paid to be friendly, anyway, and after talking so much business business, they'll probably enjoy a few minutes talking show business.

Karen Garber, who represents some of the best talent in the industrial arena, provides this concluding bit of advice:

> Treat this part of the industry as purely *business*. Behave like a business person. Show up on time. Actors who are late for an audition with me will never get a second audition. Be responsible, be prepared, do your homework. This isn't something you can fake your way through. If you handle yourself as a business commodity, you'll have a little bit of an edge in the industrial market.

For a list of business theatre producers that are signatory with Equity, see the Appendix, page 268.

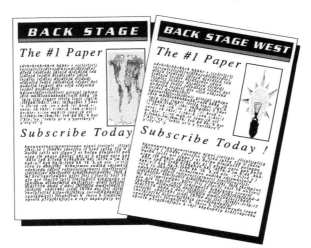

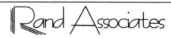

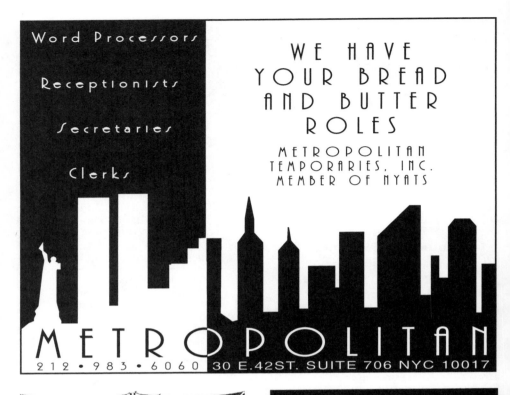
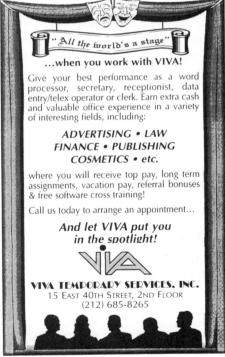
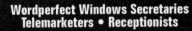
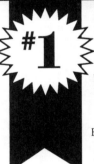

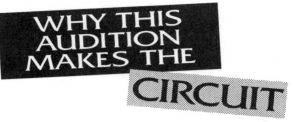

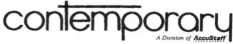
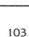

12

Non-Broadcast Media:

They're Not Just "Industrials" Anymore

JONATHAN ABARBANEL

They used to be called industrials—a good Rust Belt catch-all term that covered a variety of film and video situations. But the word seems as outdated today as an aging Ohio factory. It certainly lacks glamour, which has led too many actors to perceive industrials as a limited and limiting field. Actually, the field is expanding as never before, encompassing the latest in communications technology. For smart actors, industrials (and educational films and videos) are not only a money machine but a way to acquire or sharpen some useful technical tools. This broad area of opportunity for performers seems far less limited when labeled "non-broadcast." That's the term used by the unions under whose jurisdiction it falls: the American Federation of Television and Radio Artists (AFTRA) and the Screen Actors Guild (SAG).

Today, "industrials" includes corporate image pieces shown to a broad general public, traditional training films, motivational and sales projects, point-of-purchase videos, product demos, employee benefits programs, interactive videos, tape cut-ins for live teleconferences (sometimes global via satellite uplink), and recordings on laser discs, CDIs, and CD-ROMs—in short, anything and everything that can go on tape, film, or disc but isn't made for broadcast television or for theatrical release. (Music videos fall under the non-broadcast label, although they won't be covered here.)

CD-ROM (Compact Disc—Read Only Memory) and CDI (Compact Disc Interactive) are burgeoning technologies with enormous potential for performers. They are computer-compatible compact discs, including laser discs, that can deliver both audio and video. CDIs are used in consumer products, such as virtual reality games, which can include live actors. CD-ROMs are used in the new generation of computers capable of reproducing full-motion video.

Many (but not all) CDI and CD-ROM uses are covered by AFTRA's 1994 Interactive Media Agreement and SAG's 1993 Interactive Multimedia Agreement.

105

However, the field is enlarging so rapidly that contract law with regard to performers (and copyrights) can scarcely keep pace. Says Chicago actor Rick Elliott, a high-tech maven: "It's hard to describe what the use of CD-ROM is and what value to place on the exposure for the performer. The marketplace is so robust with all these new technologies, it's difficult to put a finger on them."

Performers' opportunities in this field include not only on-camera work but voice-overs and narration also. Given the size of the non-broadcast arena, it's amazing how few actors take time to explore it deeply.

"It's very disappointing the way actors are educated," comments Sharon C. Wottrich, president of Voices Unlimited, a Chicago talent agency. "They're never really told of all the ways actors can make a living. You can make as much money in a day in non-broadcast as in a week in most regional theatres or Off-Broadway."

The Money

How large and how rich is the non-broadcast field? It's almost impossible to quantify because the field is so diverse. Also, at least 50 percent of non-broadcast work is nonunion, making reliable tracking difficult. Union jobs under just the SAG codes covering industrial non-broadcast work, earned Guild performers $8,852,595 in 1993. (The two unions' codes are titled, specifically, the "1993–1996 AFTRA National Code of Fair Practice for Non-Broadcast/Industrial/Educational Recorded Material" and the "Producers/Screen Actors Guild 1993 Codified Industrial and Educational Contract." Both non-broadcast codes predate by many years the interactive media agreements which cover more advanced technology.)

What does non-broadcast pay? The codes at publication time (in effect through April 30, 1996) have a one-day minimum of $380 for on-camera work (tape or film) in general industrials and $472 for point-of-purchase film or tape. Weekly rates are $1,333 and $1,651, respectively. A half-day rate (four hours or less) is 65 percent of the day rate. Under both unions' interactive media agreements, on-camera scale is $504 for a day, $1,276 for three days, and $1,752 for a week. As with other AFTRA and SAG contracts, pension and welfare payments and agent's percentage are added to—not subtracted from—the minimum.

As for nonunion work, reputable producers will pay at or near union scale, but without union benefits and usage protections. In nonunion cities or states with "right-to-work" laws, you'll find commensurately less protection, as well as much greater regional variations in rates of pay.

But why be satisfied with scale? Non-broadcast offers tremendous opportunities for above-scale pay for experienced performers or those with special skills. Says Bill Bilowit, president of The Show Works, Inc., New York: "The typical speaking role will range from double scale up to $2,000 a day. The people we want can demand that much." Agent Wottrich has a voice-over performer who gets $500 an hour for industrial narration in a highly technical field.

The Skills

What does it take for actors to be good at non-broadcast? "They have to get it fast, they have to get it right, and they have to get it on the first take," answers Joan Greenspan, SAG's national director of industrial contracts. Particularly in the area of corporate communications, they have to be "very sharp technicians": "The issues they are explaining today are far more complex than they were 10 years ago. They have to tell a very simple story about very complex things," she says. Wottrich concurs: "They have to be extremely good cold readers."

Bilowit observes: "One of the hardest things is to find actors who can deliver a 10-minute speech and also learn to operate or demonstrate a piece of equipment or a product." He suggests that in the corporate communications field, "any computer skills are a plus."

In most situations, you won't see the script until the day shooting begins or perhaps a day or two in advance, if you're lucky. Do ask for it in advance, especially if the project involves any specialized vocabulary or high-tech terminology. "You'll have to correct regionalisms that won't be understood everywhere. If you have the script beforehand, you should do your homework in learning terms and pronunciations," advises Midwest actress Jill Shellaberger, who derives one-third of her income from corporate and point-of-purchase narration.

Another absolute must for success in non-broadcast is experience with teleprompters and ear prompters. Everyone interviewed emphasized that performers in industrials work with both devices, especially the ear prompter. AFTRA and SAG offer periodic training seminars in these areas through all their regional offices. Private training through commercial acting classes also is available. The only way to be good at ear-prompting is to practice. Actor Ray Bradford, president of AFTRA's Chicago local, says, "You have to work at it constantly. If you leave it behind for a month or two, you lose your edge." (For more on ear prompters, see Chapter 11.)

Other special skills that can lead to above-scale incomes include fluency in foreign languages, knowledge of a technical field, and variety skills such as comedy, singing, juggling, and dialects—although 75 percent of non-broadcast work is straightforward stuff.

Foreign language fluency is more in demand for voice-overs and narration than for on-camera work, but it is growing in each of these areas. Spanish is the tongue most in demand, followed by other Romance languages. The increase in international teleconferencing and the need for multilingual educational/training films and tapes and point-of-purchase materials has helped fuel the demand.

Two cautions about foreign language work: First, don't let the producer hand you a script in English and ask you to translate it. That's not what you're being paid to do. A script translated from English to a Romance language will lengthen by 10 to 20 percent. It is the producer's and client's job to provide a correct, properly timed translation. Second, highly skilled artists can do dialects and regionalisms within a foreign language, which are particularly useful for dramatizations and role-playing. Myrna Salazar, perhaps Chicago's most successful Latina performer in the field, speaks Spanish in Puerto Rican, Mexican, Cuban, and Bolivian accents.

In the creative arena, comedy skills are probably most often looked for. Several years ago in Chicago, the improvisation troupe The Second City organized a division called The Second City Business Theatre, which takes on live and film and tape projects. Members of the troupe generally write or co-author the scripts for, as well as perform, these projects. If you are a member of an improv troupe or comedy collective, it might be worthwhile to explore group non-broadcast opportunities.

The skill or special knowledge most readily translatable into cash is mastery of a technical field or vocabulary, especially computers, medicine, and the pharmaceutical industry. If you actually understand high-tech terminology or Latin-based medical terms, it will increase your marketability.

Both SAG's Greenspan and producer Imero Fiorentino, president of New York City's Imero Fiorentino Associates, emphasize opportunities in pharmaceuticals. Because of increased government scrutiny, Fiorentino suggests, the big drug companies are constantly revamping their training videos. Greenspan says that the pharmaceutical industry has taken the lead in satellite teleconferencing, putting it on the cutting edge of interactive communications. "Whatever they manufacture has global applications," she comments.

The Shoot

What should you expect on an industrial shoot? Typically, you'll be called for one to three days of work; shooting schedules of a week or more are rare. You may be the single "talking head" in a point-of-purchase video, or you may have one or two scenes in a longer training film. In most cases, the wardrobe is contemporary and standard, so you'll be expected to supply your own. Shooting is as likely to be on location as in a studio, and the former might call for odd hours. (In busy retail stores, shoots will almost always be at night; in hospitals, they'll be held during the slowest normal cycle of activity.)

If you're already in a live show, you potentially have a scheduling conflict to resolve before you sign a contract. In theatre-heavy cities like New York and Chicago, a so-called theatre release is standard practice. But it is a *verbal* agreement that is *not* part of the written contract. Chicago-based actor–musician James Sie advises: "If you have a theatre conflict, you *must* tell them at the audition, at the callback, and when you sign the contract. A theatre release guarantees you'll be finished up by an agreed-upon time. Since it isn't a written thing, you have to remind them all the time."

You should also be aware of, and forthcoming about, potential conflicts of interest. This is especially important if you're asked to serve as an on-camera spokesperson. It's just like doing on-air commercials: You should not do two breakfast foods at the same time.

The "rules" in non-broadcast industrials really are a matter of common sense more than anything else, and they are well worth observing. One of the rewards of the field is frequent return business. Production houses often cast actors in project after project if they know them to be reliable. Clients, too, will call for a particular performer, especially in a spokesperson role. "Clients tend to get comfortable and use the same people all the time," reports Bill Bilowit.

Your Job Search

How do you find jobs in non-broadcast? It varies a bit by region. New York City and Chicago have more non-broadcast work than any other markets. In New York, you'll need a good commercial agent. In Chicago, where one agent covers all fields, the non-broadcast area is so big that most agencies have an "Industrials Department."

In Los Angeles, most commercial agents aren't interested in pursuing non-broadcast work for their clients. As the president of one top commercial agency put it: "For one day's work, we don't break our backs to make $30. Our main area is commercials." He adds that, in L.A., film and TV agents deal with industrials.

Non-broadcast producers there and in New York frequently bypass casting directors and work directly with agencies when seeking talent. This is particularly true in New York; virtually all producers interviewed said they find talent that way. In Chicago, too, using casting directors for non-broadcast is the exception, not the rule.

The non-broadcast field is not limited to the three major production centers. San Francisco, Seattle, Denver, Dallas, Detroit, Minneapolis, Atlanta, Miami, Washington, Boston, Nashville, and many points between have multiple producers working in non-broadcast. Perhaps the essential difference is that smaller regional production centers will have lower rates of pay and much higher frequencies of nonunion work.

One final note: The non-broadcast field offers ample opportunities for minority performers. Imero Fiorentino says his clients just assume that a cast will look like America. Asian-American James Sie and Latino Ray Bradford confirm that large corporations such as McDonald's and Allstate, which both do a great deal of non-broadcast work, definitely want an ethnic mix in their projects. Lisa Shanks, executive producer for SMS/Casablanca Productions in Los Angeles, agrees, citing particular West Coast opportunities for minority performers.

The proviso, of course, is that ethnicity alone won't get you the job. Non-broadcast is no different from stage or broadcast work: You've got to be able to deliver the goods. Whoever you are, in this business, you have to get it right, get it fast, and get it on the first take.

13

Children's Theatre Comes of Age

MARCIA ANNE WOOD

Theatre for Young Audiences—or TYA, as it is known—is theatre performed by adults for children, teens, and family audiences. TYA productions are usually shorter than adult productions, ordinarily running about an hour and not more than 90 minutes. In addition to playing in traditional theatres, TYA is often performed in schools and often has a pronounced message regarding education and growth. Sometimes productions are targeted to specific age groups (for example, ages 4–7, or 8–11, or 12–17), but many of the people involved in TYA regard their work as being not just for children but for teens and adults as well.

The Repertoire

TYA productions include classical and contemporary plays, musicals and straight dramas, presentational and interactive theatre. There are four kinds of shows often produced for youth. First, adult plays may be shortened and adapted for young people—for example, a 90-minute *Romeo and Juliet*. This category also includes shows for family audiences, such as *A Christmas Carol*.

Second, adaptations of classic fairy tales such as *Cinderella* or *Rumpelstiltskin,* are usually produced as musicals. These often call for period sets, costumes, and theatrical styles.

Third, adaptations of children's books, such as *Winnie the Pooh* or *The Velveteen Rabbit,* may be full-length dramatizations or a series of several short dramatizations telling several stories in one production.

Fourth, plays may be educational or deal with current social issues such as teen pregnancy, cultural differences, or ethnic identity. Study guides to accompany such plays are often provided to teachers in advance, and frequently the cast will discuss the play with a young audience after the performance.

An Expanding Field

In a profession where employment opportunities are scarce, there is a great deal of work available in TYA for both Equity and nonunion actors. Equity's Theatre for Young Audiences contract ranks a surprising fifth among Equity's

20 contracts in the amount of income produced for actors. In 1994, TYA contracts generated $4 million in income and 14,583 workweeks. This area of theatre is in a period of tremendous expansion, both in the amount and in the kinds of shows produced. There are now 69 producers of Equity children's shows in the United States, up from 50 in 1991. Of these, 45 are in Equity's Eastern region, 14 are in the Midwest, and 10 are on the West Coast.

Nellie McCason, in her book *A History of Children's Theatre in the United States,* counts 450 nonunion producers of children's theatre. This includes university and community theatres and other categories not under Equity jurisdiction, such as puppeteers or musicians performing opera for youth. At any given time, some percentage of these are developing into Equity companies.

"The market hasn't even been tapped," says Dick Natkowski, Eastern region TYA representative at the Equity office in New York: "Independent producers could find a market almost anywhere in the U.S." For both Equity and nonunion actors who want to create work by producing their own shows or starting their own companies, TYA is a promising and dynamic area.

Advantages for Actors

"The bottom line is that TYA is *work*; it pays the bills. You're making a living while getting experience, and it can be a good showcase," says Steve Sterner, a New York actor, composer, pianist, and musical director who has worked both on Broadway and off. Work often leads to other work, and TYA is no exception. Many people involved in TYA are simultaneously involved in projects in other areas of show business, and the more people know a performer's work, the more often the performer's name will come up when a role is being filled. Because TYA companies are often small, low-budget repertory companies, members have the opportunity to play a variety of roles and wear many hats, from writing to directing to choreographing. TYA, in short, is a chance for the beginning actor to get steady work and develop skills.

"Our long tours give the actors a chance to work on their roles over a period of time," says Jay Harnick, artistic director of Theatreworks/USA, which employs about 180 actors in 12 shows a year and is the largest producer of children's theatre tours in the United States. "I like to see the shows before they go out, and again at the end of the tours; the growth in the actors is amazing!"

Sterner agrees: "It's a wonderful honing ground. Working for the Gingerbread Players & Jack, I have played many different kinds of roles. I also made lots of connections. I've been able to recommend people for jobs and other people have recommended me for jobs."

A Gateway to Equity

Many people do not realize that one of the main advantages of working in TYA is that there are more chances for nonunion actors to get into Equity through a TYA contract than any other way. TYA is primarily a touring contract, and often more established or older actors either can't afford to leave town for tours at TYA's lower salaries, or they don't have the stamina for the rigors of touring with a TYA contract. Tours, of course, can include long periods away from home, long hours traveling in vans, multi-performance days, and assistant stage manager duties. Therefore, producers frequently open TYA auditions to nonunion performers. These are often young actors who will be unflagging on tour and who may be hoping in that way to become Equity members.

Under the current Equity TYA contract, which expires November 17, 1996, actors are guaranteed a minimum wage on either a weekly, or per-performance basis. In the weekly contract, minimum salaries are, for an actor, $300 and, for a stage manager, $400. A per-performance TYA contract guarantees an actor a minimum of $45 to $60 for each show, and a stage manager $65 to $75, depending on the size of the theatre.

Nonunion companies sometimes do not pay up to Equity scale and often do not include benefits, overtime, per diems, and other guarantees required by Equity. You should be aware of what is expected of you before you sign a contract.

The TYA Experience

TYA tours may be as short as a few days or as long as six months. They are often linked to the school year and to school hours. Your shows may be in the morning, at 10 and 11:30 or earlier. In order to get to the theatre and set up, you may be up at 5 or 6. It can sometimes feel like going on stage in your pajamas.

As a TYA actor, you will perform in every imaginable venue, from small auditoriums to huge stadiums where body mikes must be used. You will learn to find your light on stage and adjust your blocking in all situations. As with any tour, you will be in close quarters with the same people for a long period of time. For a flexible person who gets along with others and can "go with the flow," TYA tours can be a great deal of fun, involving new experiences and friendships. Sometimes the local sponsors of the productions are on hand before or between shows, with coffee and food for the cast and crew.

Not all TYA involves touring. You may work in a resident theatre where you will be playing repertory: contemporary one day, classical the next. You can gain firsthand experience of theatre history, for TYA often employs troubadour-like characters and period styles like commedia dell' arte. Pantomime and puppets also come into play.

Ticket prices average $5 to $7 for children and families. Therefore, most TYA companies don't have big budgets. In many cases, you will be singing with an audiotape accompaniment rather than with live musicians.

Children are an honest, responsive audience who will be spellbound and will shriek with delight and excitement when they are involved in the show. Or they will talk with each other and grow quickly disruptive if bored. They will not cut you any slack. If anyone will, they will teach you how to hold an audience.

Making It Happen

In the past, most U.S. children's theatre producers have been located in the East, especially in New York. However, over the last 10 to 15 years, dynamic centers of children's theatre have developed in Chicago, Louisville, Milwaukee, Minneapolis, and Seattle. Another trend has been an increase in resident children's companies, as compared to touring companies. Each of the above cities has *several* children's theatres at least one of which is heavily subscribed and producing new shows each season. Some examples are The Drury Lane Children's Theatre, in Chicago; Stage One, in Louisville; The Great American Children's Theatre Company, in Milwaukee; Milwaukee Children's Theatre; The Children's Theatre Company of Minneapolis; and The Seattle Children's Theater.

Other theatres actively producing plays for youth are the Mark Taper Forum, in Los Angeles, the Honolulu Theatre for Youth, in Hawaii, and the Kennedy Center, in Washington, D.C. The old Victory Theater in New York's Times Square will soon become a home for nonprofit and children's theatre, where Theatreworks/USA will perform.

Many diligent, committed producers and several other organizations are contributing to the growth of children's theatre. The New York–based Producers' Association of Children's Theatre (PACT), formed in 1968, continues to sponsor a large annual TYA Showcase, which takes place each January in New York. The Producers' League of Theatre for Young Audiences (PLOTYA) emerged from this group. The New Generation Play Project (formed by a group of Midwestern and Western children's theatres) and New Visions, New Voices (sponsored by The Kennedy Center) are two of several organizations that promote playwriting for young audiences.

These organizations, along with various national and international youth theatre festivals and conferences, are examples of what is happening in many communities. TYA is enriching the lives of young people and becoming a vital part of developing a theatre-going audience for the future.

For a list of Equity TYA producers, see the Appendix, page 270.

14

Putting It Together:
How to Create Your Own Cabaret Act

JOHN HOGLUND

What do Woody Allen, Harry Connick, Jr., Bette Midler, and Barbra Streisand have in common? These stars all started out playing in small clubs. So did Michael Feinstein, Whoopi Goldberg, Peggy Lee, David Letterman, Barry Manilow, and many more. Cabaret could be your springboard to fame as well.

Just what is cabaret, and what makes it unique?

Unlike theatre, cabaret is small. *Intimacy* is the operative word. Imagine cabaret as a performance for a few guests in your own living room, where you can let down your guard and share your innermost emotions with them through your songs, gestures, and speeches. This unique art form allows you to hold onto your individuality even after the lights dim. You are the star for one hour in a spotlight that belongs to you.

Long associated with the performance of musical treasures by Irving Berlin, Cole Porter, and the Gershwins, among others, cabaret today includes many diverse, contemporary songwriters. The key to choosing your material is to find the lyric you can make your own, be it a familiar standard or a new and original comic riff. Using your imagination as your guide, the sky's the limit.

If approached with savvy, perseverance, and the right sense of fun, cabaret can be unbelievably rewarding. Unfortunately, all too many artists plunge into this arena with too little knowledge and too much vanity. Putting together a cabaret act begins with commitment and common sense.

Know Who You Are

As you prepare to enter the world of cabaret, it is important that you understand exactly who you are. Be aware, too, that in recent years this milieu has grown more diverse, with impersonators, magicians, ventriloquists, and comics joining a crowded field of singers.

Unlike theatre, in which you play a character, cabaret requires you to be yourself—to be open and entertaining. You need to bring your passion and true personality to what you are presenting. In a club, there's no fourth wall, so you must be confident that you have something special to offer an audience.

Ask questions of performers whose work affects and inspires you: Who helped you prepare for your show? What made you decide to put together your first cabaret act? What was the hardest part of the process? What first steps would you recommend that a cabaret newcomer take? Have you any other suggestions for someone starting out?

The more you learn at this "entry level," the more likely you will be to master the business and artistic aspects of cabaret. That mastery will keep you focused and in control of your career.

The theatrical world offers many rules and precedents for your guidance, but cabaret is idiosyncratic and highly personal—what triumphs for one performer may spell disaster for another. A great singing voice or comedic skill won't of themselves guarantee success. While the success stories which have emerged from cabaret are impressive, the failure rate is staggering.

If you have many doubts about where you are going, perhaps you need to reorganize your thoughts and consider taking another road. Such questions require difficult, sometimes painfully honest, answers. However, you will never make it to first base without being truthful.

Is Now the Time?

Are you ready to make this move into cabaret? This is, by far, the most important question to ask yourself before going further. Lead up to it with these: Why am I doing a cabaret act? Am I willing to work hard to get it right? Am I willing to accept a degree of failure as part of the learning process?

Again, be honest with yourself. If you have any doubts about the aforementioned, you aren't truly ready.

Watching as well as talking to cabaret performers will also help you decide whether this field is for you. Catch as many shows as time and money allow. Set your standards early and take notes. Here are some things to consider: How well does the performer connect with the audience? Can you relate to the material? Does the show move well or are there weak spots that lose interest? Are the musical arrangements complementary, overbearing, or lacking imagination? What do you like most about this show? What do you like least?

With careful observation and scrupulous candor, you can avoid pitfalls that all too many performers fall into because of inflated egos. Remember, few singers are more memorable, more effective, or more impressive than those who interpret an honest lyric straight from the heart. It's that simple.

Auditions

As the Sondheim song goes, ". . . everything you do is an audition." Be prepared. Some club owners or operators will ask for a video or audiotape if they are unfamiliar with you. The tape should not only reflect your vocal style but be representative of your act. Three selections are usually the safest bet. These should include one upbeat song, a serious ballad, and, if possible, a novelty or original tune. Submit the tape with a recent photo and a succinct, professional résumé. (Avoid an overwrought résumé with too many details and a lack of focus.)

If a live audition is necessary, be prepared to sing two songs. Though a beautiful voice is a plus, it is just as important that you demonstrate your interpretive skills, your phrasing. What makes your rendition stand out from someone else's? At most auditions, patter is not necessary unless it is an integral part of your act or you are doing a performance piece or characterization.

Preparedness cannot be emphasized enough, so unless otherwise advised, bring your own pianist. If an accompanist is to be provided (you'll learn this when scheduling the audition), bring music written in your key. Never ask for a transposition on the spot.

Also, be familiar with the club. Arrive having already seen at least three acts there. Know the technical advantages and limitations of the space.

If you are offered a booking, be sure that the dates allow you enough time to prepare. Do not accept any date(s) if conflicts or other problems are possible. Most club owners are understanding and will work with you on this.

Unfortunately, there may be a few clubs that will book performers solely on the strength of their drawing power rather than on their talent. Some require a performer to guarantee that a certain percentage of seats will be filled; that is, he or she must agree to pay for the empty seats. Granted, this is not a common practice, but it is an economic reality that must be noted.

Preparing a Budget

Expect to spend money. From inception to encore, putting together a cabaret act can cost as little as a few hundred dollars or several thousand dollars, depending on the route you choose and your own financial situation.

There are many variables to consider. Figure out how many performances you can afford to do. If you're a beginner, you'll probably be working for the door—that is, you'll get the cover charge (or, in some cases, a percentage of the cover). Estimate the costs of, among other things, financing rehearsals and accompaniment, photo and reproduction fees, flyers (graphics, postage, and other distribution expenses), and paid advertisements. Although you are just starting out, you can present yourself as a skilled professional. If you outline a budget in advance and stick to it, you will avoid major pitfalls.

Picking Your Musical Collaborators

Putting an act together requires much more than choosing songs interspersed with clever banter. In cabaret, few things are more important than picking the right music director and accompanist. A music director is usually the person responsible for helping you with song selections, tailoring intricate arrangements, and, in some cases, researching specialty material. The music director is also the one who will chart your arrangements, thereby enabling others to accompany you if necessary.

The role of the accompanist, who rehearses and plays for you on stage, is to put you in the best possible light, while being musically intelligent and comfortable with the material. Very often in cabaret the roles of music director and accompanist are filled by the same person.

Where do you find musical collaborators? You can ask cabaret booking managers to suggest those with good track records. Talk to other singers or simply approach an accompanist who's played a show you've enjoyed.

A singer and his or her music director must work as a team, and getting off on the right foot in cabaret begins with the right partnership. Veteran singer Rosemary Clooney sums it up best: "My confidence [in music director–arranger John Oddo] allows me to be what I am up there and to be honest with my audience. That's the greatest gift a performer can share."

Do You Need a Director?

There are well-defined differences between a music director and a director. The former guides you musically and, if accompanying, shares the stage with you. The latter remains behind the scenes.

In rehearsals, a director can provide you with the perspective of a "third eye," seeing what an audience sees when it watches you perform. Aside from working out blocking, stage business, the use of props, and so on, a director can help tailor, structure, and pace your act. (Most cabaret shows are an hour long; this means you can count on doing about a dozen songs and an encore.)

At what point do you decide whether you need a director? Can you afford one? How do you find the right one? If a director is not in your budget, consider simplifying the show and making it easier on yourself. You can always try something more ambitious once you get your feet wet.

Though hiring a director has become *de rigueur*, it's no crime not to have one; performers have been doing cabaret without directors for decades. If you do decide to use a director, remember that you must find a professional with whom you can develop a rapport.

Probably the best way to judge a director's work is to see it. Catch another act he or she worked on. Did the performer's own identity come across, or did the act seem too slick or overrehearsed? A good director's work is never obtrusive. You don't want your act to turn into a "director's show" with little of your individuality shining through.

Choosing the Right Material

There are endless sources to find the right material: racks of sheet music in music stores, songwriters who compose special material, and libraries, such as the New York Public Library for the Performing Arts at Lincoln Center. Decide first on the kind of show you want to offer. Ideally, you would find a unifying theme or through-line that tells something about yourself without being too overt. People in the room should leave your show feeling they know you better. If you can define this through-line, you are well on your way.

A strictly autobiographical show, however, is one of the most difficult acts to pull off successfully. Few people are interested in all the milestones of your life. Misguided, many beginners choose this formula, and such shows often become exercises in self-indulgence. This format can work if you have an exceptional flare for timing and a gift for entertaining, but these attributes usually come only with experience.

What should you sing? Cabaret nowadays encompasses every kind of music: show tunes, country, pop, jazz, blues. You can mix and match or do a theme show devoted to one composer or period. If you fully know where your talents lie, you will instinctively gravitate toward the ideal songs best suited for your voice. Be careful not to overdo one thing, though: A soprano, for instance, while impressive in coloratura passages, should not attempt to fill an hour with such vocal flights. This is a cabaret act, not a concert recital. A performer with a limited range can turn in a terrific show by choosing the songs that complement his or her vocal range. Again, it begins with knowing who you are.

Getting Noticed

Besides doing your show, you must market yourself and build your press kit. Getting noticed in cabaret should be part of a carefully thought-out plan to advance your career to the next level.

How do you do that? First, get the word out. Mail out flyers, put up posters, take out ads, offer to perform at benefits. Stop by piano bars, sing a song, and schmooze with the customers while distributing your flyers; this can be most helpful. Go to other singers' shows. In New York, the Manhattan Association of Cabarets & Clubs offers periodic seminars as well as songwriter showcases. Perhaps other cities offer similar programs. They are opportunities not only for learning but for mingling and networking as well.

Most cabaret performers have had little or no experience in dealing with the press. One of the best ways to learn the fundamentals of promotion is to do it yourself. If you handle this job properly, you'll be able to evaluate the pros and cons of hiring a press agent when the time comes.

Conversely, if you don't know how to handle public relations—if you don't know when and how to effectively notify the right people about your performances and progress—you'll never be in control of your own career.

Few newcomers should spend their money hiring press agents for their first cabaret outings. Fees for press agents vary from $1,200 to $1,500 for an average run. Upscale publicity firms command $2,000 and more. (Such agents are usually working with established performers.) Here, too, there are many variables. Occasionally, a staggered payment fee can be worked out. In any case, never work without a basic written contract. Do not accept a verbal agreement.

Above all, know when you are ready to be reviewed. Premature press coverage might harm rather than help you. Critics don't like to have their time wasted, and you won't get a second chance to make a first impression. Early in your cabaret career, you don't have to be great; this is the time to give yourself room for failure. It's not the time to be raked over the coals in print.

If you *are* ready for reviews, here are some basics: A flyer with a brief note to the critics will usually suffice at this level. If you send out a press kit, include a recent 8 x 10, a résumé, and an announcement containing all the pertinent details of your engagement (collaborators, cover charges, drink minimum, and so on). It should all be as neat and simple as possible. To pique a writer's interest in a newcomer is, at best, a challenge. But word of mouth travels fast in this community, so if you have something exceptional to offer, chances are that an astute critic will hear about you.

Looking to the Future

The late cabaret legend Sylvia Syms had high hopes for cabaret's future when she said in 1990: "It's going to be better; it's going to be greater; it's going to be wilder and more colorful than it ever was." While perpetuating the treasures of the musical theatre, cabaret now incorporates newer forms of expression, fulfilling Syms' vision. Indeed, talented cabaret performers are making the future happen now. It's staying on that intimate scale, but it's sizzling.

For a list of cabaret venues in New York, Chicago, and Los Angeles, see the Appendix, page 274.

15

Advice for the Fledgling Comic

DONNA COE

While still in his teens, the late comic Freddie Prinze asked comedian David Brenner how to tell if a particular routine was going over well with a crowd. "Listen to the silence," Brenner told him. "In the pauses, if they're not shuffling their feet, coughing, or stirring, you've got them."

Of course, silence throughout a stand-up routine is anathema to a comedian. After serious consideration, most comics would rather hear a heckler yell "Get off the stage!" than hear a pin drop. In at least one instance, the fear of silence was instrumental in shaping a beginning comic's persona: Deadpan comic Steven Wright, a *Tonight Show* regular, explains, "I didn't want to be just standing there if the audience wasn't laughing. That's why I tell five jokes a minute—the silence makes me too nervous."

A crowd can seize on a neophyte's anxiety like a mongoose on a cobra. Paul Reiser, star of NBC-TV's *Mad About You,* agrees that this can present problems for new "stand-ups." He cautions, "The audience gets shaky if they see you panic for no reason."

This can sometimes lead to a performer blaming an audience for his or her inadequacy. Says Richard Belzer, one of the ensemble on the NBC series *Homicide*, "Some comics mistake their own ineptness for indifference or stupidity on the part of the audience."

Some comedians make their living underestimating the intelligence of the people they play to. But successful comedians believe that if the anticipated response isn't there, it's *not* the fault of the audience.

Confidence plays a major role in the way a comic is perceived by the crowd. It's tough to fool an audience into believing you're terrific if you don't think so yourself. The more comfortable you are on stage with your material, the better a performer you will be. We've all seen a comic get enthusiastic responses with hack material and the intelligent but unassertive comic go begging for a laugh. This is where image comes into play.

Assessing your persona as a comedian takes years. Some, like Steven Wright, stumble across theirs early on, but the perfecting of this sometimes elusive quality is an ongoing process. Unless you're very lucky or have been blessed with some marketable neuroses, it's a long, grueling effort. Those who are successful hone their craft on a nightly basis.

A comic needs to recognize the power of comedy as being more than just a series of jokes strung together. The best material comes from the heart and has that personal twist unique to a given performer. Stand-up is a form of comedy in which the creator is sole writer, performer, and editor. For those who feel passionately about it, it's a powerful medium wherein you can express ideas, entertain, or simply have fun.

Jerry Seinfeld, star of the long-running *Seinfeld* on NBC, advises, "If you think something is funny, and you think that no one else could possibly think it's funny, that's exactly the direction you should go in . . . assuming that it gets a laugh." Elaborating, he says, "I always start with me. I don't think, 'Here's something people will like.' I start with what I like."

Talent, though intangible, is a palpable cause for sweat. Frank Gannon, former talent coordinator for CBS-TV's *Late Night with David Letterman,* believes, "There are only so many funny people in the world. It's a gift." But it's not a free one, he warns: "It's a gift that requires a lot of hard work."

And it doesn't end there. Just being a good comic isn't enough anymore. With the proliferation of comics on TV and in films, acting skills are fast becoming a necessity.

What to Do and How to Do It

Gannon's advice is to "struggle, suffer, starve, go on the road, make yourself worthy, and kneel all night before the god of comedy." He believes that the pursuit of stand-up is Darwinian. The rigors of being on the road—missing travel connections, staying in notoriously heinous comedy condos, and playing clubs that would make better tool sheds—winnow out the weak.

Adrianne Tolsch, a veteran of 18 years in the business, is a three-time comedy award–winner for Best Female Stand-Up in New York, and she has also appeared on Broadway. Her philosophy: "When buzzards start circling the stage, go sit down." In other words, "Get on stage wherever you can and for as long as you can."

Don't, however, perform predominantly for friends and family, she adds. "You won't get the correct feedback. They won't be there in the room when you're on the road in Kansas City."

Seinfeld discovered the art of crafting a joke by sitting in the back of dingy clubs watching other comics go through their acts night after night. "I learned that a particular set-up didn't work because maybe one word wasn't clear, or the timing was off by this much. You listen and study and eventually get to understand what makes people and premises funny."

Sometimes, however, you can do everything right and still be passed by. A case in point: Years ago, the talent agency William Morris overlooked Jim Car-rey, a young comic who went on to success in the Fox network's *In Living Color,* and subsequently became a major box-office draw. Such things happen. The point is: Don't allow letdowns to discourage you.

Mistakes and How to Avoid Them

Pandering to an audience was one error nobody ever accused the late, brilliant Bill Hicks of committing. To him, that would have been demeaning because he considered himself one of them. "Only those who are arrogant enough to think that they're better than the audience would talk down to them," he said.

In general, people come to a comedy club to be entertained. They don't walk in expecting to hate the show, and they certainly don't expect to be treated badly by the people they have paid to see.

One error made by comics is seeking out television appearances before they're ready. The best strategy is to work on your act for four or five years before taking it to TV. This advice may be too cautionary for many, who after only a year or two in the business are aggressively courted by television's myriad cable shows, which gobbles up comics the way whales eat plankton. It might help to remember that after overexposing your "A" material on several cable shows, it's going to be much more difficult to get on *The Tonight Show* with the same act.

Naturally, no comic wants to wait tables or do word processing instead of making a living as a stand-up, but performing in front of important industry people before you're ready is another unadvisable move.

As already implied, cookie-cutter comedy is no way to get noticed. Be distinctively yourself. Whether or not you like the abrasiveness of someone like Roseanne, her different persona caused her to stand out—and succeed. Yet novice comics often neglect to develop their own performing identities. Many top comics have some outstanding characteristic—Judy Tenuta, Richard Lewis, and Louie Anderson, to name a few.

Don't forget that there's also room for good, hard-working monologists like Jay Leno or Paul Reiser. As Seinfeld points out, "I'm a hookless act. There's nothing odd about me—no screaming, no props, no strange wardrobe, and my name isn't catchy either." The important thing is to be aware of and to define your identity—a brand of comedy that is you.

Addressing the need also for beginners to establish a good, solid comedy foundation, Seinfeld asserts, "Whatever success I've achieved has been done almost solely on technique. It's not like you'd just look at me and laugh. If I didn't have good technique, there'd be nothing funny about me at all."

Generic comedy, or the overuse of certain premises, is just one of the hazards of a business where, until recently, supply and demand were on equal footing. It will always be a seller's market, however, for those with a fresh, quality product.

The Future of Comedy

There are approximately 4,000 working comics (to greater or lesser degrees) in the United States today. By all accounts, the comedy boom of the 1980s has leveled off, heralded by a slight decrease in the number of comedy clubs. Because there are more performers now than the market can bear, the vast majority of them will, through attrition, go on to other vocations.

But what about those who are fortunate and talented enough to withstand the decline? And what about the newcomers who are joining the comedy ranks every day? Where will the future of the art take them?

Club activity is cyclical. Comedy, at its apex in the mid-1980s, has now leveled off to some extent, and some industry insiders believe that clubs will turn to more varied programming, as cabaret has done. Their evenings will feature singers, magicians, and more variety acts. Television can't capture the excitement of live entertainment, so people will start going back to clubs in search of that all-important live theatre experience.

The tide will turn away from reality-based comedy, some predict, and toward the ridiculous. The popularity of Michael Richard's eccentric character, Kramer, on *Seinfeld,* leads some to believe that people want a change from comedy based on negatives, such as domestic abuse, in sitcoms. The pendulum, they say, will swing back to an older, arrow-through-the-head silliness; it may come back in a revised form to be sure, but its return is inevitable.

Obviously, no one in decision-making positions knows exactly what's going to happen. At the end of the day, all one can do is follow his or her own vision. If you're compelled to go on stage, suffer rejection, and see your determination through to a not-so-bitter end—you have much of what it takes. And if you happen to fall by the wayside, at the very least you'll have some good memories and a lot of funny stories to tell.

For a list of comedy clubs in New York and its environs, Los Angeles, San Francisco, and Chicago, see the Appendix, page 277.

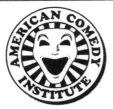

16

Summer Stock:
Working in the Straw Hat Season

THOMAS WALSH

Summer stock is many things, but most of all it's an invaluable and rewarding way to advance a career as a performer. In many stock situations, the production quality can be top-grade professional; so can the working and living conditions, the pay and benefits, and the experience.

"Summer stock is really *the* perfect place to hone your craft," says Patrick Quinn, first vice president of Equity and an actor who has excelled on Broadway and elsewhere but values his years of stock work above almost anything.

"In general, summer stock is the best learning place in the world," adds Norman Duttweiler, producer at the Forestburgh Playhouse in Forestburgh, New York, a fixture on the stock map for 50 years.

"It's very, very good training in how to sharpen your craft, your focus, and your technique," notes Judy Blazer, another Broadway pro with dozens of stock credits.

Summer Venues

The major theatre directories list summer stock venues in 45 of the 50 states—which amounts to more than 300 houses nationwide. Companies come in all sizes and styles, and the average stock operation hires 20 or so performers per season. Some hire many more.

More than 30 theatres operate under Actors' Equity Association's five "traditional" summer stock contracts, and several dozen others use smaller Equity agreements, such as Letters of Agreement (LOA) and Small Professional Theatre (SPT) deals. Then there are the hundreds of nonunion facilities thriving under the summer sun.

What is generally on summer stock schedules is a mix of three to ten mainstage productions per venue each season, plus the occasional in-house cabaret presentation and/or a young-audience show. The fare is predominantly light, with a strong accent on musicals and comedy. The summer audiences come, after all, to relax.

For actors, however, the work pace in stock is fast, faster, and fastest!

The Audition Picture

Most stock theatres conduct their auditions from January to April. Heavily attended open-call auditions are still very common in this arena.

Then there are "combined auditions," the 20 or so convention-like gatherings where many producers and presenters can see and hear thousands of actors and technicians at one central location in a few days' time. Held by state, by region, and on a national scale, these events include the Southeastern Theatre Conference, the StrawHat Auditions, and the New England Theatre Conference. (For more on combined auditions, see Chapter 17.)

In summer stock auditions, producers shop for the basics: singing, dancing, and acting. A few hundred performers contend for jobs that may last from six to twenty weeks, encompassing at least four very different shows.

"Never forget that those of us behind that desk are seeking a cast of people whom we're going to *trust*, who are going to justify our production," says Carleton Davis, who for 30+ years has been a veteran packager and a producer of stock mini-tours and is now general manager of the Cape Playhouse, in Dennis, Massachusetts. "We want to see security, something that says they've earned their square foot of that stage."

"Temperament is very, very important," adds producer Duttweiler. "If I see a real "attitude" at an audition, I start to think about what they might be like come mid-August. . . . A company has to quickly become a family. They'll be living, eating, and working together. They have to be team players."

At the audition "actors need to be very well prepared," states Robin Farquhar, executive artistic director of the Flat Rock Playhouse in Flat Rock, North Carolina. "I've got three minutes to see somebody; that might mean I'm seeing 125 or so people a day. On 'chorus day,' I might see another 200."

"When going on stock auditions, always check into who was in the original cast and get the cast album," says Quinn. "What they want basically is what the original looked like. We're talking about having one week to prepare each show." And Davis, who also hopes to see actors showing a secure knowledge of their material, advises:

> There's a great fallacy among actors who approach auditions and say that they want to appear as a "blank page." I'd much rather have them try to fit in with what they do best. They'll get their share of work if they do that. They need to be familiar with the shows they're auditioning for and to do something in the style of those shows. If I'm doing an operetta, don't do rock or rap in your audition.

"Types" Means Versatility

Your auditioners are recruiting for a big musical with a cast of 14, most of whom will be going into the next show and the next on the season schedule—say, a comedy and then a murder mystery. You're a young character actress who sings and moves well, and you're looking for stock. What do they want you to be? Knowing your "sub-types" within your overall "type" can be crucial. Will you play the "efficient secretary" as potently as you do the "neurotic younger sister?"

Your audition material should reflect more than just one sub-type. You'll want to show nuances of those sub-types and be ready for anything, so choose more material than you might need. "If you're lucky enough to be asked to do a second piece, you should pick the most contrasting piece," notes Blazer. "You'd like them to want more."

When a Broadway or Off-Broadway show is casting, thousands of performers may be submitted for each role. "In those auditions," observes Farquhar, "people are too often 'typed out'—as in: 'You're two days too old,' or 'You're two inches too tall.' In summer stock, sometimes the age range of an actor we're seeking might be 35 all the way to 55. With a little gray in the hair and a mustache, he might pull it off."

Davis comments on the need for versatility this implies:

> It's unbelievable how well singers dance and dancers sing today. They're far better at being all-around performers, because they have to be. One reason is that we can't afford separate choruses. In the old days, there was little crossover. For example, "I'm a singer who moves" was a whole category. They weren't really required to dance. Now they are.

How Tough?

Summer stock is hard work for everyone. Generally, daytime rehearsals and production meetings for upcoming shows are followed by evening performances of the current production. The post-show clean-up may lead to a late-night cabaret performance; then it's back "home" to study lines and grab some food, a shower, and sleep.

Provisions in Equity's stock contracts protect members in every area. Limits are strict as to how much actors can be asked to do in rehearsals and performances. But in both nonunion theatres and Equity venues permitted to hire a percentage of non-Equity people, the picture may change considerably.

"It can be bone-crushing," agrees Duttweiler, who assembles a five-show Forestburgh season that runs from mid-June to Labor Day, using an Equity SPT agreement. "The talk of 14-hour days for the nonunion people is often absolutely correct. When you're 19 or 20 years old, it seems terrific—at least it did for me. But someone who doesn't really love the work and doesn't have a great attitude—I would tell them to not do it."

Having done at least 30 stock shows since his early twenties, Quinn states:

> There are, indeed, some unpleasant jobs in summer stock. There are [non-Equity] companies that take advantage of actors. There are places where they make *you* pay to work as an apprentice. It's like

going to camp. That is abusing actors. It's taking advantage of the fact that these people want to work. But as a result these actors may never want to do it again.

"It's a dismal summer for someone who gets into it and doesn't understand what he's getting involved in," says Lynn Archer, who has chaired Equity's Stock Committee since 1980 and is a long-time stock performer herself.

"It's never very hard," counters Davis. "Eight shows a week means about 24 hours of performing in a week. And we don't rehearse a show much once it's open. How tough is that really?"

"Sometimes, in fact, it's very easy," admits Archer. "You may have a total of six weeks working on a show, and that's not too difficult. But I'm very proud of the work that the Stock Committee has done. Among the main things we have to keep abreast of is what makes our actors comfortable."

Adjusting

"So much of it is about trusting your instincts," says Blazer. "Sometimes when you work on a production for a very long time, you 'layer' it." By contrast, summer stock offers little opportunity to try different approaches to a role or to explore subtleties. "Here, the first choice is the one you go with—so you learn to trust that. By the time you finish your last performance in a week of stock, you say to yourself, 'Wow, I'm beginning to really get this character'— and it's closing night."

Summer stock is about a lot of strangers bonding together offstage as well as on—another thing you may need to adjust to. "Some people have stronger nesting instincts than others. Sometimes it's necessary to find a place of your own . . . where you can tune out," says Blazer. Given the close quarters in which you must function, she observes:

> If you need to vent, it's important to find a safe outlet for it—a friend, a place to go for a walk, your family. A newcomer is bound to get frustrated or scared. But you can't bring too much panic into the workplace, because people are always watching you. The top rule, I feel, is "Don't panic." What seems like a problem will eventually work itself out.

Economic Realities

One reason many Equity members seek summer stock jobs is to keep their health benefits alive by accumulating work weeks. The months of a summer contract can crank up the benefits again for a year or more after employment ends. "Performers definitely do take stock work to get the health coverage," says Archer. "It has gotten so terribly urgent for some of them."

The motive doesn't put off Duttweiler: "If some terrific Broadway actor needs six more weeks of work to get coverage, and he can get them from me and is willing to work for a lower salary than he's accustomed to, who loses by that?"

Summer stock jobs are getting harder to find, a subject of concern for many. Recalls Davis, "Thirty years ago, when I started as a performer, everybody was getting work. But all through the 1960s and the mid-'70s, we started losing theatres." Archer agrees: "There was a period when there was a tremendously higher number of stock theatres, and it has dwindled down. Those who are operating them now have settled into their operations; if we lose them, we generally lose them to other, less-expensive Equity contracts."

"My audience seems to have leveled off in terms of growth, and that's something I want to attack," says Duttweiler. "We're trying to reach out to audiences, especially to younger audiences and to those who weren't raised with the habit of going to the theatre. Summer stock is always a wing and a prayer."

"There just aren't as many theatres, and that's the problem," Quinn adds. "On talk shows, I'm asked about how an actor should get started, and I often have to say that I don't know. At one time, there were three times as many stock theatres as there are now."

Pros and Cons

Summer stock has been good to Quinn, and he has found it "a lot of fun." His biggest surprise early on was that "established actors and stars in this business treated me as equal to everyone else. That was really nice," he recounts. "It made me feel like I was a part of the business. I expected to be an underling for many, many years, but I was just accepted."

In the big picture, how rewarding is summer stock, really?

"On the plus side," says Blazer, "there are the great friendships you make. And, of course, there's the fun of having so many different roles to play. On the negative side, I feel it's easy to be surprised by the lack of attention that may be paid to you in stock. That, along with the amount of material that's thrown at you."

"It can be like working in a vacuum," Quinn responds, "but it's a lovely vacuum. Also, actors who aren't as seasoned as others can do a lot of roles that they might not normally do. I was doing character roles at age 20 that I might not ever play on Broadway. That allowed me to really stretch as an actor."

Blazer agrees that summer stock's reward is its opportunities for big forward steps:

> Suddenly, in a few weeks, you've added seven shows to the résumé. And usually, these are shows that are done repeatedly, so casting people who see that you've done this or that might easily think, 'Great, let's hire him.' You learn to ask a selected number of questions; you learn how to make a moment yours on stage; you learn how to develop a character by yourself, without the full assistance of the director, who's busy focusing on getting the whole piece up. And since you're probably fresh from training, you're adaptable. And you gain a lot of stamina. It is incredible.

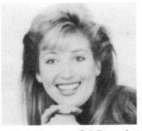

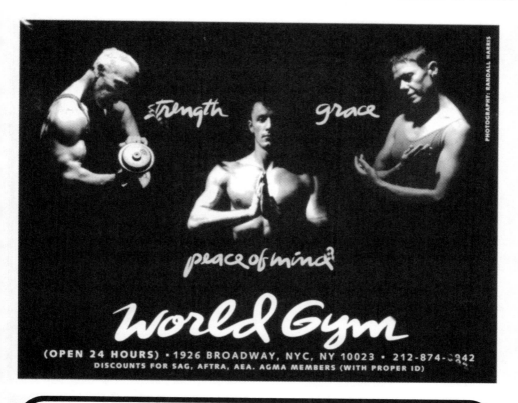

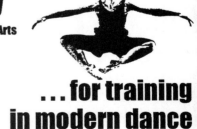

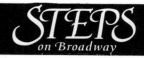

STEPS
on Broadway

Dance with the best. At Steps.

BALLET
Kim Abel
Dick Andros
Robert Atwood
Jefferson Baum
Wilhelm Burmann
Emilietta Ettlin
Andra Corvino
Alexander Filipov
Dawn Hillen
Lori Klinger
Elena Kunikova
Peff Modelski
Kathryn Sullivan
Alexander Tressor
Michael Vernon

**ZENA ROMMETT
FLOOR BARRE
TECHNIQUE**
Douglas Bolivar
Zena Rommett
Lonne Moretton
Maguerite Wesley
Dawn Hillen
Robert Atwood

FLAMENCO
Victorio Korjhan

**MODERN/
MODERN JAZZ**
Milton Myers
David Storey
Val Suzrez
Guido Tuveri
Kevin Wynn
Jolea Maffei

JAZZ
Carol Abizaid
Robert Koval
Debra Zalkind
Sarah Zimmerman
Michele Assaf
Fred Benjamin
A.C.
Arlene Erb
Nancy Koch
Joe Lanteri
Roberta Mathes
Michael Owens

Richard Pierlon
Larry Post
Gary Restifo
Max Stone
Suzi Taylor
Patricia Wilcox

**MODERN
BRAZILIAN**
Rosangela Silvestre

HIP HOP/FUNK
Jay T. Jenkins
Levi Claiborne

GUEST TEACHERS:
Andrew Asnes
Terry Beeman
Fernando Bujones
Geta Constantinescu
Robert Denvers
Simon Dow
Jean-Yves Esquerre
Christopher Huggins
Irina Kolpakova
Molly Molloy

Mia Michaels
Maya Plisetskaya
Ann Reinking
Dwight Rhoden
Desmond Richardson
Margo Sappington
Lynn Seymour
Daniel Tinazzi

TAP
Mark Goodman
Sharon Heller
Darrin Contessa
Barbara Duffy
Charles Goddertz
Mary Beth Griffith
Lisa Hopkins
Jimmy Kichler
Herve Le Goff
Nick Leone
Lesley Lockery
Alan Onickel
Robin Tribble

FITNESS PROGRAM

THEATRE DANCE
Mary Rotella
Lisa Hopkins
Alan Onickel
Bob Rizzo
Randy Skinner

**YOUNG
PEOPLE'S
PROGRAM**

YOGA
Eva Grubler
Lygia Lima

**ARTISTIC
DIRECTORS:**
Carol Paumgarten
Patrice Soriero

**MANAGING
DIRECTOR:**
Diane Grumet

2121 Broadway @74th — (212) 874-2410

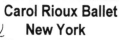

Carol Rioux Ballet New York
"Discover Your Possibilities"

Absolute Beginner to Professional

For all types of dancers, actors, singers,
etc. Learn how to minimize stress
for maximum results & easier movement
quality. Experience the "joy of learning"!
Locations Midtown & Downtown

Call (212) 631-1013

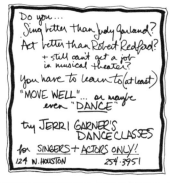

Do you...
Sing better than Judy Garland?
Act better than Robert Redford?
+ still can't get a job
in musical theater?
You have to learn to (at least)
"MOVE WELL"... or maybe
even "DANCE"

try JERRI GARNER'S
DANCE CLASSES

for SINGERS + ACTORS ONLY!
124 N. HOUSTON   254·3951

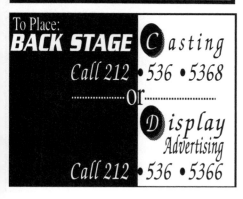

To Place:
BACK STAGE *Casting*
Call 212 • 536 • 5368
····················· or ·····················
Display Advertising
Call 212 • 536 • 5366

17

Combined Auditions:
Maximum Exposure,
Minimum Expense

JILL CHARLES

The performing opportunities which present themselves in the summer vary widely. There are Shakespeare festivals, Renaissance fairs, outdoor dramas, showboats, theme parks, non-Equity companies that run on a shoestring, and Equity package shows with major stars as a drawing card. If any actor were to try to approach all these venues individually, the cost, in time and money, of getting a job—sending out pictures and résumés, lining up auditions, traveling to those that don't hold open calls in New York—would be overwhelming.

Fortunately, for the last twenty years or so it has been possible to audition for many summer companies at once, through more than a dozen regional combined auditions held throughout the country. On one spring weekend an actor might be seen by producers of as many as 90 different companies.

The actor seriously looking for summer work must begin in winter—December or January—writing for applications for the audition weekends he or she might want to attend. Since many of these auditions receive more applications than available time slots, they must screen applications by as much as 50 percent. Thus, applying early will greatly increase your chance of receiving an audition time. Once accepted, you will be sent a time slot, instructions for your two- or three-minute audition, and information on the companies that will be attending the auditions.

Each audition has a callback system by which producers can contact the performers they are interested in, to see them again on the same weekend or to set up a callback elsewhere at another time.

Many actors who attend combined auditions each spring mistakenly equate the entire experience with the two minutes they spend on stage. Granted, these are probably the most important two minutes of the experience, but there's much more going on. The wise performer will make the most of it all. So here are some tips for creating your own opportunities at these marathons.

The Right Attitude

It all begins when you walk in the door. All day long you will be dealing with people: those working at the registration table, the monitors and timekeepers, the producers and casting people you'll meet at callbacks or casually around the canteen truck parked outside. The atmosphere might be tense, and you might be tense too, but the attitude to project is one of confidence, efficiency, and professionalism. All those people running the audition are trying to make things go smoothly, but there are inevitable crises. The accompanist is late getting back from lunch, no one can find the janitor to unlock the callback rooms, the auditions are running late, and the coffee is running out. So the first tip is simple: *Be nice.*

By their very nature, these auditions can bring out the worst in people. Many actors become completely self-involved, totally focused on the two minutes they have onstage, and closed off to all around them—as if they were tight little boxes anxiously waiting in line, sometimes bumping into other boxes. They cut themselves off from any communication with others and then complain about how inhuman the whole process is.

In a situation with so many people crammed together, the trick is to make yourself stand out, but always in the most positive sense. You can be the considerate actor who stops to help the harried assistant who just dropped 800 picture/résumés in the hallway. You can be the actor who pauses after finishing the audition to tell the accompanist, "Thanks, your tempo was perfect." You can be the actor who tells the producer at the callback, "I know you must be exhausted, and I appreciate your taking this extra time with me. What can I show you that you didn't see in my audition? Or, would you rather get together at another time when we're not so rushed?"

The payoff for you is twofold: The whole experience becomes at least more bearable, if not actually pleasant, and you are remembered in a positive light by those you come in contact with. You never know if the person assisting at the registration table might be casting for someone the next year, or if that accompanist is also the music director for a summer theatre.

Networking and Being Organized

Some of these auditions happen in the context of an annual convention: The Southeastern Theatre, East Central Theatre, and Rocky Mountain Theatre Association conferences are three examples. Usually, you have to register for the convention in order to attend the auditions. The convention organizers, no fools, create a captive audience for their events so they can be sure to cover costs. Many auditionees simply grumble, pay the fees, and go only to the audition anyway.

Yet it's at least worth looking over the convention calendar to see what workshops are being offered and by whom. If you're pursuing a Shakespeare festival that operates on a university campus, and the chair of that university's theatre department is offering a workshop on Shakespearean texts, how could it hurt to sit in? You could perhaps mention when you interview with the casting people from the festival that you enjoyed the workshop. In high school we called this "brown-nosing"; now we can call it "networking."

One thing to be sure of as you work these auditions is to stay organized. Bring plenty of extra picture/résumés, and write everything down. You will receive a listing of all the theatres attending and what their casting needs are. Read about a theatre before you go to its callback, so you come across as an actor who's genuinely interested in that particular company. Know what shows it is doing so you know which roles you could play in its season. And "bone-up" a bit so you avoid asking stupid questions like, "So, your theatre is in Maine, right—or is it New Hampshire?" Have your datebook with you, to confirm on the spot any callbacks you might set up for a future time. Write down the name of everyone you meet, with his or her title if possible, and after a callback make notes on what was said—so you can remember which producer wanted to see you juggle and which was interested in your Scottish dialect.

Non-Equity performers should be aware that many non-Equity companies are looking for multitalented personnel. So an actor who can also work in the shop, stage-manage, or write press releases frequently has the edge over others. If you have such nonperforming experience, don't hide this on your acting résumé, and do mention it when you get into an interview or callback. In fact, if your skills are very strong in a nonperforming area, it might be worth your while to do a completely separate résumé in that area and apply for tech/staff interviews as well as the auditions. Most combined auditions have a day or an afternoon devoted to putting producers together with potential design, technical, and management staff. In many cases it doesn't cost any more to attend these interviews in addition to performing your audition. If you can do both, you may be able to interview as staff for the theatres that called you back as an actor, and you may find that your extra skills make you more desirable than your competition.

Helping Out

The way to learn what these auditions are really all about is to experience them at least once from the other side—that is, assist a producer who goes to these things. If you have worked for a summer theatre that attends any of these combined auditions, call the staff there—now!—and ask if they would like some help at upcoming auditions. Since you're planning to attend anyway, could you sit in with them and help them keep track of callbacks, make notes, get them coffee—anything at all, for a significant chunk of the time when you're not auditioning? If you're really smart, you'll arrange to do this for them for a whole day, before the day of your scheduled audition.

For starters, you will learn more about auditioning after watching a day of it than you ever imagined you could. You will see good actors blow their shot at a callback through nervousness, lack of preparation, self-indulgence, or just having a lousy attitude. You will understand how important it is to walk into an audition with confidence instead of an apology, and to maintain that confidence not just through the audition but all the way out of the room. You will see green actors make poor choices in material, using pieces that are too youthful or too old or against their type. You will become angry with actors who look like they just don't care or who even project hostility across the footlights. You will share the anguish of a young actor who goes up on lines or who is clearly terrified. And ultimately, you will understand that, yes, as much as actors hate the idea, you do know if you're interested in a performer within the first 20 seconds of his or her audition.

Meanwhile, you will learn a lot about the producers who are watching the auditions. Hearing their comments to each other about actors, you will realize that they're not sitting in judgment or waiting for people to fail—they're just trying to cast their plays. The more good actors they see, the better; that way, producers won't have to fight each other over the top performers. You'll hear producers complain about pieces they hate, songs they can't bear to hear one more time, how they're offended by actors who won't take the trouble to dress decently, how they resent having obscenities screamed in their faces, even if the selection is from Mamet. You will share the experience of complete numbness, as time stands still at four o'clock, with 45 more actors to see before dinner break. You will feel how exhausted producers and directors are by the time they finally get to callbacks, and realize it's a miracle they can still remember their own names, much less anyone else's.

And the final bonus is more networking time. When you stand around at coffee breaks you can introduce yourself to other producers and fall into casual conversations about their seasons, their theatres, mutual friends—the usual stuff, but it can make you a recognizable person to them, so when you audition the next day you'll stand out among the masses. And you can check them out at the same time, deciding which producers you'd enjoy working for, and which not.

To paraphrase the old proverb: You'll never truly understand a producer until you've jogged a mile in his Reeboks. So now that you're on the inside track, send off for those applications, and let the marathon begin!

For a list of regional combined auditions nationwide, see the Appendix, page 280.

18

Student Films:
Experience in Front of the Camera
SIMI HORWITZ

Thinking about appearing in student films? Or wondering just what they are, anyway? Well, they are precisely what their name suggests: Films made by students at film schools nationwide, and they're a wonderful opportunity for learning on the job, especially if you have little or no film experience.

The range of actors who have performed in student films is striking. This is where Alec Baldwin and Bridget Fonda launched their careers, and a handful of others, such as James Earl Jones and Jerry Stiller, still lend their services to these films from time to time.

Obviously, most actors involved in student films are not "big names" like these, but they're not newcomers, either. Some have substantial theatre credits but want the opportunity to expand their acting repertoires. Other performers who have film credits galore, like 45-year-old actress Holgie Forrester, just want to keep on acting and honing their craft between jobs. Student films are a good way to do it. And though you won't get paid, short of carfare and free lunches, the things you'll learn about the whole movie-making experience will be invaluable.

"I perform in student films to continue acting and working with all kinds of directors," says Forrester. "I also do student films to learn about film-making. There's more opportunity to talk to the crew and ask questions than on a professional set. And I have found that student directors love to talk about films with their actors. I enjoy that!"

The Benefits
There are other bonuses, too: The networking possibilities are considerable. You never know who today's student director might become tomorrow. Spike Lee, George Lucas, Martin Scorcese, and Steven Spielberg were *all* student directors once. If you impress the directors you work with now, they may remember you when they work for the major studios.

For some actors, this route may lead directly to a professional-level acting job, especially when student films win national exposure as award-winners. (The Academy of Motion Picture Arts and Sciences presents a Student Academy Award.) A fair number of student films end up in international festivals (Toronto, Sundance, Cannes), where producers, agents, and studio heads are all too eager to find that "hot" new property.

There's even a chance, admittedly slim, of earning a few dollars for your efforts. While the Screen Actors Guild's "letter agreement," created exclusively for student films used in classrooms or student festivals, allows SAG members to work for reimbursement of expenses, the agreement also states that SAG actors must be paid if a student film they've performed in goes on to commercial release. It requires Workers Compensation insurance on each project, coverage that protects all the actors involved—union and nonunion—in case of accident.

While the SAG agreement provides for future pay for members, it does not extend to nonunion performers. Still, there's nothing to prevent an actor— any actor—from negotiating independently with a student director for additional monies.

Another major reason to consider appearing in student projects is that you are usually promised a free videotape of the completed product. If the film and your performance are good, you can effectively incorporate clips into a demo for submission to casting directors and agents. Most agents are not turned off by demos that include quality student film work. Many actors, however, despite the promise made to them, do not get their tapes. In some instances, the project is never finished; in other, rarer instances, student directors just don't fulfill their obligations. (Extra videos cost them extra money, which is in short supply). On other occasions, with no malice aforethought, directors and actors simply lose touch and the performers end up sans tape. Still, if the videos do exist, most performers get copies—it just sometimes takes planning and persistent inquiry.

What's Out There?

At any one time, dozens, if not hundreds, of student films are being shot coast to coast. You can find out who's casting what in your area by reading *Back Stage* and any local trade publications and by contacting nearby university film departments. In New York City, the major film schools include New York University, Columbia University, and the School of Visual Arts; nearby, there's the State University of New York's film school at Purchase. Prominent on the West Coast are the University of Southern California and the University of California at Los Angeles.

The kinds of films being made run the gamut from 8mm black-and-white experimental shorts to 35mm full-color Hollywood-style features. Most of the scripts for these films are written by the student directors themselves.

Undergraduate as well as graduate students produce films; the most professional-looking work is typically in the hands of seniors and graduates, whose movies represent thesis projects. Accordingly, seniors and graduates are the most likely to complete their films—something to keep in mind if you're counting on getting that video.

Cast sizes can vary, but they're usually small because of the enormous cost of shooting. (Even unpaid actors need meals, transportation, costumes, and makeup.) A budget of $100,000 is not unheard of, and expenses are often paid out, at least in part, from the student director's own pocket. Shooting schedules also cover the spectrum—from several hours on just one day to 12 hours daily over the course of several weeks.

The big surprise is that the competition to get into these student films is heavy-duty. "For every lead I advertised for in *Back Stage,*" recalls Gary Nadeau, a former NYU film student, "I got over 1,000 headshots and résumés." The thirty-year-old Nadeau, who won the 1994 Student Academy Award for his picture *Red,* currently has a movie deal with Disney. No doubt it's a seller's market, and directors can pretty much get whomever they want, within limits.

Choosing What's Right for You

Of course, actors can pick and choose, too. Obviously, not every student film that comes down the pike is right for every performer. Determining which project might be worthwhile for you depends on a variety of factors, not the least of which is the appeal the material holds for you. If there is *any* indication, either in the casting-call notice or your initial interview with the director, that the style of the picture or subject matter is off-putting, you shouldn't get involved. All our interviewees agree that the script is the bottom line. It's important to remember that the films with the good scripts are more likely to be the award-winners.

Darrel Adelman, a 52-year-old actor–playwright who has appeared in four student films, offers this advice:

> I believe it's legitimate for an actor to know as much as he can about a student film before he gets involved in it, including the director's vision, his budget, and exactly where you'll be shooting. You have a right to know if you'll be going into a dangerous neighborhood that doesn't have much police protection. If that's the case, you might not want to do it.

Most important is the person directing. Get a sense of him or her before you commit to the project. Does he seem to know what he's doing? Is she articulate and willing to answer questions? Is he comfortable with you? Is she comfortable with herself? The rapport between director and actor is key, and instinct is the only way to go. Although flexibility is essential in an actor, if you're not really at ease with the director during the early interview and audition stage, maybe this is not the project for you.

Tips on Preparation

Once you're involved in a student film, you should, of course, behave professionally. Be on time, be prepared, and don't be a prima donna. Nothing turns off a director, crew, or fellow actors more than a bragging, self-indulgent performer and/or actor who believes he or she is there to teach the director.

Working with a student director, from audition to rehearsal, from shooting to "wrap," shouldn't be all that different from working with a professional— with several notable exceptions. For example, many student directors are not well-versed in the acting process. Not knowing how to work with actors, they may want immediate results—for example, a novice might command: "Go to that chair and burst into tears!" Then there are directors who have definite ideas about acting that may seem distasteful to some actors—calling for endless improvisations, for instance. Actors who have been there stress the point that one must be prepared for the young director's quirks. Be tolerant and patient.

That leads to another important point: Student directors, on occasion, seem to spend a great deal of time on technical issues—lighting nuances and production values—as opposed to spending enough time with actors. Technology often takes precedence, performers report. But that's not necessarily a bad thing. Remember, it's those quality production values that get the films into the festivals and help them win the awards. Ultimately, that is far more helpful to the actor than a brilliant performance in a shoddily made film that nobody sees.

Rehearsing and shooting schedules should be handled professionally by the student director, meaning that you should know well ahead of time what hours you'll be working. You should also have sufficient time off between the end of a shoot and your next call.

Accommodations, however, are often adequate at best. Even the SAG letter agreement does not address working conditions. There are no formal dressing rooms or trailers; costume changes frequently take place in hallways. During out-of-town shoots you may find yourself sleeping, with 20 other actors, on the living room floor at the director's parents' house. (Since this can go on for weeks, you had better be good-natured and maintain your sense of humor. At the same time, don't allow a student filmmaker and a low budget to become an opportunity for exploitation.)

Of course, taking responsibility for yourself is generally a good idea, but it has special application in working on student films. If you're going to be shooting near the ocean in February, bring extra layers of clothing that can be peeled off quickly and then put on again. It's a detail, but no one else is going to think about it.

Be super-vigilant about transportation. Yes, it's supposed to be provided, but there can be slip-ups. It's common sense to address these issues before there's a crisis. Say you've finished your scene in Stamford, Connecticut, at midnight, and no one you want to drive with is returning, and there are no trains back to Manhattan at that hour. Do you have a contingency plan?

Also, be prepared with your own costumes and makeup. You rarely have the kind of wardrobe set-ups that you would on a professional picture, emphasizes Holgie Forrester: "I always make it my business to bring the right clothes. For example, if in the last scene I was wearing black, I'd have my black stockings with me. I also bring my own makeup and rollers, just in case they're necessary."

After the Shoot

At no time is it more necessary to take responsibility than after the wrap. It's over. It's been a ball, or a bust, but in either case you're going to want a video-tape. It may be months before tapes are forthcoming, if not a year or more. Nonetheless, you have a right to know the film's status and to call the director and ask about it. Sometimes, of course, it's hard to track this filmmaker down—especially in this business, people move on.

One good way to avoid this kind of frustration is to obtain the director's and assistant director's permanent home addresses and phone numbers before the conclusion of the project. If they don't get back to you, get back to them. That doesn't mean be a pest. (Yes, there's a thin line.)

If, after a reasonable amount of time, there's still no videotape or information forthcoming, you can always contact the head of the school's film department. A responsible administrator will be committed to meeting any written or oral agreements that promise actors videotapes.

Is There a Time to Stop?

When have you done enough student films? At what point are your appearances in these projects counterproductive?

This is a judgment call; there are no easy answers. There's always the possibility that the next student film you appear in will get the awards, make the festival circuit, and land you that dream contract. You must ask yourself, then, if the possibility is real in the case of each new student film opportunity. Like anyone in any profession, unless you have moved on after a certain point, you face the danger of being identified with particular kinds of projects and thus being seen as out of the running for more prestigious ventures. Try not to let the possibility of "the next time" become an excuse for neglecting that step that could put you on a new footing in your career. Student films are valuable experiences, but there could be a fully professional film role lying in store for you.

19

Theme Parks:
Job Opportunities Are the Main Attraction
THOMAS WALSH

Once upon a time, the term "theme park" may have evoked a magical land of kids clad in mouse ears riding jungle river boats and choo-choo trains, but for performers today, the term suggests a land of performance opportunities. Disneyland, Busch Gardens, Sea World, and numerous other attractions draw over 200 million visitors each year for diversions of all kinds. What this adds up to is a great need for performers with a wide range of talents.

While rides, games, and food are at the core of theme parks' entertainment, there is another constant which provides work for performers: Most parks offer entertainment in the form of theme-based live performances, especially musical revues about the Wild West, the Roaring Twenties, Hollywood, and Broadway, to name a few. There are also dance spectaculars, stunt shows, live music, singalongs, and shows filled with popular cartoon, television, and movie characters. In a world where performing jobs are hard to come by, theme parks hire thousands of actors, singers, dancers, circus performers, storytellers, impressionists, and musicians every season.

Highs and Lows

What can young performers gain from such employment? To begin with, there's the experience itself—rehearsing and staging perhaps three or more shows a day, learning how to take direction, maybe playing more than one role, and meeting new people. Then there's being "away from it all," pulling a steady and sometimes very attractive paycheck, and acquiring a real sense of working in a professional environment.

"Our entertainers take the stage more than 600 times during the season," says Marie Cronenwett, manager of park attractions at Cedar Point, a 125-year-old legend in Sandusky, Ohio. "It's comparable to being in a Broadway show that runs for a couple of years—only our entertainers pack it all into one summer."

To be honest, it's a life that's not for everybody. The material isn't exactly highbrow in nature, the rehearsal and performance schedules can be grueling, and the lower-end salaries unimpressive. Many people hired at the parks have to travel long distances to get there and must commit to three-month to one-year (or longer) contracts. But particularly for young up-and-comers who want to get some seasoning, theme parks offer potential: travel to new places, lighthearted material, a consistent salary, and, most important, the chance to perform in front of large, new audiences every day, honing their craft as entertainers.

While several parks do acknowledge that some of their full-time people may earn salaries barely in excess of $6 an hour, others start employees at $360 or more per week, and the numbers can climb to about $600 weekly for specialty performers. The figures are generally based on a standard 40-hour work week, as offered at most parks.

There are also benefit possibilities. Many of the facilities have huge companies behind them—Disney, Six Flags, Paramount, Busch—and even those without corporate parents may offer strong incentive packages to employees. Bonus payments based on meeting a contract's terms are sometimes given to performers and technicians. For more than 20 years, Walt Disney World, through its intensive orchestra and band programs, has been arranging college credits for young musical talent through special agreements with various schools.

The perks may also include company profit-sharing, full pay for rehearsals, some health insurance coverage, master classes, coaching sessions, seminars, and workshops with professional entertainers and technicians. Housing is often quite good (many places deduct small lodging fees from paychecks), or help is provided in finding affordable accommodations. Travel fees to and from parks, before, during, and after the seasons are sometimes supported by the companies. General admission to the parks is usually a given, along with guest passes.

When and How to Audition

For most theme parks, auditions and interviews are held in the December through February period. Multi-city national auditions are common, particularly for Disney, Busch, and independent companies like Show Biz International and Cedar Point. Others, like Six Flags, generally search for talent on a local level, but they'll do it several times a year. And some do it both ways, holding major auditions in key cities and regular calls at, or near, the home park.

Musical performers in various combinations (singer–actors, dancer–singers, actor–dancers) are by far the most sought-after. For actor-only types, comic monologues are almost always requested by producers, and improvisation skills are generally helpful, particularly for stand-up comics, street entertainers, jugglers, and impersonators. Directors, choreographers, designers, conductors, stage managers, emcees, announcers, and technicians of all abilities are also hired by the score through audition tours and at the home park. These people often stand a better chance of getting hired at other times during the year because most parks solicit tech résumés year-round and report

that they do a lot of hiring that way. Technicians are sometimes asked for letters of recommendation as well as résumés and are then interviewed.

The basic requirements for auditionees and interviewees don't change
much from year to year. Singers are usually asked to prepare an up-tempo
number and a ballad, and they might be asked to dance. Dancers, often expected to have some training in jazz, tap, and ballet, could be taught dance
numbers and also asked to sing. (Accompanists are almost always provided.)

Since music is such a hot commodity at the parks, musicians who audition
need to be especially sharp. The ability to sight-read and to play more than
one instrument are often minimum requirements.

When it comes to performers, some places make no bones about what kind
of people they want at the tryouts: A common refrain in the audition guide-
lines is something like, "Don't forget to look happy," or "Wear a smile!"

Casts of Hundreds

Some of the bigger parks, such as Disneyland, hire more than 500 performers
and crew members in a year, while the relatively small ones, like Worlds of
Fun in Kansas City, Missouri, might top out at 50 to 100. At the 365-day-a-
year operations, a full-year commitment is commonly asked of employees,
but the parks with finite seasons generally hire on a season-only basis.

Since there are so many genres and styles of performance at theme parks,
the shows themselves run the gamut. Some performers, such as jugglers, street
entertainers, and roving costumed characters, might be on for less than a
minute or up to 10 minutes; others will be on for 20 minutes to well over an
hour in full-scale Broadway-style song-and-dance productions. Some performances may be presented 10 to 20 times a day, others three to six times.

Over time, this schedule can prove exhausting. Seasons at most theme parks
are long—from March or April to after Labor Day, sometimes extending into au-
tumn. For quite a few sites such as Disney World, the season is year-round.
(Nine of the top 10 parks in California and Florida are year-round operations.)

All Eyes on You

In 1994, Disney World's Magic Kingdom in Florida maintained its perennial
status as the foremost theme park, as 11.2 million customers passed through
the gates, according to *Amusement Business* magazine. It was followed by Disneyland, the pioneer park that basically started it all in the 1950s; it pulled in
10.3 million visitors in 1994.

Naturally, every one of those parkgoers has access to shows at the venues
every day. In other words, no matter what kind of presentation you're a part of
at a theme park, the potential size of your audience is tremendous. And the more
exposure you have, the better your chances of telling the world just who you are.

*For a list of theme parks and theme park show producers, see the Appendix, page
287.*

20

Actors Aweigh

JEFFREY ERIC JENKINS

Imagine riding the high seas to such exciting places as Spain, Italy, Russia, and India. Now imagine being well paid to make the trip. It's certainly possible. It's also possible that when you finally land in an exotic locale after ten days with a too-talkative roommate and that passenger who swears he loves you madly, you'll want nothing more than to hop a plane back home.

Formerly the domain of the wealthy leisure class, cruise ships have become the theme parks of the briny blue. Thousands of travelers are squeezing more enjoyment from their vacation budgets by turning simple trips into fun fests aboard these floating palaces—and most cruise lines use entertainers to help make the voyage more enjoyable.

Cruise entertainment staff range from revue singer–dancers who may perform additional duties to headliner variety artists who are treated like passengers and perform once or twice a week. While revue performers share dormitory-style rooms with other staff, headliners are allowed to bring a guest to share passenger-style quarters at no extra charge.

Variety Artist Heaven

Over the past 20 years, work in the burgeoning cruise business has become the successor to the vaudeville and Borscht Belt circuits. With this expansion has come an ever-growing need for singer–dancers in Broadway- and Las Vegas-style shows, lead singers for revues, solo singers, comedians, and specialty acts.

For variety artists such as Karen Saunders, a New York–based nightclub singer who is considered a cruise headliner, the ships seem like heaven. "The first time I did a cruise," she recalls, "I thought, 'Will I get claustrophobic?' But the ship was so big, I actually got lost." She quickly adapted. "It's work, not stardom. You need to be on land to build a career. But the cruise lines treat headliners royally, like a passenger, and with your food and expenses paid, it's easy to save money."

Saunders performed her solo act of new renditions of older popular music for about five years on cruise ships. "You really need two different shows of about 45 minutes to an hour," she says, "and the material has to be very commercial—similar to what you might hear in the Catskills or in Atlantic City."

By definition, variety artists do self-contained acts for which the ship provides a minimum of staff support. All medium and large ships have an orchestra for the solo performers, but it is the artist's responsibility to provide musical charts for, say, a 14-piece group. "That's an investment of $10,000–$20,000," Saunders says, "which is an enormous expense for someone trying to start an act. And you also have to know, or learn somewhere, how to rehearse an orchestra." Also, she explains, it is also hard to break into the business as a solo act these days because revue productions, which are very popular, are cheaper to do.

The Long Chorus Line

In a world that makes careful class distinctions between headliners, lead revue performers, and chorus people, the majority of cruise line performers earn their living in revue-type productions. The musical shows range in quality from full-scale Broadway productions and upscale revues featuring established Broadway artists to lively musical offerings performed by young professionals trying to build their careers.

Peter Grey Terhune, of Peter Grey Terhune Presents, in Cape Canaveral, Florida, currently produces musical revues for Royal Caribbean Cruise Line, Royal Cruise Line, Regency Cruises, and Cunard Line Limited. "We look for the most talented, presentable people we can find," he states. Regarding multiracial casting, he says, "On the *Nordic Prince*, our show features a cast of 10 with one Hispanic and two African-American performers. Most important to us is that our entertainers are the human link between the cruise line and the passengers."

While performers are helping make vacations memorable for cruise passengers, they earn pretty good money for their trouble. "Compared to theme parks or non-Equity shows," Terhune says, "cruises pay revue performers quite well." Though pay rates are guarded like state secrets, estimates range from $400–$800 per week for chorus people.

Terhune said he is "very bullish" on the expanding cruise market. "There is a lot of work for talented people," Terhune affirms. "Of course, the catch is that the supply of people outweighs the demand, and our hardest job is matching the right people with the right positions."

Perks and Privations

As with any job, cruise work has its perks and privations. You may see Kathie Lee Gifford dancing and singing in a TV commercial for Carnival Cruise Lines that makes a cruise look like total fun. Or you may see a chorus line strutting as an announcer intones that these Broadway performers are appearing nightly on the high seas. You may think, "Now that's a job for me." But what does that job *really* entail? How many times a week will you perform? Four, six, eight? Will you emcee a matinee-style game of *What's My Line?* for 300 passengers or lead exercises in the swimming pool? How do you feel about running the ship's library for a couple of hours a day? On some smaller ships, space is at such a premium that being an entertainer takes on a very broad meaning.

Former cruise performer John Allen, who now heads the New York City–based Interborough Repertory Theatre, spent several years working the ships before his land-based theatre career demanded full attention. Allen reflected on some of the responsibilties he had had on board:

> Some people resent the cruise staff duties that are often assigned to revue performers. We would be asked to work in the ship's library, checking out books for a couple of hours. Or maybe we would help with Bingo games. But the only staff duties that were particularly odious involved shepherding passengers at embarkation and dis-embarkation. We could be standing for four to six hours trying to keep passengers calm and relaxed while negotiating customs—and we really didn't know what was going on anyway. For the most part, though, cruise work involves a light work schedule. In fact, there probably isn't enough to do.

When the Nashville-based husband-and-wife team of Andy and Tammy Heath began working as revue performers on cruise lines in 1986, they couldn't get enough. "We worked constantly, 10 or 11 months a year, for three years," Andy Heath says. Now, though, "six or seven months is about our limit." Even so, he goes on to say:

> We love the travel and the people we've met. We've seen some-thing like 105 countries, and we've done all this while working to-gether, which was our goal all along. Unfortunately, you miss a lot when you're on a ship. When my grandfather died, for instance, it took a couple of days for my father to reach me, and there was no way I could go home for the funeral.

Andy also remarks that, among all the other qualifications necessary for cruise work, it doesn't hurt to have a strong stomach and a sturdy pair of sea legs. "We spent nine days in a hurricane on a ship's maiden voyage," he remem-bers. "The captain held position for four days to conserve fuel. Our Thanks-giving turkey flew out of the oven and the soup was on the wall, so we ate pastrami sandwiches and wore our life jackets."

Modern meteorology helps captains avoid the worst storms, but when you live on a ship for months at a time, you're going to get some bad weather and rough seas. Individual cruises vary in length from three to fourteen days, but once a performer signs on, he or she usually remains with the ship for the length of the contract—up to six months.

Of course, you have an eager and captive audience all that time, but the audience has a captive performer, too. Even when you aren't performing, you are always "on stage." When your show is over, you can't just duck out the stage door and head home to your cats and your answering machine—but you can drop by the midnight buffet for a snack with your audience. And when that chorus diva who always tries to upstage you finally sends you over the edge, you have no one to complain to, because she's your roommate.

Not the Lap of Luxury

Life for a revue performer on a ship does vary from line to line, and accommodations are comfortable, generally, if not the lap of luxury enjoyed by headliners. On Norwegian Cruise Line, for instance, principals in full-scale Broadway productions—which are, reportedly, as close to actual Broadway shows as you can get without being in New York—are given passenger cabins. Chorus people on Norwegian have staff-area accommodations, some of which are in the less-desirable passenger areas.

While headliners enjoy the passenger dining facilities, revue performers are generally relegated to the staff dining areas. However, Joanne Maiello, vice president of Jean Ann Ryan Productions, in Ft. Lauderdale, Florida, says, "Soloists generally use the staff mess as well, because it's less formal and easier to deal with just before a show." And Peter Terhune adds, "The staff eats the same food as the passengers; it's just served in a less fancy manner—cafeteria-style, for instance."

The Search Continues

"We are always looking for well-trained dancers, singers, and singer–dancers," Maiello explains. She tours the country twice a year, auditioning performers in such uncommon places as Oklahoma and South Dakota. "We go where the résumés come from," she says. The audition tour visits nearly 20 cities in the United States and Canada to fill the casts for full-scale productions of *The Will Rogers Follies, Grease, Dreamgirls* and *George M!* on Norwegian Cruise Line. The company also creates Las Vegas-style shows around themes such as Hollywood, Broadway legends, current Broadway shows, and the circus.

"Our three- to six-month contracts are a lot of hard work," Maiello adds, "but it is a wonderful opportunity to travel and save money."

Compensation

So what does it pay to be isolated from the outside world for weeks on end, to live in comfortable accommodations and eat well, to work about four hours a day, and to ride out the occasional storm?

None of the people we spoke to were very forthcoming about pay scales, but, as mentioned above, it was generally agreed that revue performers earn $400 to $800 per week based on experience and cruise line. For instance, Carnival Cruise Lines—which, because of its mass-marketing approach, is known as "the Holiday Inn of the cruise industry"—tends to hire less-experienced chorus people at the lower end of the pay scale and "really work them," as one headliner attests.

Performers are paid aboard ship on a regular basis, either monthly or bi-monthly, and payment is always in U.S. dollars. One producer said he makes direct deposits to his performers' bank accounts every two weeks.

Performers who are not "name" solo singing artists earn in the range of $1,000 to $1,200 per week, while a specialty act such as a magician will make around $1,500. Top money is earned by comedians—that is, comedians whose material is "clean"—at $2,000 to $3,000 per week.

"Comedy clubs are closing all over the country," observes James Abramson, president of Bramson Entertainment Bureau, in New York City, the largest booking organization for cruise work. "I have comics calling for jobs all the time. But to work on a ship," he says, "comics must work 'clean.' Those comics are very hard to find."

Abramson advises novice performers to try the lower-priced cruise lines because they "are more willing to break new people in." However, he cautions that those lines are not automatically stepping stones to more prestigious cruise work.

Staying Afloat and More

Working as a performer on a cruise ship may sound like a vacation for a head-liner, but it isn't. With the expanded privileges of being treated as a passenger comes responsibility and a loss of anonymity. All the headliners we spoke to felt that they had to be on guard as representatives of the cruise lines and that they were "performing" continuously. However, these performers are working and earning good money—most of which can be saved during the cruise.

As for revue performers, chorus work can sometimes be a bridge to leading roles and to developing a solo act. One performer taking that route is Ken Prescott, a New York City–based singer–dancer-choreographer. Prescott has worked as a singing actor for about 20 years and began performing leading-man roles in floating Broadway shows, such as *George M!* and *42nd Street*, on Norwegian Cruise Line three years ago.

"It's called show business," Prescott says. "Work is work." And this work, he said, "pays well, the schedule isn't hard, and we get good accommodations."

While doing the cruise shows, Prescott is busy developing his own solo act. "I have a cabaret act, but I'm trying to build it up so I can make a recording. With so few musicals playing on Broadway these days, cruise ships are a great opportunity for singer–dancers to learn their craft in shows with full production values. Where else can that happen—and for such good pay?"

For a list of sources—agents, producers, and cruise lines—to contact for opportunities in this field, see the Appendix, page 291.

21

Producing Your Own Showcase

BEN ALEXANDER

W hen you're an aspiring actor, director, or playwright, your greatest need is to get your work seen on the stage. The quest for exposure, even when no pay is involved, usually means standing in one long line after another or endlessly submitting scripts or résumés. There is, though, one alternative to the exhausting process of marketing your talent to producers: producing something yourself in the form of a showcase.

"Showcase" is the standard word for a short-run production that's mounted primarily to gain exposure in the business. Like any theatrical production, it requires both time and money, neither of which the typical artist has much of. If you think of all the necessities that somehow seem to get taken care of behind the scenes when you're working for an established company—things like rehearsal space, performance space, costumes, props, scenery, electricity, publicity, insurance—and then imagine yourself being solely responsible for all these, you have a taste of the word "producer."

Laying the Foundation

The first step toward producing a showcase is defining clearly for yourself the *raison d'etre* for your project. The motive may be the sheer exercise of your craft. Even more important may be attracting the interest of an agent, a producer, or a casting director. Getting the whole production picked up for an extended run at a larger venue is also an aim. For many who mount their own productions, still another objective is to get reviewed—favorably, one hopes.

Next comes the planning: making a budget, figuring out where the funds will come from, getting legal advice, plotting a timetable, deciding how to find the best actors to join you in the venture, sorting out where the rehearsals and the performances will happen, and lining up the necessary help.

One basic decision at the outset is whether to do the showcase with or without members of Actors' Equity Association in the cast. What Equity policies allow its actors to do differs from city to city. In New York, the key to using Equity performers is the union's Approved Basic Showcase Code, which must be followed if even one Equity member is involved. This code involves transportation reimbursement, insurance, rehearsal and performance limits, and conditions, and a copy of it can be obtained from the Equity office in New York. Other major cities have their own Equity agreements. In Los Angeles, it's the 99-Seat Theatre Plan; in Chicago, it's the Chicago Showcase Code (for use by Equity actors and producers only).

The performer unions discipline their members with fines for taking part in projects that are not union-sanctioned. Doing a play with all nonunion actors will eliminate a host of regulations and stipulations but will also greatly reduce the pool of talent available to you.

Making a budget is an absolute necessity. Showcase costs can range from $100 to $15,000, the maximum that Equity allows. A major cost will be the theatre rental, which can range from $1,000 to $2,500 a week. Once you've ascertained the cost of your performance rentals, work backward to how many hours of rehearsal the project will need and choose your rehearsal space. In New York, these rates run in the vicinity of $10 to $25 per hour. Many people have connections for free rehearsal space in church basements, college classrooms, and so on. The budget-making stage is also the time to go through the script and figure out what scenery, props, and costumes will be needed. Insurance is a factor to budget, as well. If Equity actors are involved, it's a requirement; even otherwise, it makes good sense to insure the production.

Plays are often subject to royalties, which must be checked with the licensing agent at the outset. If royalties are due, budget for them and pay them to avoid legal problems that can be quite serious.

Publicity is vital, and one should allow several hundred dollars for it—postage and photocopying costs add up quickly. In budgeting, estimate receipts from ticket sales conservatively.

At about the same time you compile your budget, you should make a timetable. The standard run for a showcase is 16 performances within a four-week period. Assuming that you want industry professionals (including reviewers) to see your showcase, the performance dates need to be chosen carefully, avoiding times that conflict with multiple Broadway openings, Tony Awards, holidays, and so on. Summer months and January–February are the optimal months for small productions. Once the performance dates are in place, a schedule for everything that will lead up to opening night must be set. By such and such a date, the show will be cast. Rehearsals will begin at *this* point; props and furnishings will have been gathered by *that* point; the press releases will have been sent out . . . the flyers . . . the invitations to industry professionals—and so on.

Getting Started

Especially if this is your maiden voyage as a producer, trying to be Superman or Wonder Woman is not advisable. If you're producing and acting, somebody else should be directing. Also, the more hats you're wearing in the creative department, the more help you'll need with business management. Be realistic about how much you can do well yourself and line up the appropriate help.

It's a good idea to give your group a production company name and, in your publicity, not to be obvious about the fact that you're not an established theatre troupe. You don't want to blare out to agents: "Hey, I'm an aspiring actor who can play Tom Wingfield better than anybody I know, so I've gotten my friends together to play Amanda, Laura, and Jim, and we're putting on a show!" You want a name with a professional, stable ring.

Getting the most capable and dedicated people onto your team will greatly affect how successfully the show and your own talent come across. You want to work with others whose artistic vision and work style are compatible with yours. The director is pivotal to the success of the show, so choosing one can't be done lightly. A good stage manager can be a key player in the show's success as well. You also need to have a solid corps of helpers, for jobs ranging from running lights to keeping track of reservations. And choose your technical personnel wisely: they are crucial to your production.

When working with other people, even friends, written agreements are always a good idea. The purpose of securing a contract is not to accuse the other party of any treacherous intents, but to make sure that each party understands what can be expected in the working relationship. You should have a documented accord with landlords at both rehearsal and performance spaces, spelling out schedules, rates, and liabilities. Unfortunately, producers at the Off-Off-Broadway level are less likely to make written agreements with their actors and technicians.

Among the earliest and most important steps in the process is choosing a performance space. Location is crucial: Friends and industry professionals should feel safe leaving your theatre at 10:30 PM. You'll also need to choose a theatre whose size, shape, and general ambiance are suitable for your play. Book it well in advance, and when you negotiate, get all the terms in writing.

While low price is a consideration in deciding where to rehearse, it's also true that clean, comfortable, well-constructed, well-lit rehearsal rooms are most conducive to high morale. And take note: If Equity actors are involved, the production can get into trouble for using spaces that are not union-approved.

To cast the play, assuming that you want to reach as many actors as possible, the standard practice is to place a casting notice in the trade papers. This notice needs to state as clearly as possible what the project is and whom you're looking for. You can announce an audition for which performers are invited to show up at a site during a specified period, or you can give a phone number for people to use to get time slots. Many casting notices have an address to which prospects can mail their pictures and résumés. This gives the director a chance to screen actors in advance. Whatever method you follow, any effort you make to keep the audition from turning into a mob scene will be to everyone's benefit. Alternatively, you can sidestep the audition process completely by casting people you know.

The Road to Opening Night

The show is cast, rehearsals have started, and you can see your dreams shaping up beautifully. Congratulations are in order, because getting this far at all is a victory. Just one little caution, though. This is also the time when important managerial tasks can easily be overlooked or done late. And you can't afford to let this happen.

Publicity takes center stage among the administrative duties to be done between the first rehearsal and the first performance. Press releases must be sent out to newspapers to solicit announcements and reviews. If you've hired a publicist, this will be taken care of for you; if you're handling publicity yourself, it's imperative that you do it right.

An effective press release puts all the vital information on one page, with a professional-looking letterhead and an easy-to-read layout. It has no typographical errors. It's usual to have two to three press mailings—one must announce the show in detail, including listing information, and one must formally invite reviewers. In addition, you can also send production photos to the photo editors of your local papers. Your press mailing list should include the prominent papers and various neighborhood papers and trade publications—most of these run reviews and carry listings. Plan at least a three- to four-week lead time between the day these places receive your material and your opening. The review request may be followed up by one phone call—emphasis on the word "one"—to each theatre editor.

Most of the time, a showcase is intended to make one's talent visible to agents, managers, casting directors, commercial theatre producers, and so on. (Part of the homework leading up to inviting such people is having already met some of them in the essential process of "networking.") An attractive invitation can easily be printed up for industry professionals. Most of the rules for such a mailing are good common sense: Make it attractive, accurate, concise, interesting, and prompt. Be realistic about the fact that it's being addressed to a person who is (1) busy, (2) swamped with invitations to other showcases, (3) wary about going to substandard shows, because of painful experiences in the past, and (4) eager, even so, to take a chance on discovering new talent.

In addition to critics, agents, and the like, you want to attract as many paying customers as possible. (The usual ticket price for a showcase is $12; if it's Equity-approved, that's the maximum.) You, and all others involved in the project, should be calling upon your personal friends to come. Outside this circle are those acquaintances you've met in the course of doing other shows, auditioning, and working temp jobs. All these people should be on your mailing list to send flyers to—*at least* a week before your first performance—with personal notes saying you'd love for them to attend. (It's not a bad idea to reciprocate by going to their shows, too.) If you're actively involved with an established theatre company, you may be in a position to buy or borrow its larger mailing list.

Posters and flyers for your show should be all over town. If you know of any theatre lobby that displays flyers, deposit a stack of yours there. People will sometimes go to a play because they've seen the title in several places over just a few days, and it's got them curious. You may or may not choose to advertise in newspapers. As early as the publicity begins, a reservation phone line has to be active. Having a separate number for press contacts is a good idea if it's feasible. Where an answering machine is being used, it's imperative that it be functioning correctly, able to handle a heavy volume of incoming messages. The weeks leading up to the performances are also the time for gathering materials and ironing out logistical problems. The better you've chosen your support crew, the less of this you'll have to be concerned with yourself.

Another Opening, Another Show

Thousands of Off-Off-Broadway showcases have opened and closed, but this one is special—it's yours. Opening night is another point at which to congratulate yourself. No matter what else happens, the opening of a show that you've produced is a victory.

From the reservations line, you should have some estimate of how many paying customers to expect on opening night and beyond. Here, another consideration comes to the fore: Any seat that can't be filled with a paying customer is better filled with a nonpaying customer than left empty. Thus, if you know that 20 seats will be vacant, it will cost you nothing to make that number of seats available on a complimentary basis to some affinity group (such as Actors' Equity, the Dramatists Guild, or any organization that will be interested in the subject matter of the play). Actors need an audience to do their work well, and it's just plain humiliating to have an industry professional come to your show and watch it with a minuscule audience.

If audience members enjoy seeing an out-of-this-world product on stage, they also appreciate all the courtesies and comforts that you can afford them off stage. Therefore, serve refreshments. Make sure that the restrooms are clean, operational, and stocked with soap and paper goods. Don't have the theatre either too hot or too cold. Open the house at a reasonable time, not five minutes before curtain, and keep the lobby looking as nice as possible.

Programs don't have to be done extravagantly to look professional, but they should be neat and typo-free. The actors' headshots need to be on prominent display in the lobby and available to industry professionals. A guest book should be prominent in the lobby, to gather names and addresses for your future mailing lists.

Above all, no matter how small the space and no matter how simple the production values, you want to create an atmosphere of serious, professional theatre: at the door, in the lobby, and on the stage.

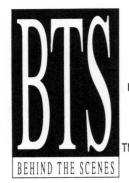

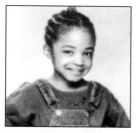
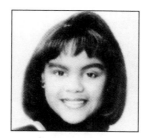
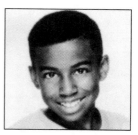

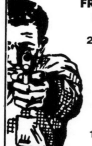
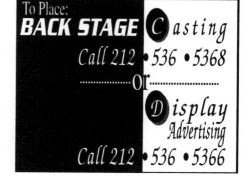

22

Creating a One-Person Show

MICHÈLE LaRUE

There are as many pitfalls to creating a one-person show as there are subjects, sources, and styles of shows. For advice on selecting, scripting, developing, mounting, and trouping a solo effort, we turned to some experts.

A Perfect Match

First, you'll need to find your material. Or, rather, you'll need to keep looking until it finds you. A one-person show is not something you can take on half-heartedly. If you're not fully committed to your subject and your character, then you're going to find your months of research, writing, rehearsals, and performance a chore. If you don't believe that your show is special, then you won't work hard enough to hone it, you won't care enough to sell it, and your audiences won't like it enough to recommend it.

Anna Deavere Smith and Viveca Lindfors are veterans of the form who have perfectly matched their material and their personal interests. *Twilight: Los Angeles, 1992* is the latest-produced installment of Smith's *On the Road: A Search for American Character*, a series of 14 pieces that she began evolving 11 years ago. In each piece, the actress–teacher portrays denizens of a specific neighborhood or organization she cares about. Smith edits and arranges tape-recorded "texts of real people" whom she has personally interviewed, exploring "how the spoken word works as a way of revealing character and emotional state."

Anna, the Gypsy Swede is Lindfors' third solo outing. It's been over 30 years since she discovered the germ of the show—a brief diary entry written by Anna Olesdotter-Wing, a native of Sweden who came to Minnesota in 1872. Herself a Swedish immigrant, Lindfors found Anna amazing: "She took such initiative. She was such an unfearful person." The theme of *Anna*, "home is within," is one she believes homesick immigrants of any generation must learn.

An Outside Eye

Even strong-minded, seasoned performers need an outside eye. You may be an experienced director and/or writer, as well as an actor. But during rehearsals you'll want feedback from someone who can see your show from the audience's perspective.

"There are moments when you wish you had somebody out front whom you could trust," says Lindfors. "You need somebody you can at least ask, 'What did this look like? Did it come across?'" Sometimes that somebody is hard to find. "Most directors don't like to work on one-person shows. It's such an ungrateful position," continues Lindfors, who consulted with several short-term directors over her eight-year developmental period.

For Smith, prior to *Twilight* (directed by George C. Wolfe), only three short-term directors were involved in her *Road* series. "In the beginning," she recounts, "it was hard to find people with the same sensibility as me." Back then, however, as part of her development process, Smith directed other actors in the monologues before performing them herself. That director's perspective helped her in her own solo rehearsals.

As a writer–adapter, director, and/or actor, Warren Kliewer has been involved in a dozen one-person shows for his New Jersey-based East Lynne Company. He excerpted and adapted his *Uncle Dan's Financial Tips—Or, Sunday Is Sunday, but the Other Six Days Is for Business* from an alleged autobiography of stock exchange and railroad wheeler-dealer Daniel Drew (1797–1879). "The fact that I did *Uncle Dan* without a director is a violation of my own principles," states the 63-year-old Kliewer. "It's just that there was nobody else who was interested in doing the kind of homework that was needed for that show."

When rehearsing *Uncle Dan*, Kliewer, too, called on other professionals for their perspectives. Further, when doubling as actor and director, he has "always relied on recalcitrant material that does not permit any self-indulgence." For instance, "in *Uncle Dan*, there are the facts of history that must not be violated, and there is the text of the book from which this came which cannot be changed—except in minor ways. You need to fence yourself in. Otherwise you end up going all over the map."

Avoiding Pitfalls

In writing a one-person show, you'll encounter two inherent, fundamental problems. First, your character has to get somewhere. He or she has to grow or change or discover something important. (Watching an actress in a pretty period costume recount "autobiographical" anecdotes about her character is *not* innately dramatic, however expert the actress.) Second, your character must have a legitimate reason for talking at length to this particular audience. Notes Kliewer:

> The kinds of one-person shows I find most satisfying are plays which happen to have only one character. The story progresses just as it would in any other play. Something is happening there, on stage, right now, before the audience's eyes. If you're doing a one-person show, you have to figure out a way to justify the fact that

one person is up there alone talking to somebody. Somehow, you have to create a listener.

In Kliewer's piece, for example, Uncle Dan immediately establishes why he is here: His audience has asked him for tips on getting rich.

Thinking About Design

Once you've established your dramatic convention and your script is in the works, you'll need to consider the design elements; set, props, costume, lights, and sound will all affect your staging. When you're on your feet, off book, and on the boards alone, you may find many places where (metaphorically speaking) you'd like a prop to lean on. Yet if your script is solid you won't need many of those. Trust your material. If the prop isn't essential to the action, omit it.

Each prop, costume, or set element that you adopt lengthens your set-up time, requires storage space backstage, and increases risk of theft, "borrowing," or breakage. It is also troublesome when traveling, especially by plane. Try to keep things compact enough to be carried on the plane with you. No matter how carefully you label and pack anything to be stowed as cargo, one day it will get lost or broken. (Really. This is a rule).

The only set element that Lindfors travels with is a wheeled trunk full of smaller objects; she scrounges in the theatre for additional commonplace items. Kliewer's bookers supply him with two chairs and a table; he travels with his costume and one hard-to-find prop, a spittoon.

Although Smith's characterizations are enhanced by a variety of defining small props and costume pieces, these have always been minimal. Recreating 29 interviewees in *Fires*, she wore one basic costume because she didn't want "to spend lots of time changing clothes; I need to move fast from one thing to the next." In rehearsals, she didn't give her characters a prop "unless it insinuated where they were or was incorporated in what they were doing."

Be sensitive from the inception of your project to its space, lighting, and sound (if any) requirements, especially if you hope to tour. If you expect to do your show in only one venue for a single, solid run, you can block for that space only. You can create a simple light plot, and your sensitive sound equipment will suffer only one round trip.

On tour, conventional blocking can get you into trouble. Says Kliewer:

> When you direct a show for a box set, that box set provides you with a certain set of dimensions. You can direct spatially, from the outside in—for example, "four steps toward the door." When you're directing for variable spaces, you can't know what all those dimensions are going to be, so you have to treat your center line as your point of reference: "four steps away from the center line."

This writer has learned a hard lesson about stage lighting: What you hope for often isn't there. In the 20 years I've toured as an actress, I've found that this applies to fully equipped theatres as well as to "gymnatoriums" and adapted spaces. You'd expect to find a college theatre well lit on your arrival. Unfortunately, you're just as likely to discover that the lights have been inalterably focused for an in-house production or are strewn over the shop floor for inventory.

To protect yourself against such surprises, avoid elaborate lighting requirements. Your priority is simply to be seen. Don't rely on "design"; your presenter may not have the equipment or personnel needed to provide it. Be flexible. Lindfors' rather complex *I Am a Woman* has two light plots: One requires a four-hour set-up for weeklong engagements; the other is a simplified version for one-performance venues. My own solo show takes place over a three-month period and at varying times of day, so my suggested plot designates warm and cool areas. But general stage lighting will work, and I get that half the time.

These days, many bookers expect you to need amplification: Whether you asked for it or not, you may find a microphone awaiting you on stage. "Real" theatres will probably provide tape decks and sound systems which can handle your prerecorded music or sound effects. If, however, you require directional sound, you may have to troupe your own stereo equipment.

You needn't buy everything at once. Design elements can be added and improved in sensible, affordable phases. My one-woman show *The Yellow Wallpaper* dramatizes Charlotte Perkins Gilman's classic American short story of the same name, written in 1892. A library and a college booked and paid for my first two performances. *Wallpaper* debuted with two chairs and a table, and I rented my dress cheaply from the nonprofit Costume Collection in New York City. Audience and sponsor response indicated that the show merited further investment. For a second series of bookings, I paid a designer–carpenter to build two collapsible window seats and a folding screen. For the third, I hired a designer–seamstress to create my own period costume.

The Actor as Producer

Once you believe that your show is ready, you can seek a paying audience in one of two ways: Either produce or co-produce yourself in one or more venues, or sell your show as a package to a booker who will present you.

Your obligations as self- or co-producer differ from your responsibilities as a jobbed-in event. As your own producer, you'll have to find, negotiate for, and rent a space; provide your own equipment (including lighting and sound if it's a "four-walls" rental); hire a press agent or create, distribute, and follow up on your own promotional materials to the media and audience (press releases, flyers, posters, and reviews); and handle ticket sales and reservations, front-of-house and backstage operations, bookkeeping, and payroll. Alternatively, you could, in effect, co-produce the show with the owner of a venue. Any number of options are negotiable here—the venue might provide virtually everything listed above in return for a favorable box office split.

If, instead, you're selling your show as a package for a flat fee to a presenter, other rules apply. You'll be absolved of a lot of responsibility—and be at the mercy of any ineptitude on your sponsor's part. For instance, unless you've contracted for a fee plus a percentage of the box office, a small audience will not decrease your earnings one bit. However, you'll have no say in how thoroughly your show is publicized. You may go home happy with your bank balance, but disappointed by your audience of 12.

Whatever your relationship to your venue, there are two things you can do in advance to prevent many regrets: Make sure you have a contract—*in writing*—and keep on communicating. Let's assume that your presenter is a department in a college or university. In the simplest scenario, you'll have mailed information about your show to the school's or department's booking person. That person will have called you back, asked some questions, and (we hope) offered to buy your show. In response, you'll send a contract confirming and further defining what you've agreed to on the phone.

It is standard practice in the business to attach to your contract a "tech sheet"—a list of technical requirements—so that your sponsor knows well in advance of your arrival just who is providing how much of what, and when. Both parties should consider this tech sheet to be an integral part of the contract. Make sure by phone that what you need is clear to your presenters and to their technical staff. Your chief aim here is to avoid surprises.

Generally speaking, your tech sheet should specify those elements that are crucial to your production and cannot be compromised—the minimum dimensions required for your acting area, for instance. You should also list those items which can be compromised, noting to what extent. If you need a room in which to change and can cope with either a private dressing room or a public restroom, say so. Be specific whenever necessary and adaptable whenever possible.

The information you send your sponsor should probably include a light plot. If your set is complicated, and/or the playing area is critical, consider adding a simple floor plan. A sophisticated sponsoring organization will include a diagram of its stage when mailing you its own introductory material.

Be sure to get accurate phone numbers and precise directions from your sponsor not only for traveling to the campus but for finding the theatre, the parking lot, the loading dock, and your contact person's office. You can easily spend an hour just getting your bearings, parking, and locating your sponsor. When you're negotiating a set-up schedule, allow ample time for these and other preliminaries. Finally, don't forget to bring along copies of your contract, tech sheet, and light plot in case your sponsors lost theirs. It happens.

That's it—from the glimmer of an idea to getting out and doing it. Take it away: This show's all yours.

23

Hit the Road:
Booking a Small Show
AMY HERSH

You've got a one-person or small show that you love. You want to create work for yourself. You're organized, and you enjoy making scores of phone calls and sending out dozens of mailings. Now it's time for you to think about how you can start booking your own show—around town, around your area, or around the country.

The list of venues where you can present your work is only as limited as your imagination. In addition to theatres and performing arts centers, almost any organization can be a presenter. That includes cafés, cabarets, resorts and hotels, parks and recreation departments, libraries, museums, town halls, community centers, public and private schools at all educational levels, English and history departments, hospitals, nursing homes, retirement communities, country clubs, churches, synagogues, monasteries, camps for adults, civic organizations such as Lions and Rotary clubs, bridge clubs, corporations, and any group that has regular get-togethers.

Before you make your first phone call, you need to seriously ask yourself these questions: Am I ready for the touring world, and are audiences out there ready for me? When you start out, you're going to have to do a lot of the work yourself, because very few booking management companies deal with single artists or small touring groups.

There are advantages to serving as your own manager and booking agent, according to Emma Palzere, who writes, produces, and performs one-woman shows. You'll work harder for yourself than someone else will. And if you hire an agent or manager to do your booking, he or she will take a big chunk out of your performance fee as a commission. Palzere advises, "Tell everybody you know that you have a show." Tell friends of the family and notify your college alumni club. If your show is appropriate, tell your church and the administrators of your elementary and secondary schools. When Palzere auditions for regional theatres, she mentions her show, just in case.

Staying organized is important when making contacts, as many performers will attest. Some keep separate file cards on each person and organization they contact. Every time you perform, take along your business card and brochures for your next event so that you can distribute them.

It helps if your material is flexible enough to be changed for different age ranges, and if you've written a few versions that vary in running times. Depending on the needs of the group for which you're performing, you may need (for example) a 90-minute, an hour, and a half-hour version.

Several performers suggest that you have more than one show in your repertoire, because it makes you more employable. Presenters who like you may want to have you back, but they probably won't want a repeat of the same show.

Getting to Know You

Over the last few years, actor Stuart Warmflash has performed his one-man show *A Map and a Cap . . .* more than a hundred times around the country. The play, which is about a man coming to terms with his father's legacy from the Holocaust, has found audiences at theatres, synagogues, public libraries, and many other organizations. Warmflash comments:

> The first thing to do is try to objectively evaluate the audience for your show: Who is the audience that your show is correct for? You can't sell something to someone who doesn't want what you're selling. Find where it fits. For example, suppose it's a show that deals with women's issues. Find every organization that has anything to do with women's issues. If your show is more specific, such as women in history, then you can be more specific about the people you contact, such as women's historical societies, college history departments that have a women's division, and women's history museums. The sources are endless.

The Yellow Pages are an essential source; so is your public library, which has many vital resource directories. State and local arts councils also have lists of potential presenters for you to contact. If you're in New York City, says Warmflash, the New York Public Library for the Performing Arts is "a gold mine."

"The next step is to give the show away for free," Warmflash continues. This serves many functions: It tests your material, it allows you to rehearse the show on your feet, and it gives you the opportunity to request a letter of reference from the person who hired you.

Before you make phone calls about *paid* performances of your production, Warmflash recommends creating a brochure:

> Brochures should be simple and clean, with the title of the show, your name, a brief paragraph on what the show is about, a brief bio, possibly a picture, and a contact number. If you call an organization, and they say, "We're not interested," don't hang up. Say, "Thank you for your time. Can you suggest another organization or person that may be interested?" Good leads can happen as a result.

National and Regional Conferences

Once you've had some experience touring locally, you might consider participating in a conference of presenters. These conferences take place on the regional and national levels annually and are a combination of trade shows and arts festivals. They're held in large hotels, convention centers, and exhibition halls where artists of all disciplines and artists' managers rent space in booths. Arts presenters from all types of performing arts centers visit these booths to get information about the productions that are available.

If you're very lucky, says Evan Kavanagh, executive director of the Western Alliance of Arts Administrators, you can "catch fire" at a conference. He advises that, when you're starting out, it's best to take part in one regional conference. That way, if you begin to book shows, you're traveling within one region, rather than around the whole United States.

Showcasing has also become more much important in recent years at these booking conferences, Kavanagh adds. One conference may feature as many as 200 different live performances, so that presenters may see the work of artists they're considering for appearances on their series. Showcasing can be expensive but, if done well, it can pay off in the long run. Kavanagh also notes that showcasing is different at every conference, so you should ask the conference sponsor several months in advance about the role showcasing plays at his or her event.

Make sure that you have a good video of your performance to show at the conference. "A bad video is worse than no video at all," says Kavanagh.

Conference participation is an investment of time and money, and that expense should be taken into consideration in your long-range planning. First you must join the association sponsoring the conference; then you must rent a booth, pay your travel and hotel fees, and bring or rent video equipment to show a tape of your work. For more information on how to become involved in national and regional conferences, contact: The Association of Performing Arts Presenters, 112 16th St. NW, Suite 400, Washington, DC 20036; (202) 833-2787.

Aiming for Younger Audiences

If your act is geared for audiences of children and teens, Ken Arthur, education and marketing director for Theatreworks/USA, recommends: "Always attend as many conferences as possible." Based in New York City, Theatreworks/USA is the largest producer of children's theatre in the country and serves as a booking agency for artists who are placed nationwide.

When contacting schools or performing arts centers for educational and entertainment-oriented programming, Arthur advises that you prepare a videotape that's at least 10 to 15 minutes long that was "not made in a cold studio setting." Also, he says, "It's preferable to have an interactive setting with kids, so the presenter doesn't have to use his or her imagination about how kids will react."

When you describe your work, specify the age range for which it's appropriate. You should also supply these potential bookers with a list of performances you've done in their region, with a publicity packet with evaluation forms from principals, arts coordinators, or other school-based administrators, and with letters of endorsement. It's very important that you give the presenter access to people who have booked you in the past, because the presenter will want to make a lot of phone calls to those people to hear their opinions of your performance.

"Give away shows, invite local schools and arts coordinators to see you, network as much as possible with other arts-in-education professionals, and develop a respect for your audience," concludes Arthur. "It's the most unforgiving audience there is."

The College Circuit

Colleges and universities have special needs when they book shows, says Mims Harris, the director of campus activities at Colorado State University. Even if you're not interested in reaching these presenters specifically, Harris' advice applies to contacting any presenting organization. "If you call me, the first thing I'm going to ask is for you to send a package of information," she states. That package should contain lots of "clear, factual information," along with a description of the show. "How much do you cost? When you quote a fee, what does that mean? Is it all-inclusive? What is the presenter paying for? If there's a range, say what that range is. If you have specific technical needs, be able to articulate those needs."

If you're just getting a foot in the door, you may want to offer a free master class or do some outreach to the community for free. Also, you should explain how long you've been doing this, what your expertise is, the kinds of audiences you've played to, and where you've been well-received.

Include a list of places where you've performed and any reviews of your work. If you get reviewed after your initial contact with a presenting organization, send those new reviews out as a reminder with a note that might say, "I know you're still considering your season. Here's a review of my most recent performance."

Harris says that videotapes are especially useful. "I like to see pieces that are going to give me a real sense not only of the quality but also the meaning and substance of this particular presentation," she explains. That can be conveyed in 10 minutes of tape with several short vignettes or sections of the show.

Get information about the season at the university or college and about how booking decisions are made, Harris advises. The director of a performing arts center might be able to make an independent decision, but in many instances, he or she decides as part of a committee. Most series are planned out for an entire year and some a semester at a time.

It's also reasonable to ask your contact person at the university to pass your information package to someone else in the community—for example, an arts center—if the university is not interested in booking you.

If you have a performance that falls through, you can still use it to advantage. "I appreciate when an artist says, 'I just had a cancellation. I'm routing through your area, and I can give you a special fee,'" Harris comments. "Sometimes, I need last-minute fill-ins. I would urge artists to make these kinds of follow-up calls."

More and more museums around the United States and beyond are using innovative theatre to educate patrons, according to Catherine Hughes, a member of the theatre company at the Museum of Science in Boston and executive director of International Museum Theatre Alliance. (The Alliance, by the way, does not represent artists.) What's being done at museums ranges from storytelling to original musicals, dramas, mime, and puppetry. "Sometimes it's like street theatre, but often there's a full set, with lights and sound," observes Hughes. "There's such a wide variety of theatre in museums, and it's presented at a high caliber. It's an alternative theatre world."

This type of theatre consists of original work written expressly for museums and their exhibits and collections, and museum administrators are looking to the theatre community for playwrights, directors, and actors to fill the need. If you'd like to do this kind of work, Harris suggests contacting the education and interpretation departments at museums and asking if their administrators are interested. There's no reason to send big packets of information, she notes. A brief cover letter and résumé will do. (For more on museum theatre, see Chapter 24.)

Single-Performance Slots

Other opportunities for one-person and small shows exist in single-performances that you can book for a theatre's dark nights or as special matinees at road houses and regional theatres. First, you'll need to locate those companies that do have such slots. Then you'll want to send a general information kit, possibly with a videotape, to the theatres' administrators.

Flexibility is important here. You must be able to adapt to different rooms and to stages of varying sizes. Also, you may have to do your show on a set that's already up for another play and be able to work with the technical and artistic team regarding your requirements for staging, lighting, and sound.

Booking your show takes a lot of motivation and dedication, but in the view of performers who have done it successfully, it's enormously rewarding and fulfilling. "The sense of accomplishment is overwhelming," says Warmflash. "The artistic fulfillment is ideal."

For a list of national and regional presenters' conferences, see the Appendix, page 296.

24

Museum Theatre

ESTHER TOLKOFF

Over the past 20 years, many museums throughout the United States, Canada, and Great Britain have turned to theatre to convey the messages of their exhibits. National parks, historic homes, zoos, and aquariums are also hiring actors, singers, dancers, and other artists. The trend is growing rapidly, offering opportunities in the biggest cities and the smallest hamlets.

"Actors bring to life the human stories behind the pictures on the gallery wall, the signs, the historical and scientific objects," says Bob Marion, an actor and managing director of the Seattle Public Theatre, which works with that city's Museum of History and Industry. By seeking out nearby cultural sites, an enterprising soul may be able to create an excellent opportunity right in his or her own backyard.

Engaging the Audience

Today's public is used to getting information from watching people on television and in films and from using computers, which make learning into an activity. As a result, performers have come to play an important role where cultural institutions are concerned. Many museums have found that putting actors on the gallery floor strongly engages visitors. The legacy of a historical figure, the destruction of the rain forest, the technology which affects our lives, the amorous intrigues of families depicted in Renaissance art—these are a few of the topics that have been portrayed recently in museums. Actors often pose as yesteryear's political leaders, scientists, artists, or ordinary folks, such as freed slaves, immigrants, housewives, and workers. Singers and dancers may convey the forms the arts took in a given culture or period. There are many possibilities—playing modern, everyday people with a problem to solve or Martians asking earthlings—the audience members—to explain how they live.

Museum theatre performances are usually interactive. The key artistic goal in performing at cultural sites like museums and parks is conveying information or stimulating thought by drawing visitors through the power and immediacy that only live theatre can provide. And it works; the public responds.

After the show, visitors often start to talk about the issues the exhibit or historic site raises. They look at the displays and read the signs more closely.

The message gets across as it never has before, which is why more and more museums are jumping on the bandwagon and reaching out to performers.

That there is a serious message does not mean that the work atmosphere in this kind of theatre is somber. Some productions are emotionally strong, and others are quite playful. Because this genre is so new, it is often extremely creative, especially because it brings actors into direct contact with the public. Performers must be ready for anything while being careful not to sacrifice accuracy, a word which crops up often in conversations with artists in this field.

Growing Opportunities

Museum theatre—or gallery theatre, or "living history," as this work is sometimes called—is different, employment-wise and artistically, from more established theatre markets. In fact, seeing themselves as a "market" is sometimes a leap for museum staffers. These are scholarly people with a great love of their subject matter and sometimes a bit fearful of lending "their baby" to what they perceive as a commercialization of the knowledge they are devoted to preserving. But those who do hire actors usually become converts all the way. Several build up in-house repertory companies or actively seek ongoing working relationships with local artists. Others with low budgets or far from theatre centers turn to university drama departments for their casting needs—providing an excellent starting point for a young artist.

In the 1970s, before he became a Pulitzer Prize–winner, August Wilson was a (then unknown) staff playwright at the Science Museum of Minnesota, in St. Paul. At that time, few parks, museums, and historic homes hired actors or playwrights. But now many institutions are in regular contact with one another, and every year increasing numbers of museum staffers take the Minnesota museum's workshop, long headed by actress Tessa Bridal, to learn how to bring theatre to their own institutions. That means more work for performers.

What's It Like?

The types of places that make use of museum theatre include science museums and their "cousins," zoos and aquariums, which often focus on environmental and animal care issues; historical museums and sites, where theatre is sometimes controversial but is rapidly growing; children's museums; and to a lesser extent, art museums and national parks, which often have "interpretative" departments that hire people to portray historical figures.

In describing this work, directors most often mention that the exhibit area is usually the set, so actors are often physically very close to the audience. Lighting, as a demarcating device, is rare. Directors look for actors who can adapt to this.

The audience is the visiting public strolling in or out throughout the performance. They may be talking, particularly if they are with children.

The plays are very short and are performed several times a day; actors are usually involved in several such short plays in repertory fashion, so local talent or actors committed to staying on get strong preference. This can mean steady work as part of an in-house repertory troupe or as an independent performer who regularly returns to a given park, museum, zoo, or historic home. Sometimes specialized one-person characterizations or troupes portraying a given culture are "booked," and several theatre companies have ties with museums. The troupe often plays area libraries and schools as well.

Audiences are often families, so performances must play to both children and adults. Pieces are frequently interactive—some address the audiences throughout, and others break the fourth wall to elicit audience responses, even pulling audience members into the show. This calls for both flexibility and politeness in encountering the occasional boorish adult or a young child wandering in while maintaining one's character's authenticity. Many places use "roving theatre"—where actors in character and in costume walk up to members of the public and engage them in conversation. Sometimes it's the other way around, with actors in a fixed setting; as visitors rove in, they initiate relatively unscripted interaction.

Diane Stillman of the Walters Art Gallery, in Baltimore, says, "Actors tell me the immediate, direct feedback they get from the audience is incredibly exciting. They feel that after this they can do anything."

The importance of authenticity means that role preparation is real research on the issue and/or period in question. Playwrights work with curatorial staff, and performers must stick to the language of the era portrayed—no slipping into modern slang if you're Leonardo da Vinci or a Mayan folkdancer. Background training is often provided during rehearsal, along with help in dealing with questions, for after a skit breaks, actors stay in character and may be approached by their audience.

Landing Work

The casting process varies widely. Those museums, national parks, and similar venues that have long been involved in theatre work follow "regular" casting routes, such as placing casting calls in trade papers. Many work with nonunion professionals or drama students. But several hire Equity performers at wages and working conditions negotiated with the union for the specific engagement.

As with most nonprofit theatre, there are enormous opportunities for creative growth but, except in the largest, most established venues, pay is not high. But these are, by and large, honest and steady employers. Directors say they look for performers who are persuasive and who can think quickly on their feet yet keep in mind the messages they ought to be conveying. They also look for people who can perform in the extremely close-up situations they may find themselves in and refrain from "projecting to the third balcony with stage gestures," as Stillman puts it. On the other hand, outdoor venues do want actors who can project their voices on a windy day and be heard despite background distractions.

All the theatre directors we spoke to say they look for evidence of a serious commitment. It's good to do your homework about a particular museum's or park's focus, checking what kinds of exhibits and events it has mounted before approaching it with an idea. "I won't even consider a picture or résumé that arrives without a cover letter explaining why the performer wants to do this and why here," says Stephen Diamond, director of the Smithsonian's Discovery Theatre and creator of the highly praised resident theatre company, The Treehouse, at the Philadelphia Zoo. This sentiment was often repeated.

Along the same lines, follow-up in this milieu is better done through conventional letters than cheery monthly postcards, which in many cases would be unheard of, if not the kiss of death. Quite a few historical sites and national parks employ individuals known as *character interpreters* who have devoted extensive time to developing what they view as a portrait that is as exact as possible. Many of these people do not consider themselves to be actors, and there are those in the museum world who only hire such interpreters for live presentations. On the other hand, there are professional actors with a deep knowledge of a given person or topic—having played an individual for years, perhaps from sheer interest—who work as interpreters or as actors according to the situation. There are also museums and cultural sites who use costumed nonprofessionals. But many places that started this way changed their minds when they saw what professional actors could do and understood that the actors are serious about the institution's goals.

Initiating a Project

Several performers have approached museums with the idea of introducing theatre and succeeded in landing jobs performing regularly or even starting entire theatre programs. Amy Feinberg was a working actress who'd gotten a day job at Ellis Island National Park, located in New York harbor, and had the idea of creating a theatre piece from immigrant oral histories. She convinced her employers to try it and went on to direct a play, *Ellis Island Stories,* employing 10 professional actors, which played three consecutive summers and now runs seven months a year. The piece has proven so popular that the Park Service now plans to build a theatre there. Feinberg also works with the Tenement Museum in New York City, which has long employed actors in plays and as in-character guides.

Robert Richter was an actor who, while working in a nonacting job at the Mystic Seaport Museum in Connecticut, saw that the museum employed (and still does) costumed nonprofessionals. He was persistent in making his case and convinced the institution to hire professionals as well. He went on to direct its theatre program, mounting regular interactive plays about the whaling industry and coastal New England life of the 19th century. Richter holds auditions for actors for every summer season. He also worked with the City Stage Company of Boston to put together *Tale of a Whaler,* a participatory play about a woman who disguises herself as a man and goes to sea. Audience members, both adults and children, are picked out to join the crew, help with chores, and weather storms.

For lists of cultural sites that incorporate theatre on a regular basis, write to the following organizations to obtain their membership directories (each charges a different nominal fee) and copies of their newsletters, which list several new member locales and networking events in every issue:

• The International Museum Theatre Alliance (IMTAL) includes many museums, parks, zoos, and aquariums throughout the U.S., Canada, and Great Britain. Their address is: Museum of Science, Science Park, Boston, MA 02114-1099.

• The Museum Theatre Professional Interest Committee of the American Association of Museums can be contacted in care of Tessa Bridal, Science Museum of Minnesota, 30 E. 10 St., St. Paul, MN 55101.

• At the U.S. National Parks Service, contact the Division of Interpretation, P.O. Box 37127, Washington, D.C. 20013-7127.

25

Actors' Alert:
Avoiding Scams, Rip-offs, and Unethical People
MICHÈLE LaRUE

There's a sucker born every minute," show biz entrepreneur Phineas T. Barnum reportedly declared back in the 1800s. He might well have added, "And there's a scam artist born every two or three." Of course, neither show biz nor scam artistry originated with Barnum; both were thriving long before he arrived on the scene. And, more to the point, both continue to do so now.

Acting is a craft that fosters high expectations and emotions, leaving its practitioners vulnerable to dashed hopes and dashing con artists. Because you're not a performer if you're not performing, you'll do almost anything to land that role; you'll believe almost anyone who swears he or she can lead you to success. This chapter is aimed at the rational, intelligent human being you are when an acting job is *not* at stake. If you're one of the few thousand novices newly arrived in New York, Los Angeles, or Chicago, here's your introduction to the darker side of the business—some basics in how to beware.

Promises and Lures

There are subtler come-ons than "Stick with me, baby. I'll make you a star." Have you ever seen those ads seeking models, promising big money and easy hours for "real people" types with "no experience"? Or those casting notices offering "bit parts and extra work" in "major feature films and commercials"—again, "no experience needed"? Don't believe them for a minute. You'll find these lures in the "Classified: Help Wanted" sections of suburban newspapers, in supermarket tabloids, and even in major dailies.

Such ads target novices and daydreamers. Advertisers aim not to get you work, but to take your money. Give them a call, and they'll love you at the interview, where they'll try to sell you pictures or classes or "how-to" books. Coincidentally, the photographer or the teacher or the bookseller will be a close relative who works next door. You'll never see that modeling job or extra role, but you'll have a stack of second-rate pictures for a souvenir.

What's in a Book?

Photos are a popular rip-off in the business, because a picture is a tangible product. You may be disappointed in the quality of the final print, but the photographer *did* give you something for your money. The same holds true for a "how-to" book. Many fine ones have been written by knowledgeable professionals and published by respected presses. But anybody with a word processor and a photocopier can write a "book." It may be just a couple of introductory paragraphs followed by 20 pages of out-of-date lists of casting directors who work through agents only. But if it's titled "How to Meet New York Casting Directors," and if that's the title you ordered—well, you got what you paid for.

Variations on the headshot pitch are the portfolio pitch and the headsheet books pitch. A professional portfolio is built up over time as a model accumulates diverse and improved samples of his or her work with various photographers. So it's pointless for a neophyte who is still not entirely at ease with the camera and still learning the fine points of makeup and hair to buy a full portfolio from a single (possibly inadequate) photographer. Young models should beware bogus agents or personal managers trying to sell them these in their initial interviews.

Headsheet books compile photos of scores of would-be models or actor/models. For a fee, the publisher will include your pictures in the book, which will be sent to modeling agencies and casting directors. Legitimate modeling agencies distribute these books selectively and effectively. But beware the "agent" or "manager" who *requires* you to be in such a book. And don't fall for phony publishers of headsheet books. In recent years, many have cashed models' checks but have never gone to press. Others have indeed published and distributed their books as promised to hundreds of modeling agents and casting directors—many of whom were not in the least bit interested.

Reference Checks

Lana Turner and Schwab's Drugstore are long gone, but actors everywhere still dream of "getting discovered" in the most mundane situations. It *can* happen, especially in Los Angeles' film community, where physical attributes are so important. But not every "producer" or "manager" or "director" who stops you on the street and hands you a business card is legit. And not every agent you find in the phone book has a direct line to Steven Spielberg. Most performers, even the "overnight successes," have had to cultivate their careers for a long time. And that cultivation has included careful, time-consuming research.

The legitimacy of potential employers and representatives can be checked through a variety of sources. Throughout the year, *Back Stage* runs updated and verified rosters of everyone from producers of outdoor theatre companies to agents specializing in child talent. Theatre bookstores in Manhattan carry the monthly *Ross Reports*, which lists independent casting directors and casting directors who work for advertising agencies in the New York City area. A related quarterly, *Ross Reports USA*, bills itself as a guide to talent agents and personal managers nationwide and covers franchised agents in 27 states. Both publications are available from Television Index, Inc. 40-29 27th St., Long Island City, NY 11101.

The unions—notably, Actors' Equity Association, the Screen Actors Guild, and the American Federation of Television and Radio Artists—regulate talent agencies by granting them franchises. Members can pick up lists of these approved agents at their union offices. Nonunion actors can find similar listings from time to time in *Back Stage* or can find out from Equity if a given agent is franchised and in good standing. Generally, the performer unions don't allow those they've franchised to advertise for clients. New York Actor's Equity business rep Gareth May states that a reputable agency shouldn't have to solicit actors. (Of the New York area's 16,000 Equity members, 12,000 are not signed with agents and most of those 12,000 are probably seeking representation.)

Some states—California, Illinois, New Jersey, and New York, for instance— license talent agencies. In such states, any talent agency that is *not* licensed is operating illegally. In California, licensing is handled by the Labor Commission of the State of California. In New York, it's done by the State Department of Labor. In New York City, the municipal Department of Consumer Affairs issues such licenses.

Union franchises and state licenses regulate several facets of representation; for example, AEA, SAG, AFTRA, and the states of New York and California limit a talent agent's commission to 10 percent.

It's harder to evaluate personal managers. States don't license them because they are not "employment agencies," and unions don't franchise them. What a personal manager and a performer have is "a private services agreement between two individuals," according to May. The best you can do is contact the National Conference of Personal Managers (NCOPM). In order to join this association, potential members must earn their main source of income through personal management and must have been personal managers for at least one year or have an extensive knowledge of the entertainment business, reports Joseph Rapp, executive director of the East Coast chapter [1650 Broadway, Suite 705, New York, NY 10019; (212) 265-3366]. Agents and casting directors have their own professional organizations: The Association of Talent Agents [in Los Angeles: 9255 Sunset Blvd., Suite 318, Los Angeles, CA 90069; (310) 274-0628], the National Association of Talent Representatives, Inc. [in New York: (212) 262-5696], and the Casting Society of America [c/o 311 W. 43rd St., New York, NY 10036; (212) 333-4552]. They too, could be part of your research.

While membership usually implies professionalism, a firm or individual may have a perfectly good reason for choosing not to join up. It's also conceivable that a solid, ethical manager or agent may not yet qualify for NCOPM membership or union franchising (just as you may not yet be eligible for SAG or Equity). And it's equally conceivable that an unscrupulous firm could slip past the rules and regulations of even the most stringent association. So membership in a professional organization should not be the sole criterion in your evaluations.

Another way to check out a firm's legitimacy is by calling your local branch of the Better Business Bureau, a national nonprofit organization which keeps on file complaints against specific firms (and offers general tips on common scams and problems to avoid). You can also investigate on your own: As you make the rounds, ask friends and acquaintances who their representatives are; listen to reasonable complaints, and keep an ear out for news of current scams. Talk to agents' or managers' current clients; ask representatives, directors, or casting directors for references and credits. Do your homework. For models, who have no unions, guilds, or associations (and are more often represented by management firms than by agencies), this kind of reference checking can be critical.

Back to School
Teachers, too, can harm you if you don't do your homework. Finding your mentor among scores of reputable instructors is hard enough, but determining who is reputable should be your first step. Your tools as a performer include your body and your psyche; an inept or immoral teacher can abuse either or both—with far-reaching, long-lasting consequences.

Licensing requirements for acting and modeling schools vary from state to state. New York, for example, exempts schools of acting, music, dance, and fine arts from licensing, but its State Education Department licenses modeling schools as trade schools. In any case, do some research. If you're seeking a teacher, talk to his or her former and current students, audit some classes and/or interview the teacher. Check out teachers' résumés and read any texts they may have written before you head for school.

Rules to Live by
Whatever professional relationship you're considering, there are some basic rules you should always follow in this (or any) business. Rule Number One is: "Get it in writing." Never rely on a verbal agreement. Even with a best friend, a little, honest misunderstanding can cause a lot of grief. Whether it be a contract, a simple letter of agreement, or a receipt, write it out and keep a copy. Also, don't be pressured into signing anything on the spot. Take the time to read carefully and ask questions, and don't hesitate to consult elsewhere for answers.

This is not to say that all your transactions require a lawyer. Many need only common sense and patience. Inexpensive advice can be obtained from one of the more than 40 branches of Volunteer Lawyers for the Arts, a nationwide, nonprofit network. (The New York City office's "Art Law Line" can direct you to the Volunteer Lawyers for the Arts nearest you—for more about their services, see Chapter 4.)

Rule Number Two: Beware of demands that you pay up front. It's one thing for a reputable school to ask you in advance for partial payment that is documented by a receipt. It's quite another for a "manager" whom you met an hour ago to demand $300 on the spot, with no contract, to guarantee your placement in a headsheet book.

Speaking of guarantees, here's Rule Number Three: Nobody can guarantee you a job. (Well, a *select few* may have the clout to do so, but that doesn't mean that they'll follow through on their promises.) If you "sign up with me"; if you "get these headshots"; if you "buy my book," or if you "let me see you with your blouse off"—you're not assured a role, much less a career.

And that leads us to Rule Number Four: Use your common sense. If this were a word-processing job, wouldn't you think 10 PM in the personnel director's hotel room a strange time and place to interview? Sure, in the theatre we work on strange schedules and in odd places; and, sure, a penniless student who's toiling at two jobs to pay for graduate studies in drama may have to hold auditions after dark. But a stage manager or assistant director should be present there, too. A "producer" who promises you a feature film job can certainly afford a real office and daytime casting hours. Don't let your own acute need to be employed as an actor overpower your common sense and survival instinct.

Finally, if the scam artists (and your own high hopes) do get the better of you, there are several ways to redress your grievances or, at least, to make it harder for a con artist to rip off the next person. Report disreputable firms to the Better Business Bureau.

If you haven't been paid as promised, especially if you have a written contract to back you up, call, write, and/or visit the delinquent party till you are paid. (Keep copies of your letters.) Failing that, notify the Better Business Bureau; *Back Stage*, which runs periodic scam alerts; and the appropriate unions and associations. Failing that, take the person who owes you to small claims court. It will take some time, but it isn't difficult.

If the company that ripped you off disappears after cashing your check, or if you've been defrauded in any way, contact the local Better Business Bureau and the state's Attorney General's office. If the scam in any way used the U.S. Postal Service, contact the Mail Fraud Division.

If you've been subjected to sexual abuse or harassment, notify the Better Business Bureau, the state's Division of Human Rights, and/or (in New York City) the City's Commission on Human Rights, and the sex-crimes unit of the police department, plus applicable unions and associations.

In New York City, the Department of Consumer Affairs investigates complaints about fraudulent practices by talent agents and personal managers. AEA, SAG, and AFTRA members are advised to contact their union representatives first, but nonunion performers should write directly to the Department's Complaint Division.

However much you want that part—however desperately you want acting to be your career—when it comes to looking for work, keep a clear head. Remember: "There's a sucker born every minute." If you're careful, there won't be a minute with your name on it.

Appendix:
Resource Listings

Equity, SAG, and AFTRA Agents

New York, Los Angeles, and Chicago
Casting Directors

Personal Managers

National and Regional Union Offices

League of Resident Theatres

Dinner Theatres

Off- and Off-Off-Broadway Theatre Companies

Los Angeles 99-Seat Theatres

Chicago Theatres

Acting Schools and Teachers

Commercial Print Agencies and
Management Firms

Business Theatre Producers

Equity Theatre for Young Audiences Companies

Cabaret Rooms

Comedy Clubs

Regional Combined Auditions Nationwide

Theme Parks and Show Producers

Cruise Line Agents and Producers

Conference Resources

Equity, SAG, and AFTRA Agents

The following agencies in the New York, Los Angeles, and Chicago metropolitan areas are franchised with Actors' Equity Association, Screen Actors Guild, and/or the American Federation of Television and Radio Artists, indicated by (E) for Equity; (S) for SAG; and (A) for AFTRA.

NEW YORK

ABRAMS ARTISTS & ASSOCIATES, LTD.
420 Madison Ave., 14th fl.
New York, NY 10017
(212) 935-8980 (E) (S) (A)

THE ACTORS GROUP AGENCY
157 W. 57th St., Suite 604
New York, NY 10019
(212) 245-2930 (E) (S) (A)

BRET ADAMS LIMITED
448 W. 44th St.
New York, NY 10036
(212) 765-5630 (E) (S) (A)

AGENCY FOR THE PERFORMING ARTS, INC.
888 Seventh Ave.
New York, NY 10106
(212) 582-1500 (E) (S) (A)

AGENTS FOR THE ARTS, INC.
203 W. 23rd St., 3rd fl.
New York, NY 10011
(212) 229-2562 (E) (S) (A)

ALLIANCE TALENT, INC.
1501 Broadway, Suite 404
New York, NY 10036
(212) 840-6868 (E) (S) (A)

ALLURE ASSOCIATES
811 Church Hill Rd., Suite 206
Cherry Hill, NJ 08002
(609) 486-9000 (A)

MICHAEL AMATO THEATRICAL ENTERPRISE
1650 Broadway, Room 307
New York, NY 10019
(212) 247-4456 (S) (A)

AMBROSIO/MORTIMER & ASSOCIATES, INC.
165 W. 46th St., Suite 1214
New York, NY 10036
(212) 719-1677 (E) (S) (A)

AMERICAN INTERNATIONAL TALENT
303 W. 42nd St., Suite 608
New York, NY 10036
(212) 245-8888 (S) (A)

BEVERLY ANDERSON AGENCY
1501 Broadway, Suite 2008
New York, NY 10036
(212) 944-7773 (E) (S) (A)

ANDREADIS TALENT AGENCY, INC.
119 W. 57th St., Suite 711
New York, NY 10019
(212) 315-0303 (E) (S) (A)

ARTIST'S AGENCY, INC.
230 W. 55th St., Suite 29D
New York, NY 10019
(212) 245-6960 (E) (S) (A)

ARTISTS & AUDIENCE ENTERTAINMENT
83 Riverside Dr.
New York, NY 10024
(212) 721-2400 (S)
Handles clients of celebrity status exclusively.

ARTISTS GROUP EAST
1650 Broadway, Suite 711
New York, NY 10019
(212) 586-1452 (E) (S) (A)

ASSOCIATED BOOKING
1995 Broadway, Suite 501
New York, NY 10023
(212) 874-2400 (E) (S) (A)
Handles singers, musicians, musicals for major recording artists.

RICHARD ASTOR AGENCY
250 W. 57th St., Suite 2014
New York, NY 10107
(212) 581-1970 (E) (S) (A)

AVENUE TALENT LTD.
315 W. 35th St., Suite 12B
New York, NY 10001
(212) 628-1380 (S)

BARRY, HAFT, BROWN ARTISTS AGENCY
165 W. 46th St., Suite 908
New York, NY 10036
(212) 869-9310 (E) (S) (A)

BAUMAN, HILLER & ASSOCIATES
250 W. 57th St., Suite 2223
New York, NY 10107
(212) 757-0098 (E) (S) (A)

PETER BEILIN AGENCY, INC.
230 Park Ave., Room 923
New York, NY 10169
(212) 949-9119 (S) (A)

THE BETHEL AGENCY
360 W. 53rd St., Suite BA
New York, NY 10019
(212) 664-0455 or 0462 (E) (S)

N.S. BIENSTOCK INC.
1740 Broadway, 24th fl.
New York, NY 10019
(212) 765-3040 (A)
*Newscasters, sports announcers, and sports
players only.*

J. MICHAEL BLOOM & ASSOCIATES
233 Park Ave. So., 10th fl.
New York, NY 10003
(212) 529-6500 (E) (S) (A)

J. MICHAEL BLOOM & ASSOCIATES
344 E. 59th St.
New York, NY 10022
(212) 688-8628 (S) (A)

BOOKERS, INC.
150 Fifth Ave., Suite 834
New York, NY 10011
(212) 645-9706 (E) (S)

DON BUCHWALD & ASSOCIATES
10 E. 44th St.
New York, NY 10017
(212) 867-1070 (E) (S) (A)

CARRY COMPANY
1501 Broadway, Suite 1408
New York, NY 10036
(212) 768-2793 (E) (S) (A)

CARSON–ADLER AGENCY, INC.
250 W. 57th St.
New York, NY 10107
(212) 307-1882 (E) (S) (A)

THE CARSON ORGANIZATION, LTD.
240 W. 44th St., PH 12
New York, NY 10036
(212) 221-1517 (E) (S) (A)

RICHARD CATALDI AGENCY
180 Seventh Ave., Suite 1C
New York, NY 10011
(212) 741-7450 (E) (S) (A)

COLEMAN–ROSENBERG
155 E. 55th St.
New York, NY 10022
(212) 838-0734 (E) (S) (A)

BILL COOPER ASSOCIATES, INC.
224 W. 49th St., Suite 411
New York, NY 10019
(212) 307-1100 (S) (A)
*Primarily handles professional newscasters
and writers.*

CUNNINGHAM–ESCOTT–DIPENE
118 E. 25th St., 6th fl.
New York, NY 10010
(212) 477-1666 (E) (S) (A)

GINGER DICCE TALENT
1650 Broadway, Suite 714
New York, NY 10019
(212) 974-7455 (E) (S) (A)

DOUGLAS, GORMAN, ROTHACKER &
WILHELM, INC.
1501 Broadway, Suite 703
New York, NY 10036
(212) 382-2000 (E) (S) (A)

DAVID DRUMMOND TALENT
REPRESENTATIVES
21 Pomander Walk
New York, NY 10025
(212) 662-6838 (E) (S) (A)

DUVA–FLACK ASSOCIATES
200 W. 57th St., Suite 1407
New York, NY 10019
(212) 957-9600 (E) (S) (A)
*Handles clients of celebrity status
exclusively.*

EASTWOOD TALENT GROUP
214 E. 9th St.
New York, NY 10003
(212) 982-9700 (S) (A)

DULCINA EISEN ASSOCIATES
154 E. 61st St.
New York, NY 10021
(212) 355-6617 (E) (S) (A)

EPSTEIN/WYCKOFF & ASSOCIATES
311 W. 43rd St., Suite 1401
New York, NY 10036
(212) 586-9110 (E) (S) (A)

ESTEEM AGENCY INC.
1200 MacArthur Blvd.
Mahwah, NJ 07430
(201) 825-8822 (E) (A)

FAMOUS ARTISTS AGENCY, INC.
1700 Broadway
New York, NY 10019
(212) 245-3939 (A)
*Books music groups, established rock and
soul singers; no actors.*

FLICK EAST–WEST TALENTS, INC.
881 Seventh Ave., Suite 1110
New York, NY 10019
(212) 307-1850 (E) (S) (A)

FORMATION MODELS, INC.
156 Fifth Ave., Suite 515
New York, NY 10010
(212) 675-7037 (S)

FRONTIER BOOKING INTERNATIONAL
1560 Broadway, Suite 1110
New York, NY 10019
(212) 221-0220 (E) (S) (A)

THE GAGE GROUP, INC.
315 W. 57th St., Suite 4H
New York, NY 10019
(212) 541-5250 (E) (S) (A)

THE GERSH AGENCY N.Y., INC.
130 W. 42nd St., Suite 2400
New York, NY 10036
(212) 997-1818 (E) (S) (A)

THE GILCHRIST TALENT GROUP INC.
310 Madison Ave., Suite 1025
New York, NY 10017
(212) 692-9166 (E) (S) (A)

PEGGY HADLEY ENTERPRISES, LTD.
250 W. 57th St., Suite 2317
New York, NY 10019
(212) 246-2166 (E) (S) (A)

MICHAEL HARTIG AGENCY, LTD.
156 Fifth Ave., Suite 820
New York, NY 10010
(212) 929-1772 (E) (S) (A)

HENDERSON/HOGAN AGENCY, INC.
850 Seventh Ave., Suite 1003
New York, NY 10019
(212) 765-5190 (E) (S) (A)

DIANA HUNT MANAGEMENT
Royalton Hotel
44 W. 44th St., Room 1614
New York, NY 10036
(212) 391-4971 (A)

H.W.A. TALENT REPRESENTATIVES, LTD.
36 E. 22nd St., 3rd fl.
New York, NY 10010
(212) 529-4555 (E) (S) (A)

INGBER AND ASSOCIATES
274 Madison Ave., Suite 1104
New York, NY 10016
(212) 889-9450 (S) (A)

INNOVATIVE ARTISTS TALENT AND LITERARY
AGENCY
1776 Broadway, Suite 1810
New York, NY 10019
(212) 315-4455 (E) (S) (A)

INTERNATIONAL CREATIVE MANAGEMENT,
INC.
40 W. 57th St.
New York, NY 10019
(212) 556-5600 (E) (S) (A)

IT MODELS/OMAR'S MEN
251 Fifth Ave., 7th fl. PH
New York, NY 10016
(212) 481-7220 (S)

JAM THEATRICAL AGENCY, INC.
352 Seventh Ave., Suite 1500
New York, NY 10001
(212) 376-6330 (E) (S) (A)

JAN J. AGENCY, INC.
365 W. 34th St.
New York, NY 10001
(212) 967-5265 (E) (S) (A)

JORDAN, GILL & DORNBAUM AGENCY, INC.
156 Fifth Ave., Suite 711
New York, NY 10010
(212) 463-8455 (E) (S) (A)

MARVIN JOSEPHSON AGENCY
16 W. 22nd St., 7th fl.
New York, NY 10010
(212) 727-7820 (E)

JERRY KAHN, INC.
853 Seventh Ave., Suite 7C
New York, NY 10019
(212) 245-7317 (E) (A)

CHARLES KERIN ASSOCIATES
155 E. 55th St., Suite 5D
New York, NY 10022
(212) 838-7373 (E) (S) (A)

ARCHER KING LTD.
10 Columbus Circle, Suite 1492
New York, NY 10019
(212) 765-3103 (E) (S) (A)

ROSEANNE KIRK ARTISTS
730 Fifth Ave., 9th fl.
New York, NY 10019
(212) 315-3487 (E)

KMA ASSOCIATES
211 W. 56th St., Suite 17D
New York, NY 10019
(212) 581-4610 (S) (A)

THE KRASNY OFFICE, INC.
1501 Broadway, Suite 1510
New York, NY 10036
(212) 730-8160 (E) (S) (A)

KRONICK, KELLY & LAUREN
420 Madison Ave., 14th fl.
New York, NY 10017
(212) 935-8980 (S)

LALLY TALENT AGENCY
630 Ninth Ave., Suite 800
New York, NY 10036
(212) 974-8718 (E) (S) (A)

THE LANTZ OFFICE
888 Seventh Ave.
New York, NY 10106
(212) 586-0200 (E) (S) (A)

L.B.H. ASSOCIATES
1 Lincoln Plaza, Suite 30V
New York, NY 10023
(212) 787-2609 (A)
Mostly singers and musicians.

LIONEL LARNER LTD.
130 W. 57th St., Suite 10A
New York, NY 10019
(212) 246-3105 (E) (S) (A)

BRUCE LEVY AGENCY
335 W. 38th St., Suite 802
New York, NY 10018
(212) 563-7079 (E) (S) (A)

LURE INTERNATIONAL TALENT GROUP, INC.
915 Broadway, Suite 1210
New York, NY 10010
(212) 260-9300 (E) (S) (A)

LW2
9 E. 37th St.
New York, NY 10016
(212) 889-9450 (E)

MADISON TALENT GROUP, INC.
310 Madison Ave., Suite 1508
New York, NY 10017
(212) 922-9600 (S)

MCCULLOUGH ASSOCIATES
8 South Hanover Ave.
Margate, NJ 08402
(609) 822-2222 (A)

MARGE MCDERMOTT ENTERPRISES
216 E. 39th St.
New York, NY 10016
(212) 889-1583 (A)

MEREDITH MODEL MANAGEMENT
10 Furler St.
Totowa, NJ 07512
(201) 812-0122 (S) (A)

WILLIAM MORRIS AGENCY, INC.
1350 Ave. of the Americas
New York, NY 10019
(212) 586-5100 (E) (S) (A)

THE NEWS AND ENTERTAINMENT CORP.
1325 Ave. of the Americas, 6th fl.
New York, NY 10019
(212) 765-5555 (A)
Primarily handles newscasters.

NOUVELLE TALENT MANAGEMENT, INC.
20 Bethune St., Suite 3B
New York, NY 10014
(212) 645-0940 (E) (S) (A)

OMNIPOP, INC.
55 W. Old Country Rd.
Hicksville, NY 11801
(516) 937-6011 (S) (A)

OPPENHEIM–CHRISTIE ASSOCIATES, LTD.
13 E. 37th St.
New York, NY 10016
(212) 213-4330 (E) (S) (A)

FIFI OSCARD AGENCY, INC.
24 W. 40th St., 17th fl.
New York, NY 10018
(212) 764-1100 (E) (S) (A)

HARRY PACKWOOD TALENT, LTD.
250 W. 57th St., Suite 2012
New York, NY 10107
(212) 586-8900 (E) (S) (A)

DOROTHY PALMER TALENT AGENCY, INC.
235 W. 56th St., Suite 24K
New York, NY 10019
(212) 765-4280 (S)

PARADIGM, A TALENT AND LITERARY
AGENCY
200 W. 57th St., Suite 900
New York, NY 10019
(212) 246-1030 (E) (S) (A)

PAULINE'S TALENT CORP.
379 W. Broadway, Suite 502
New York, NY 10012
(212) 941-6000 (S)

PREMIER TALENT AGENCY
3 E. 54th St.
New York, NY 10022
(212) 758-4900 (S)
Established rock stars; no actors.

PROFESSIONAL ARTISTS UNLIMITED
513 W. 54th St.
New York, NY 10019
(212) 247-8770 (E) (S) (A)

PYRAMID ENTERTAINMENT GROUP
89 Fifth Ave.
New York, NY 10003
(212) 242-7274 (E) (S) (A)
Booking agents for comedy acts only.

RADIOACTIVE TALENT, INC.
240-03 Linden Blvd.
Elmont, NY 11003
(212) 315-1919 (S) (A)

THE NORMAN REICH AGENCY
1650 Broadway, Suite 303
New York, NY 10019
(212) 399-2881 (E) (S) (A)

GILLA ROOS, LTD.
16 W. 22nd St., 7th fl.
New York, NY 10010
(212) 727-7820 (S) (A)

C.V. RYAN AGENCY
1841 Broadway, Suite 907
New York, NY 10023
(212) 245-2225 (A)

SAMES & ROLLNICK ASSOCIATES, LTD.
250 W. 57th St., Suite 703
New York, NY 10107
(212) 315-4434 (E) (S) (A)

SANDERS AGENCY, LTD.
1204 Broadway, Suite 306
New York, NY 10001
(212) 779-3737 (E) (S) (A)

SCHIFFMAN, EKMAN, MORRISON, AND MARX
22 W. 19th St., 8th fl.
New York, NY 10011
(212) 627-5500 (E) (S) (A)

THE WILLIAM SCHILL AGENCY, INC.
250 W. 57th St., Suite 2402
New York, NY 10107
(212) 315-5919 (E) (S) (A)

SCHULLER TALENT, INC.,
(a.k.a. New York Kids)
276 Fifth Ave., 10th fl.
New York, NY 10001
(212) 532-6005 (S) (A)

SHEPLIN ARTISTS AND ASSOCIATES
160 Fifth Ave., Suite 909
New York, NY 10010
(212) 647-1311 (E) (S) (A)

SILVER–MASSETTI/EAST, LTD.
145 W. 45th St., Suite 1204
New York, NY 10036
(212) 391-4545 (E) (S) (A)

ANTHONY SOGLIO AGENCY
423 Madison Ave.
New York, NY 10017
(212) 751-1850 (E)

SPOTLIGHT ENTERTAINMENT SERVICES
250 W. 57th St., Suite 307
New York, NY 10107
(212) 956-4557 (A)

STEWART ARTISTS CORP.
215 E. 81st St.
New York, NY 10028
(212) 744-2272 (A)

PETER STRAIN & ASSOCIATES, INC.
1501 Broadway, Suite 2900
New York, NY 10036
(212) 391-0380 (E) (S) (A)

STROUD MANAGEMENT
1040 First Ave., Suite 273
New York, NY 10022
(212) 750-3035 (A)
Daytime soap writers only.

TALENT EAST
79 Fifth Ave., 10th fl.
New York, NY 10003
(212) 647-1166 (E) (S) (A)

TALENT REPRESENTATIVES, INC.
20 E. 53rd St.
New York, NY 10022
(212) 752-1835 (E) (S) (A)

THE TANTLEFF OFFICE, INC.
375 Greenwich St., Suite 700
New York, NY 10013
(212) 941-3939 (E) (S) (A)

MICHAEL THOMAS AGENCY, INC.
305 Madison Ave., Suite 4419
New York, NY 10165
(212) 867-0303 (E) (S) (A)

TRANUM, ROBERTSON & HUGHES, INC.
2 Dag Hammarskjold Plaza
New York, NY 10017
(212) 371-7500 (S) (A)

UNIQUE SPORTS ENTERTAINMENT
MARKETING INC.
505 Eighth Ave., Suite 900
New York, NY 10018
(212) 563-6444 (S)

UNIVERSAL ATTRACTIONS INC.
218 W. 57th St., Suite 3A
New York, NY 10019
(212) 582-7575 (A)
Pop/R&B musicians; no actors.

VAN DER VEER PEOPLE, INC.
401 E. 57th St., 2nd fl.
New York, NY 10022
(212) 688-2880 (S)

C. JAMES ROBERT VON SCHOLZ
120 Jersey Ave., Suite 206
New Brunswick, NJ 08901
(908) 828-6060 (E) (S)

WATERS AND NICOLOSI TALENT
REPRESENTATIVES
1501 Broadway, Suite 1305
New York, NY 10036
(212) 302-8787 (E) (S) (A)

HANNS WOLTERS THEATRICAL AGENCY
10 W. 37th St.
New York, NY 10018
(212) 714-0100 (S)

ANN WRIGHT REPRESENTATIVES, INC.
165 W. 46th St., Suite 1105
New York, NY 10036
(212) 764-6770 (E) (S) (A)

WRITERS & ARTISTS AGENCY
19 W. 44th St., Suite 1000
New York, NY 10036
(212) 391-1112 (E) (S) (A)

BABS ZIMMERMAN PRODUCTIONS
305 E. 86th St.
New York, NY 10021
(212) 348-7203 (E)

ZOLI MANAGEMENT, INC.
3 W. 18th St., 5th fl.
New York, NY 10011
(212) 242-7490 (E) (S) (A)

LOS ANGELES

ASA
4430 Fountain Ave., Suite A
Los Angeles, CA 90029
(213) 662-9787 (S) (A)

ABRAMS ARTISTS & ASSOCIATES
9200 Sunset Blvd., Suite 625
Los Angeles, CA 90069
(310) 859-0625 (E) (S) (A)

ABRAMS–RUBALOFF & LAWRENCE
8075 West 3rd St., Suite 303
Los Angeles, CA 90048
(213) 935-1700 (E) (S) (A)

ACME TALENT & LITERARY AGENCY
6310 San Vicente Blvd., Suite 520
Los Angeles, CA 90048
(213) 954-2263 (E) (S) (A)

AFH MANAGEMENT, TALENT AGENCY
8240 Beverly Blvd., Suite 11
Los Angeles, CA 90048
(213) 658-9152 (S)

THE AGENCY
1800 Ave. of the Stars, Suite 400
Los Angeles, CA 90067
(310) 551-3000 (E) (S) (A)

AGENCY FOR PERFORMING ARTS
9000 Sunset Blvd., 12 fl.
Los Angeles, CA 90069
(310) 273-0744 (E) (S) (A)

AIMEE ENTERTAINMENT
13743 Victory Blvd.
Van Nuys, CA 91401
(818) 994-9354 (S) (A)

ALLEN TALENT AGENCY
11755 Wilshire Blvd., Suite 1750
Los Angeles, CA 90025
(310) 474-7524 (E) (S) (A)

BONNI ALLEN TALENT
260 S. Beverly Dr., 2nd fl.
Beverly Hills, CA 90212
(310) 247-1865 (E) (S) (A)

CARLOS ALVARADO AGENCY
8455 Beverly Blvd., Suite 406
Los Angeles, CA 90048
(213) 655-7978 (S) (A)

AMBROSIO/MORTIMER
9150 Wilshire Blvd., Suite 175
Beverly Hills, CA 90212
(310) 274-4274 (E) (S) (A)

AMSEL, EISENSTADT & FRAZIER
6310 San Vicente Blvd., Suite 401
Los Angeles, CA 90048
(213) 939-1188 (E) (S) (A)

ANGEL CITY TALENT
1680 Vine St., Suite 716
Los Angeles, CA 90028
(213) 463-1680 (E) (S) (A)

CHRIS APODACA AGENCY
2049 Century Park East, Suite 1200
Los Angeles, CA 90067
(310) 284-3484 (S) (A)

APODACA/MUNRO TALENT AGENCY
13801 Ventura Blvd.
Sherman Oaks, CA 91423
(818) 380-2700 (S)

ARTIST MANAGEMENT AGENCY
4340 Campus Dr., Suite 210
Newport Beach, CA 92660
(714) 261-7557 (S) (A)

ARTIST NETWORK
8438 Melrose Pl.
Los Angeles, CA 90069
(213) 651-4244 (S)

ARTISTS AGENCY
10000 Santa Monica Blvd., Suite 305
Los Angeles, CA 90067
(310) 277-7779 (E) (S) (A)

ARTISTS FIRST, INC.
P.O. Box 7217
Beverly Hills, CA 90212-7217
(310) 550-8606 (E) (S) (A)

ARTISTS GROUP, LTD.
10100 Santa Monica, #2490
Los Angeles, CA 90067
(310) 552-1100 (E) (S) (A)

ATKINS AND ASSOCIATES
303 S. Crescent Heights Blvd.
Los Angeles, CA 90048
(213) 658-1025 (E) (S) (A)

BADGLEY & CONNOR
9229 Sunset Blvd., Suite 311
Los Angeles, CA 90069
(310) 278-9313 (E) (S) (A)

BAIER–KLEINMAN INTERNATIONAL
3575 Cahuenga Blvd. W, #500
Los Angeles, CA 90068
(818) 761-1001 (S) (A)

BALDWIN TALENT, INC.
500 Sepulveda Blvd., 4th fl.
Los Angeles, CA 90049
(310) 472-7919 (S) (A)

BOBBY BALL TALENT AGENCY
8075 W. 3rd St., Suite 550
Los Angeles, CA 90048
(213) 964-7300 (E) (S) (A)

RICKEY BARR TALENT AGENCY
P.O. Box 69590
Los Angeles, CA 90069
(310) 276-0887 (E) (S) (A)

BAUMAN, HILLER & ASSOCIATES
5757 Wilshire Blvd., Suite 5
Los Angeles, CA 90036
(213) 857-6666 (E) (S) (A)

BDP & ASSOCIATES TALENT AGENCY
10637 Burbank Blvd.
North Hollywood, CA 91601
(818) 506-7615 (E) (S) (A)

BEAKEL AND DEBORD
10637 Burbank Blvd.
North Hollywood, CA 91601
(818) 506-7615.

BELSON & KLASS
144 S. Beverly Dr., #405
Beverly Hills, CA 90212
(310) 274-9169 (E) (S) (A)

SARA BENNETT AGENCY
6404 Hollywood Blvd., Suite 327
Los Angeles, CA 90028
(213) 965-9666 (S) (A)

LOIS J. BENSON
8360 Melrose Ave., Suite 203
Los Angeles, CA 90069
(213) 653-0500 (E) (S) (A)

MARIAN BERZON TALENT AGENCY
336 E. 17th St.
Costa Mesa, CA 92627
(714) 631-5936 (E) (S) (A)

THE BIGLEY AGENCY
6442 Coldwater Canyon Ave., Suite 211
North Hollywood, CA 91606
(818) 761-9971 (E) (S) (A)

YVETTE BIKOFF AGENCY, LTD.
8721 Santa Monica Blvd.
Los Angeles, CA 90069
(213) 655-6123 (E) (S) (A)

THE BLAKE AGENCY
415 N. Camden Dr.
Beverly Hills, CA 90210,
(310) 246-0241 (S) (A)

BFL ENTERPRISES
2029 Century Park East, #600
Los Angeles, CA 90067
(310) 277-1260.

BLOOM, J. MICHAEL
9255 Sunset Blvd., Suite 710
Los Angeles, CA 90069
(310) 275-6800 (E) (S) (A)

BOP-LA TALENT AGENCY
1467 N. Tamarind Ave.
Hollywood, CA 90028
(213) 466-8667 (E) (S) (A)

NICOLE BORDEAUX TALENT AGENCY
616 N. Robertson, 2nd fl.
West Hollywood, CA 90069
(310) 289-2550 (S)

BORINSTEIN ORECK BOGART
8271 Melrose Ave., #110
Los Angeles, CA 90046
(213) 658-7500 (E) (S) (A)

BRAND MODEL AND TALENT
17941 Skypark Circle, Suite F
Irvine, CA 92714
(714) 251-0555 (S)

PAUL BRANDON & ASSOCIATES
1033 N. Carol Dr., Suite T6
Los Angeles, CA 90069
(310) 273-6173 (S)

S. W. BRANDON'S COMMERCIALS
UNLIMITED
9601 Wilshire Blvd., Suite 620
Beverly Hills, CA 90210
(310) 888-8788 (S)

BRESLER, KELLY & KIPPERMAN
15760 Ventura Blvd., Suite 1730
Encino, CA 91436
(818) 905-1155 (E) (S) (A)

DON BUCHWALD & ASSOCIATES
9229 Sunset Blvd., Suite 710
West Hollywood, CA 90069
(310) 278-3600 (E) (S) (A)

BURKETT TALENT AGENCY
1700 E. Garry, Suite 113
Santa Ana, CA 92705
(714) 724-0465 (S) (A)

IRIS BURTON AGENCY
P.O. Box 15306
Beverly Hills, CA 90209
(310) 288-0121 (S) (A)

CAMDEN ITG
822 S. Robertson Blvd., Suite 200
Los Angeles, CA 90035
(310) 289-2700 (E) (S) (A)

BARBARA CAMERON & ASSOCIATES
8369 Sausalito Ave., Suite A
West Hills, CA 91304
(818) 888-6107 (S) (A)

CAPITAL ARTISTS
8383 Wilshire Blvd., Suite 954
Beverly Hills, CA 90211
(213) 658-8118 (S)

WILLIAM CARROLL AGENCY
139 N. San Fernando Rd., Suite A
Burbank, CA 91502
(818) 848-9948 (S) (A)

CASTLE–HILL TALENT AGENCY
1101 S. Orlando Ave.
Los Angeles, CA 90035
(213) 653-3535 (E) (S) (A)

CAVALERI & ASSOCIATES
849 S. Broadway, Suite 750
Los Angeles, CA 90014
(213) 683-1354 (E) (S) (A)

CENTURY ARTISTS, LTD.
9744 Wilshire Blvd., Suite 308
Beverly Hills, CA 90212
(310) 273-4366 (E) (S) (A)

THE CHASIN AGENCY
8899 Beverly Blvd., Suite 713
Los Angeles, CA 90048
(310) 278-7505 (S)

CHATEAU BILLINGS TALENT AGENCY
5657 Wilshire Blvd., Suite 340
Los Angeles, CA 90036
(213) 965-5432 (S)

JACK CHUTUK AND ASSOCIATES
2121 Ave. of the Stars, Suite 700
Los Angeles, CA 90067
(310) 552-1773 (S)

CIRCLE TALENT ASSOCIATES
433 N. Camden Dr., Suite 400
Beverly Hills, CA 90212
(310) 285-1585 (S) (A)

CL INC.
843 N. Sycamore Ave.
Los Angeles, CA 90038
(213) 461-3971 (S)

W. RANDOLPH CLARK COMPANY
2431 Hyperion Ave.
Los Angeles, CA 90027
(213) 953-4960 (S) (A)

C' LA VIE MODEL AND TALENT
7507 Sunset Blvd., Suite 201
Los Angeles, CA 90046
(213) 969-0541 (S)

COLLEEN CLER MODELING
120 S. Victory Blvd., Suite 206
Burbank, CA 91502
(818) 841-7943 (S) (A)

CNA
1801 Ave. of the Stars, Suite 1250
Los Angeles, CA 90067
(310) 556-4343 (E) (S) (A)

COAST TO COAST TALENT GROUP, INC.
4942 Vineland Ave., Suite 200
North Hollywood, CA 91601
(818) 762-6278 (S) (E)

COLOURS MODEL & TALENT MANAGEMENT
AGENCY
8344½ W. 3rd St.
Los Angeles, CA 90048
(213) 658-7072 (S) (A)

CONTEMPORARY ARTISTS, LTD.
1427 Third St. Promenade, Suite 205
Santa Monica, CA 90401
(310) 395-1800 (E) (S) (A)

CORALIE JR. THEATRICAL AGENCY
4789 Vineland Ave., Suite 100
North Hollywood, CA 91602,
(818) 766-9501 (E) (S) (A)

THE COSDEN AGENCY
3518 Cahuenga Blvd. West, Suite 216
Los Angeles, CA 90068
(818) 752-4000 (E) (S) (A)

THE CRAIG AGENCY
8485 Melrose Place, Suite E
Los Angeles, CA 90069
(213) 655-0236 (E) (S) (A)

CAA/CREATIVE ARTISTS AGENCY
9830 Wilshire Blvd.
Beverly Hills, CA 90212
(310) 288-4545 (E) (S) (A)

SUSAN CROW & ASSOCIATES
1010 Hammond St., Suite 102
West Hollywood, CA 90069
(310) 859-9784 (S) (A)

LIL CUMBER ATTRACTIONS
6363 Sunset Blvd., Suite 807
Los Angeles, CA 90028
(213) 469-1919 (E) (S) (A)

CUNNINGHAM, ESCOTT & DIPENE
10635 Santa Monica Blvd., Suite 130
Los Angeles, CA 90025
(310) 475-2111 (E) (S) (A)

DADE/SHULTZ ASSOCIATES
11846 Ventura Blvd., Suite 101
Studio City, CA 91604
(818) 760-3100 (E) (S) (A)

MARY WEBB DAVIS TALENT AGENCY
515 N. La Cienega Blvd.
Los Angeles, CA 90048
(310) 652-6850 (S)

THE DEVROE AGENCY
6311 Romaine St.
Los Angeles, CA 90038
(213) 962-3040 (S)

DH TALENT AGENCY
1800 N. Highland Ave., Suite 300
Los Angeles, CA 90028
(213) 962-6643 (S) (A)

DURKIN ARTISTS
12229 Ventura Blvd., Suite 202
Studio City, CA 91604
(818) 762-9936 (S) (A)

EFENDI TALENT AGENCY
1923½ Westwood Blvd., Suite 3
Los Angeles, CA 90025
(310) 441-2822 (S) (A)

ELITE MODEL MANAGEMENT
345 N. Maple Dr., Suite 397
Beverly Hills, CA 90210
(310) 274-9395 (S)

ELLIS TALENT GROUP
6025 Sepulveda Blvd., Suite 201
Van Nuys, CA 91411
(818) 997-7447 (E) (S)

EMERALD ARTISTS
140 S. Beverly Dr., #202
Beverly Hills, CA 90212
(310) 271-7120 (S) (A)

EPSTEIN–WYCKOFF–LAMANNA &
ASSOCIATES
280 S. Beverly Dr., Suite 400
Beverly Hills, CA 90212
(310) 278-7222 (E) (S) (A)

ESTAPHAN TALENT AGENCY
6018 Greenmeadow Rd.
Lakewood, CA 90713
(310) 421-8048 (S)

EILEEN FARRELL TALENT AGENCY
18261 San Fernando Mission Blvd.
Northridge, CA 91326
(818) 831-7003 (E) (S) (A)

WILLIAM FELBER & ASSOCIATES
2126 Cahuenga Blvd.
Los Angeles, CA 90068
(213) 466-7629 (E) (S) (A)

FERRAR–MAZIROFF ASSOCIATES
8430 Santa Monica Blvd., Suite 220
Los Angeles, CA 90069
(213) 654-2601 (S)

LIANA FIELDS TALENT AGENCY
3325 Wilshire Blvd., Suite 749
Los Angeles, CA 90010
(213) 292-8550 (S)

FILM ARTISTS ASSOCIATES
7080 Hollywood Blvd., Suite 1118
Los Angeles, CA 90028
(213) 463-1010 (S) (A)

FIRST ARTISTS AGENCY
10000 Riverside Drive, Suite 10
Toluca Lake, CA 91602
(818) 509-9292 (S) (A)

FLICK EAST–WEST TALENTS, INC.
9057 Nemo St., Suite A
West Hollywood, CA 90069
(310) 247-1777 (E) (S) (A)

JUDITH FONTAINE AGENCY
9255 Sunset Blvd., Suite 727
Los Angeles, CA 90069
(310) 285-0545 (S) (A)

JUDITH FONTAINE KIDS AGENCY
9255 Sunset Blvd., Suite 725
Los Angeles, CA 90069
(310) 285-0905 (S) (A)

FPA TALENT AGENCY
12701 Moorpark, Suite 205
Studio City, CA 91604
(818) 508-6691 (A)

BARRY FREED COMPANY
2029 Century Park East, Suite 600
Los Angeles, CA 90067
(310) 277-1260 (S)

ALICE FRIES AGENCY
6381 Hollywood Blvd., #600
Hollywood, CA 90028
(213) 876-2990 (S)

GAGE GROUP INC.
9255 Sunset Blvd., Suite 515
Los Angeles, CA 90069
(310) 859-8777 (E) (S) (A)

HELEN GARRETT TALENT AGENCY
6525 Sunset Blvd., 5th fl.
Los Angeles, CA 90028
(213) 871-8707 (E) (S) (A)

DALE GARRICK INTERNATIONAL
8831 Sunset Blvd., Suite 402
West Hollywood, CA 90069
(310) 657-2661 (S) (A)

THE GEDDES AGENCY
1201 Greenacre Ave.
Los Angeles, CA 90046
(213) 878-1155 (S) (A)

LAYA GELFF AGENCY
16133 Ventura Blvd., Suite 700
Encino, CA 91436
(818) 713-2610 (E) (S) (A)

PAUL GERARD TALENT AGENCY
2918 Alta Vista Dr.
Newport Beach, CA 92660
(714) 644-7950 (S)

DON GERLER & ASSOCIATES
3349 Cahuenga Blvd. West, Suite 1
Los Angeles, CA 90068
(213) 850-7386 (S) (A)

THE GERSH AGENCY
232 N. Canon Dr.
Beverly Hills, CA 90210
(310) 274-6611 (E) (S) (A)

GEORGIA GILLY TALENT AGENCY
8721 Sunset Blvd., Suite 104
Los Angeles, CA 90069
(310) 657-5660 (E) (S) (A)

GOLD/MARSHAK & ASSOCIATES
3500 W. Olive Ave., Suite 1400
Burbank, CA 91505
(818) 972-4300 (E) (S) (A)

GOLDEY COMPANY, INC.
116 N. Robertson Blvd., Suite 700
Los Angeles, CA 90048
(310) 657-3277 (S)

GORDON COMPANY TALENT AGENCY
15250 Ventura, Suite 720
Sherman Oaks, CA 91403
(818) 907-0220 (S) (A)

MICHELLE GORDON & ASSOCIATES
260 S. Beverly Dr., Suite 308
Beverly Hills, CA 90212
(310) 246-9930 (E) (S) (A)

MGA/MARY GRADY AGENCY
4444 Lankershim Blvd., #207
North Hollywood, CA 91602
(818) 766-4414 (E) (S) (A)

GREENVINE AGENCY
110 E. 9th St., C-1005
Los Angeles, CA 90079
(213) 622-3016

HALPERN & ASSOCIATES
12304 Santa Monica Blvd., Suite 104
Los Angeles, CA 90025
(310) 571-4488 (S)

VAUGHN D. HART & ASSOCIATES
8899 Beverly Blvd., #815
Los Angeles, CA 90048
(310) 273-7887 (S) (A)

BEVERLY HECHT AGENCY
8949 Sunset Blvd., Suite 203
Los Angeles, CA 90069
(310) 278-3544 (S) (A)

HENDERSON/HOGAN AGENCY
247 S. Beverly Dr., #102
Beverly Hills, CA 90212
(310) 274-7815 (E) (S) (A)

HERVEY/GRIMES TALENT AGENCY
12444 Ventura Blvd., Suite 103
Studio City, CA 91604
(818) 981-0891 (S) (A)

HOUSE OF REPRESENTATIVES TALENT
AGENCY
9911 Pico Blvd., Suite 1060
Los Angeles, CA 90035
(310) 772-0772 (E) (S)

HOWARD TALENT WEST
12178 Ventura Blvd., Suite 201
Studio City, CA 91604
(818) 766-5300 (E) (S) (A)

MARTIN HURWITZ ASSOCIATES
427 N. Canon Dr., Suite 215
Beverly Hills, CA 90210
(310) 274-0240 (S)

HWA TALENT REPRESENTATIVES
1964 Westwood Blvd., Suite 400
Los Angeles, CA 90025
(310) 446-1313

INNOVATIVE ARTISTS
1999 Ave. of the Stars, Suite 2850
Los Angeles, CA 90067
(310) 553-5200 (E) (S) (A)

INTERNATIONAL CREATIVE MANAGEMENT
8942 Wilshire Blvd.
Beverly Hills, CA 90211
(310) 550-4000 (E) (S) (A)

IT MODEL MANAGEMENT
526 N. Larchmont Blvd.
Los Angeles, CA 90004
(213) 962-9564 (S)

JACKMAN & TAUSSIG
1815 Butler Ave., Suite 120
Los Angeles, CA 90025
(310) 478-6641 (S) (A)

GEORGE JAY AGENCY
6269 Selma Ave., #15
Los Angeles, CA 90028
(213) 466-6665 (S)

THOMAS JENNINGS & ASSOCIATES
28035 Dorothy Dr., Suite 210A
Agoura, CA 91301
(818) 879-1260 (S)

KENNETH B. JOHNSTON & ASSOCIATES
15043 Valley Heart Dr.
Sherman Oaks, CA 91403
(818) 907-5471 (A)

JOSEPH, HELDFOND & RIX
11365 Ventura Blvd., #100
Studio City, CA 91604
(213) 466-9111 (E) (S) (A)

KARG/WEISSENBACH & ASSOCIATES
329 N. Wetherly Dr., #101
Beverly Hills, CA 90211
(310) 205-0435 (E) (S) (A)

KELMAN/ARLETTA
7813 Sunset Blvd.
Los Angeles, CA 90046
(213) 851-8822 (E) (S) (A)

WILLIAM KERWIN AGENCY
1605 N. Cahuenga Blvd., Suite 202
Los Angeles, CA 90028
(213) 469-5155 (E) (S) (A)

TYLER KJAR AGENCY
10643 Riverside Dr.
Toluca Lake, CA 91602
(818) 760-0321 (E) (S) (A)

PAUL KOHNER INC.
9300 Wilshire Blvd., #555
Beverly Hills, CA 90212
(310) 550-1060 (E) (S) (A)

VICTOR KRUGLOV & ASSOCIATES
7060 Hollywood Blvd., Suite 1220
Los Angeles, CA 90028
(213) 957-9000 (S) (A)

L A ARTISTS
2566 Overland Ave., Suite 560
Los Angeles, CA 90064
(310) 202-0254 (E) (S) (A)

L A TALENT
8335 Sunset Blvd., 2nd fl.
Los Angeles, CA 90069
(213) 656-3722 (E) (S) (A)

STACEY LANE TALENT AGENCY
13455 Ventura Blvd., Suite 240
Sherman Oaks, CA 91423
(818) 501-2668 (S) (A)

THE LAWRENCE AGENCY
3575 Cahuenga Blvd. West, Suite 125-3
Los Angeles, CA 90068
(213) 851-7711 (S) (A)

GUY LEE & ASSOCIATES
4150 Riverside Dr., Suite 212
Burbank, CA 91505
(818) 848-7475 (S) (A)

THE LEVIN AGENCY
9255 Sunset Blvd., #400
West Hollywood, CA 90069
(310) 278-0353 (S) (A)

TERRY LICHTMAN CO.
4439 Worster Ave.
Studio City, CA 91604
(818) 783-3003 (S) (A)

ROBERT LIGHT AGENCY
6404 Wilshire Blvd., Suite 900
Los Angeles, CA 90048
(213) 651-1777 (S) (A)

KEN LINDER & ASSOCIATES
2049 Century Park East, Suite 2750
Los Angeles, CA 90067
(310) 277-9223 (S) (A)

LOS ANGELES PREMIERE ARTISTS AGENCY
8899 Beverly Blvd., Suite 102
Los Angeles, CA 90048
(310) 271-1414 (S)

LYNNE & REILLY AGENCY
Toluca Plaza Bldg.
6735 Forest Lawn Dr., #313
Los Angeles, CA 90068
(213) 850-1984 (S) (A)

MADEMOISELLE TALENT AGENCY
8693 Wilshire Blvd., Suite 200
Beverly Hills, CA 90211
(310) 289-8005 (S)

MARIS AGENCY
17620 Sherman Way, #213
Van Nuys, CA 91406
(818) 708-2493 (A)

ALESE MARSHALL MODEL & COMMERCIAL
AGENCY
23900 Hawthorne Blvd., Suite 100
Torrance, CA 90505
(310) 378-1223 (S) (A)

THE MARTEL AGENCY
1680 N. Vine St., #203
Los Angeles, CA 90028
(213) 461-5943 (E) (S) (A)

MEDIA ARTISTS GROUP
8383 Wilshire Blvd., Suite 954
Beverly Hills, CA 90211
(213) 658-5050 (S) (A)

METROPOLITAN TALENT AGENCY
4526 Wilshire Blvd.
Los Angeles, CA 90010
(213) 857-4500

MIRAMAR TALENT AGENCY
9157 Sunset Blvd., Suite 300
Los Angeles, CA 90069
(310) 858-1900 (S)

PATTY MITCHELL AGENCY
4605 Lankershim Blvd., #201
North Hollywood, CA 91602
(818) 508-6181 (S) (A)

MOORE ARTISTS TALENT AGENCY
1551 S. Robertson Blvd.
Los Angeles, CA 90035
(310) 286-3150 (E) (S) (A)

WILLIAM MORRIS AGENCY
151 El Camino Dr.
Beverly Hills, CA 90212
(310) 274-7451 (E) (S) (A)

H. DAVID MOSS & ASSOCIATES
733 N. Seward St., Penthouse
Hollywood, CA 90038
(213) 465-1234 (E) (S) (A)

MARY MURPHY AGENCY
6014 Greenbush Ave.
Van Nuys, CA 91401
(818) 989-6076 (S) (A)

OMNIPOP INC.
10700 Ventura Blvd., 2nd fl.
Studio City, CA 91604
(818) 980-9267 (S) (A)

ORANGE GROVE GROUP, INC.
12178 Ventura Blvd., Suite 205
Studio City, CA 91604
(818) 762-7498 (E) (S) (A)

CINDY OSBRINK TALENT AGENCY
4605 Lankershim Blvd., Suite 401
North Hollywood, CA 91602
(818) 760-2488 (S) (A)

DOROTHY DAY OTIS & ASSOCIATES
13223 Ventua Blvd., Suite F
Woodland Hills, CA 91604
(818) 905-9510 (S)

PARADIGM TALENT AGENCY
10100 Santa Monica Blvd., Suite 2500
Los Angeles, CA 90067
(310) 277-4400 (E) (S) (A)

PARAGON TALENT AGENCY, INC.
8439 Sunset Blvd., Suite 301
Los Angeles, CA 90069
(213) 654-4554 (S)

THE PARTOS COMPANY
Raleigh Studios
5300 Melrose, E Bldg., #217E
Los Angeles, CA 90038
(213) 654-4554 (S)

JANICE PATTERSON TALENT AGENCY
3599 Cahuenga W., #321
Los Angeles, CA 90068
(213) 876-0189.

PLAYBOY MODEL AGENCY
9242 Beverly Blvd.
Beverly Hills, CA 90210
(310) 246-4000 (A)

PLAYERS TALENT AGENCY
8770 Shoreham Dr., Suite 2,
West Hollywood, CA 90069
(310) 289-8777 (S)

PRIMA MODEL MANAGEMENT, INC.
933 N. La Brea Ave., Suite 200
Los Angeles, CA 90038
(213) 882-6900 (S)

PRIVILEGE TALENT AGENCY
8170 Beverly Blvd., Suite 204
Los Angeles, CA 90048
(213) 658-8781 (S)

PRODUCTION VALUES
606 N. Larchmont Blvd., #307
Los Angeles, CA 90004
(213) 461-0148

PRO-SPORT & ENTERTAINMENT CO.
1900 S. Bundy Dr., #700
Los Angeles, CA 90025
(310) 207-0228 (S)

PROGRESSIVE ARTISTS
400 S. Beverly Dr., Suite 216
Beverly Hills, CA 90212
(310) 553-8561 (E) (S) (A)

GORDON RAEL COMPANY
9255 Sunset Blvd., Suite 425
Los Angeles, CA 90069
(213) 969-8493 (S)

RENAISSANCE TALENT & LITERARY AGENCY
8523 Sunset Blvd.
Los Angeles, CA 90069
(310) 289-3636 (S) (A)

STEPHANIE ROGERS & ASSOCIATES
3575 W. Cahuenga Blvd., Suite 249
Los Angeles, CA 90068
(213) 851-5155 (S)

CINDY ROMANO MODELING & TALENT
AGENCY
P.O. Box 1951
Palm Springs, CA 92263
(619) 323-3333 (S)

GILLA ROOS WEST LTD.
9744 Wilshire Blvd., Suite 203
Beverly Hills, CA 90212
(310) 274-9356 (E) (S) (A)

THE MARION ROSENBERG OFFICE
8428 Melrose Pl., Suite B
Los Angeles, CA 90069
(213) 653-7383 (E) (S) (A)

NALALIE ROSSON AGENCY
11712 Moorpark St., Suite 204
Studio City, CA 91604
(818) 508-1445 (S) (A)

S D B PARTNERS, INC.
1801 Ave. of the Stars, Suite 902
Los Angeles, CA 90067
(310) 785-0060 (S)

THE SANDERS AGENCY
8831 Sunset Blvd., #304
Los Angeles, CA 90069
(310) 652-1119 (E) (S) (A)

SARNOFF COMPANY, INC.
3900 W. Alameda Ave., 17th fl.
Burbank, CA 91505
(818) 972-1779 (S) (A)

THE SAVAGE AGENCY
6212 Banner Ave.
Los Angeles, CA 90038
(213) 461-8316 (E) (S) (A)

JACK SCAGNETTI TALENT AGENCY
5118 Vineland Ave., Suite 102
North Hollywood, CA 91601
(818) 762-3871 (S) (A)

THE IRV SCHECHTER COMPANY
9300 Wilshire Blvd., #400
Beverly Hills, CA 90212
(310) 278-8070 (E) (S) (A)

SCHIOWITZ/CLAY/ROSE, INC.
1680 N. Vine St., Suite 614
Los Angeles, CA 90028
(213) 463-7300 (E) (S) (A)

SANDIE SCHNARR TALENT
8281 Melrose Ave., #200
Los Angeles, CA 90046
(213) 653-9479 (S) (A)

JUDY SCHOEN & ASSOCIATES
606 N. Larchmont Blvd., Suite 309
Los Angeles, CA 90004
(213) 962-1950 (E) (S) (A)

DON SCHWARTZ ASSOCIATES
8749 Sunset Blvd.
Los Angeles, CA 90069
(310) 657-8910 (E) (S)

SCREEN ARTISTS AGENCY
12435 Oxnard St.
North Hollywood, CA 91606
(818) 755-0026 (S)

SCREEN CHILDREN'S TALENT AGENCY
4000 Riverside Dr., Suite A,
Burbank, CA 91505
(818) 846-4300 (S) (A)

SELECTED ARTISTS AGENCY
3575 Cahuenga Blvd., West, 2nd fl.
Los Angeles, CA 90068
(213) 882-8453 (E) (S) (A)

DAVID SHAPIRA & ASSOCIATES
15301 Ventura Blvd., Suite 345
Sherman Oaks, CA 91403
(818) 906-0322 (E) (S) (A)

SHAPIRO–LICHTMAN, INC.
8827 Beverly Blvd.
Los Angeles, CA 90048
(310) 859-8877 (S) (A)

SHOWBIZ ENTERTAINMENT
6922 Hollywood Blvd., Suite 207
Los Angeles, CA 90028
(213) 469-9931 (S) (A)

DOROTHY SHREVE AGENCY
2665 N. Palm Canyon Dr.
Palm Springs, CA 92262
(619) 327-5855 (S) (A)

JEROME SIEGEL ASSOCIATES
7551 Sunset Blvd., Suite 203
Los Angeles, CA 90046
(213) 850-1275 (S)

SIERRA TALENT AGENCY
14542 Ventura Blvd., Suite 207
Sherman Oaks, CA 91403
(818) 907-9645 (S)

SILVER, KASS & MASSETTI AGENCY, LTD.
8730 Sunset Blvd., Suite 480
Los Angeles, CA 90069
(310) 289-0909 (E) (S) (A)

RICHARD SINDELL & ASSOCIATES
8271 Melrose Ave., Suite 202
Los Angeles, CA 90046
(213) 653-5051 (S) (A)

SIRENS MODEL MANAGEMENT
6404 Wilshire Blvd., #720
Beverly Hills, CA 90048
(213) 782-0310

MICHAEL SLESSINGER ASSOCIATES
8730 Sunset Blvd., Suite 220
Los Angeles, CA 90069
(310) 657-7113 (E) (S) (A)

SUSAN SMITH & ASSOCIATES
121 N. San Vicente Blvd.
Beverly Hills, CA 90211
(213) 852-4777 (E) (S) (A)

SPECIAL ARTISTS AGENCY
335 North Maple Dr., Suite 360
Beverly Hills, CA 90210
(310) 859-9688 (S) (A)

STAR TALENT AGENCY
4555½ Mariota Ave.
Toluca Lake, CA 91602
(818) 509-1931 (S)

STARWIL TALENT AGENCY
6253 Hollywood Blvd., #730
Los Angeles, CA 90028
(213) 874-1239 (S) (A)

CHARLES H. STERN AGENCY
11755 Wilshire Blvd., Suite 2320
Los Angeles, CA 90025
(310) 479-1788 (S) (A)

STONE MANNERS AGENCY
8091 Selma Ave.
Los Angeles, CA 90046
(213) 654-7575 (E) (S) (A)

SUTTON, BARTH & VENNARI INC.
145 S. Fairfax Ave., Suite 310
Los Angeles, CA 90036
(213) 938-6000 (E) (S) (A)

TALENT GROUP INC.
9250 Wilshire Blvd., Suite 208
Beverly Hills, CA 90212
(310) 273-9559 (S) (A)

HERB TANNEN & ASSOCIATES
1800 N. Vine St., Suite 305
Los Angeles, CA 90028
(213) 466-6191 (E) (S) (A)

THOMAS/ROSSEN AGENCY
124 S. Lasky Dr., 1st fl.
Beverly Hills, CA 90212
(310) 247-2727 (S)

ARLENE THORNTON & ASSOCIATES
5657 Wilshire Blvd., Suite 290
Los Angeles, CA 90036
(213) 939-5757 (S) (A)

TISHERMAN AGENCY, INC.
6767 Forest Lawn Dr., Suite 101
Los Angeles, CA 90068
(213) 850-6767 (S) (A)

THE TURTLE AGENCY
12456 Ventura Blvd., Suite 1
Studio City, CA 91604
(818) 506-6869 (S) (A)

TWENTIETH CENTURY ARTISTS
15315 Magnolia Blvd., #429
Sherman Oaks, CA 91403
(818) 788-5516 (E) (S) (A)

UMOJA TALENT AGENCY
2069 W. Slauson Ave.
Los Angeles, CA 90047
(213) 290-6612 (S)

UTA/UNITED TALENT AGENCY, INC.
9560 Wilshire Blvd., 5th fl.
Beverly Hills, CA 90212
(310) 273-6700 (E) (S)

ERIKA WAIN AGENCY
1418 N. Highland Ave., #102
Hollywood, CA 90028
(213) 460-4224 (S) (A)

WALLIS AGENCY
1126 Hollywood Way, Suite 203A
Burbank, CA 91505
(818) 953-4848 (S)

ANN WAUGH TALENT AGENCY
4731 Laurel Canyon Blvd., Suite 5
North Hollywood, CA 91607
(818) 980-0141 (E) (S) (A)

RUTH WEBB ENTERPRISES
7500 Devista Dr.
Los Angeles, CA 90046
(213) 874-1700 (E) (S) (A)

THE WHITAKER AGENCY
12725 Ventura Blvd., Suite F
Studio City, CA 91604
(818) 766-4441 (E) (S) (A)

SHIRLEY WILSON & ASSOCIATES
5410 Wilshire Blvd., Suite 227
Los Angeles, CA 90036
(213) 857-6977 (E) (S) (A)

WORLD CLASS SPORTS
9171 Wilshire Blvd., #404
Beverly Hills, CA 90210
(310) 278-2010 (S)

CARTER WRIGHT ENTERPRISES
6513 Hollywood Blvd., Suite 210
Hollywood, CA 90028
(213) 469-0944 (E) (S) (A)

WRITERS AND ARTISTS AGENCY
924 Westwood Blvd., Suite 900
Los Angeles, CA 90024
(310) 824-6300 (E) (S) (A)

ZEALOUS ARTISTS P., INC.
139 S. Beverly Dr., Suite 222
Beverly Hills, CA 90212
(310) 281-3533 (S)

CHICAGO

AMBASSADOR TALENT AGENTS
333 N. Michigan Ave., Suite 314
Chicago, IL 60601
(312) 641-3491 (S) (A)

ARIA MODEL & TALENT MANAGEMENT, LTD.
1017 W. Washington, Suite 2A
Chicago IL 60607
(312) 243-9400 (E) (S) (A)

LARRY BASTIAN
2580 Crestwood Lane
Deerfield, IL 60015
(708) 945-9283 (E)

CUNNINGHAM, ESCOTT, DIPENE &
ASSOCIATES, INC.
One E. Superior St., Suite 505
Chicago, IL 60611
(312) 944-5600 (E) (S) (A)

DAVID & LEE INC.
70 W. Hubbard St., Suite 200
Chicago, IL 60601
(312) 670-4444 (S) (A)

HARRISE DAVIDSON & ASSOCIATES, INC.
65 E. Wacker Place, Suite 2401
Chicago, IL 60601
(312) 782-4480 (E) (S) (A)

ETA, INC.
7558 S. Chicago Ave.
Chicago, IL 60619
(312) 752-3955 (S) (A)

GEDDES AGENCY
1925 N. Clybourn, Suite 402
Chicago, IL 60614
(312) 348-3333 (E) (S) (A)

SHIRLEY HAMILTON AGENCY, INC.
333 E. Ontario, Suite B
Chicago, IL 60611
(312) 787-4700 (E) (S) (A)

LINDA JACK TALENT
230 E. Ohio, Suite 200
Chicago, IL 60611
(312) 587-1155 (S) (A)

JEFFERSON & ASSOCIATES, INC.
1050 N. State St., Suite 4C
Chicago, IL 60610
(312) 337-1930 (E) (S) (A)

LILY'S TALENT AGENCY, INC.
5962 N. Elston
Chicago, IL 60646
(312) 792-3456 (E) (S) (A)

EMILIA LORENCE LTD.
619 N. Wabash Ave., 3rd fl.
Chicago, IL 60611
(312) 787-2033 (E) (S) (A)

NORTH SHORE TALENT, INC.
308 W. Huron, 2nd fl.
Chicago, IL 60610
(312) 482-9949
Other address:
450 Peterson Rd.
Libertyville, IL 60040
(708) 816-1811 (S) (A)

NOUVELLE TALENT MANAGEMENT
15 W. Hubbard St., 3rd fl.
Chicago, IL 60610
(312) 944-1133 (E) (S) (A)

PHOENIX TALENT, LTD.
410 S. Michigan Ave., PH
Chicago, IL 60605
(312) 786-2024 (S) (A)

SALAZAR & NAVAS, INC.
367 W. Chicago Ave.
Chicago, IL 60610
(312) 751-3419 (S) (A)

SA-RAH TALENT AGENCY
1935 S. Halsted St., Suite 301
Chicago, IL 60608
(312) 733-2822 (S) (A)

NORMAN SCHUCART ENTERPRISES, INC.
1417 Green Bay Rd.
Highland Park, IL 60035
(312) 433-1113 (S) (A)

HOWARD W. SCHULTZ
241 Golf Mill Court, Suite 328
Niles, IL 60714
(312) 867-4282 (A)

STEWART TALENT MANAGEMENT CORP.
212 W. Superior, Suite 406
Chicago, IL 60610
(312) 943-3131 (E) (S) (A)

SUZANNE'S A-PLUS TALENT
108 W. Oak St.
Chicago, IL 60610
(312) 943-8315 (S) (A)

VOICES UNLIMITED
680 N. Lake Shore Dr., Suite 1330
Chicago, IL 60611
(312) 642-3262 (S) (A)

ARLENE WILSON TALENT, INC.
430 W. Erie, Suite 210
Chicago, IL 60610
(312) 573-0200 (E) (S) (A)

New York, Los Angeles, and Chicago Casting Directors

The following is a list of independent casting directors. There are many other casting directors who work freelance, going from one production office to another, and do not have an office address we could include here. Casting directors request that initial contact be made by sending a picture/résumé through the mail. (Some requested that we not list their phone numbers.)

NEW YORK

AMERIFILM CASTING
375 West Broadway, Suite 3R
New York, NY 10012
(212) 334-3382

BABY WRANGLERS CASTING, INC.
500 W. 43rd St., Suite 6G
New York, NY 10036
(212) 736-0060

BAD GIRL CASTING
138-19 222nd St.
Laurelton, NY 11413-2724
(718) 712-0887

HARRIET BASS CASTING
722 Broadway, Suite 6
New York, NY 10003
(212) 598-9032

JERRY BEAVER AND ASSOCIATES
215 Park Ave. So., Suite 1704
New York, NY 10003
(212) 979-0909
Fax: (212) 460-8850

BREANNA BENJAMIN CASTING
P.O. Box 368, Lenox Hill Station
New York, NY 10021
(212) 388-2347

JAY BINDER CASTING
513 W. 54th St.
New York, NY 10019
(212) 586-6777

BORICUA CASTING
153 W. 21st St., Suite 4
New York, NY 10011
(212) 627-1789

JANE BRINKER CASTING LTD.
51 W. 16th St.
New York, NY 10011
(212) 924-3322

CTP CASTING
22 W. 27th St., 10th fl.
New York, NY 10001
(212) 696-1100

KIT CARTER CASTING
160 W. 95th St., Suite 1D
New York, NY 10025
(212) 864-3147

DONALD CASE CASTING INC.
386 Park Ave. So., Suite 809
New York, NY 10016
(212) 889-6555

CAST-AWAY! CASTING SERVICE
14 Sutton Place So.
New York, NY 10022
(212) 755-0960

CHANTILES VIGNEAULT CASTING
2 Lincoln Square, Suite 361
New York, NY 10023

ROZ CLANCY CASTING
76 Wilfred Ave.
Titusville, NJ 08560

BOB COLLIER CASTING
124 W. 18th St., 2nd fl.
New York, NY 10011-5408
(212) 929-4737

CONTEMPORARY CASTING
P.O. Box 1844, FDR Station
New York, NY 10022
(212) 838-1818

BYRON CRYSTAL
41 Union Square West, Suite 316
New York, NY 10003

SUE CRYSTAL CASTING
251 W. 87th St., Suite 26
New York, NY 10024
(212) 877-0737

MONI DAMEVSKI CASTING
4 Park Ave., #4F
New York, NY 10016
(212) 684-0477

DONNA DE SETA CASTING
525 Broadway, 3rd fl.
New York, NY 10012
(212) 274-9696

MERRY L. DELMONTE CASTING &
PRODUCTIONS INC.
555 W. 57th St.
New York, NY 10019
(212) 279-2000

LOU DIGIAIMO ASSOCIATES
513 W. 54th St.
New York, NY 10019
(212) 713-1884

SYLVIA FAY
71 Park Ave.
New York, NY 10016

LEONARD FINGER CASTING
1501 Broadway, Suite 1511
New York, NY 10036
(212) 944-8611

JUDIE FIXLER CASTING
P.O. Box 149
Green Farms, CT 06436-0149
(203) 254-7434

MAUREEN FREMONT CASTING
1001 Ave. of the Americas, Suite 1215
New York, NY 10016
(212) 302-1215

GODLOVE, SEROW & SINDLINGER CASTING
151 W. 25th St., 11th fl.
New York, NY 10001
(212) 627-7300

WENDY GOLD CASTING
39 W. 19th St., 12th fl.
New York, NY 10011

MARIA GRECO CASTING
630 Ninth Ave., Suite 702
New York, NY 10036
(212) 247-2011

CAROL HANZEL CASTING
39 W. 19 St., 12th fl.
New York, NY 10011
(212) 242-6113

HASKINS CASTING
426 Broome St., Suite 5F
New York, NY 10013
(212) 431-8405

JUDY HENDERSON & ASSOCIATES
330 W. 89th St.
New York, NY 10024
(212) 877-0225

HERMAN & LIPSON CASTING
24 W. 25th St.
New York, NY 10010
(212) 807-7706

HISPANICAST
Riccy Reed Casting
39 W. 19th St., 12th fl.
New York, NY 10011
(212) 691-7366

STUART HOWARD ASSOCIATES
22 W. 27th St., 10th fl.
New York, NY 10001
(212) 725-7770

HUGHES/MOSS CASTING
311 W. 43rd St., Suite 700
New York, NY 10036
(212) 307-6690

HYDE–HAMLET CASTING
Box 884, Times Square Station
New York, NY 10108-0218
(718) 783-9634

JOHNSON–LIFF CASTING
1501 Broadway, Suite 1400
New York, NY 10036
(212) 391-2680

ROSALIE JOSEPH CASTING
1501 Broadway
New York, NY 10036
(212) 921-5781

NANCY KAGAN ASSOCIATES
333 E. 84th St.
New York, NY 10028
(212) 794-6044

AVY KAUFMAN
180 Varick St., 16th fl.
New York, NY 10014

KEE CASTING
511 Ave. of the Americas, #384
New York, NY 10011
(212) 995-0794

JUDY KELLER CASTING
160 E. 48th St.
New York, NY 10017
(212) 751-2576

JODI KIPPERMAN CASTS
141 Fifth Ave., Suite 5 So.
New York, NY 10010
(212) 228-5551

ANDREA KURZMAN CASTING INC.
122 E. 37th St., 1st fl.
New York, NY 10016
(212) 684-0710

LELAS TALENT CASTING
P.O. Box 14
Milford, CT 06460
(212) 875-7955
(203) 877-8355

LIZ LEWIS CASTING PARTNERS
3 W. 18th St., 6th fl.
New York, NY 10011
(212) 645-1500

JOAN LYNN CASTING
39 W. 19 St., 12th fl.
New York, NY 10011
(212) 675-5595

MCCORKLE CASTING
264 W. 40th St., 9th fl.
New York, NY 10018
(212) 840-0992

ABIGAIL MCGRATH, INC.
1501 Broadway, Suite 1907
New York, NY 10036
(212) 768-3277

BETH MELSKY CASTING
928 Broadway, Suite 300
New York, NY 10010
(212) 505-5000

MATTHEW MESSINGER CASTING
129 W. 15th St.
New York, NY 10011

METROPOLITAN CASTING
208 W. 20th St., Suite 5A
New York, NY 10011
(212) 229-2694

MULTINATIONAL CASTING
119 W. 23rd St., Suite 305
New York, NY 10011

ELISSA MYERS CASTING
333 W. 52nd St., Suite 1008
New York, NY 10019
(212) 315-4777

NAVARRO/BERTONI & ASSOCIATES
101 W. 31st St., Room 2112
New York, NY 10001
(212) 736-9272

ORPHEUS GROUP, INC.
1600 Broadway, Suite 603
New York, NY 10019
(212) 957-8760

JOANNE PASCIUTO, INC.
17-08 150th St.
Whitestone, NY 11357

ELLEN POWERS CASTING
8 Fulton Dr.
Brewster, NY 10509
(914) 279-6057

SCOTT POWERS PRODUCTIONS
150 Fifth Ave., Suite 623
New York, NY 10011
(212) 242-4700

RED, WHITE AND BLUE, INC.
301 W. 57th St.
New York, NY 10019
(212) 315-5050

RICCY REED CASTING
39 W. 19th St., 12th fl.
New York, NY 10011
(212) 691-7366

RICHIN CASTING
450 W. 42nd St., Suite 2B
New York, NY 10036
(212) 243-4448

TONI ROBERTS CASTING
150 Fifth Ave., Suite 717
New York, NY 10011
(212) 627-2250

MIKE ROSCOE CASTING
153 E. 37th St., Suite 1B
New York, NY 10016
(212) 725-0014

CHARLES ROSEN CASTING, INC.
140 W. 22nd St., 4th fl.
New York, NY 10011

JUDY ROSENSTEEL CASTING
43 W. 68th St.
New York, NY 10023

SHERIE L. SEFF CASTING
400 W. 43rd St., Suite 9B
New York, NY 10036
(212) 947-7408

SELECTIVE CASTING BY CAROL NADELL
P.O. Box 1538, Radio City Station
New York, NY 10101

MARCIA SHULMAN CASTING
270 Lafayette St., Suite 610
New York, NY 10012

MEG SIMON CASTING
1600 Broadway, Suite 1005
New York, NY 10019
(212) 245-7670

CAROLINE SINCLAIR CASTING
720 Greenwich St., Suite 7J
New York, NY 10014
(212) 675-4094

ELSIE STARK CASTING/STARK NAKED
PRODUCTIONS
39 W. 19th St., 12th fl.
New York, NY 10011
(212) 366-1903
Fax: (212) 366-0495

IRENE STOCKTON CASTING
261 Broadway, Suite 2B
New York, NY 10007
(212) 964-9445

STRICKMAN–RIPPS, INC.
65 N. Moore St., Suite 3A
New York, NY 10013
(212) 966-3211

PAT SWEENEY CASTING
61 E. 8th St., Suite 144
New York, NY 10003
(212) 533-0544

HELYN TAYLOR CASTING
140 W. 58th St.
New York, NY 10019

BERNARD TELSEY CASTING
120 W. 28th St.
New York, NY 10001

TODD THALER
130 W. 57th St., Suite 4A
New York, NY 10019

VIDEOACTIVE TALENT
353 W. 48th St., 2nd fl.
New York, NY 10036
(212) 541-8106

JOY WEBER CASTING
250 W. 57th St.
New York, NY 10019

WEIST–BARRON CASTING
35 W. 45th St.
New York, NY 10036
(212) 840-7025

WILFLEY/TODD CASTING
60 Madison Ave., Room 1017
New York, NY 10010
(212) 685-3537

MARJI CAMNER WOLLIN & ASSOCIATES
233 E. 69th St.
New York, NY 10021
(212) 472-2528

LIZ WOODMAN CASTING
11 Riverside Dr., #2JE
New York, NY 10023
(212) 787-3782

WORLD PROMOTIONS
250 Sargent Dr.
New Haven, CT 06511
(203) 781-3427

LOS ANGELES
The following are all members of the Casting Society of America and can be reached at their individual mailing addresses.

DEBORAH AQUILA, VP OF CASTING,
MOTION PICTURES
Paramount Studios
5555 Melrose Ave.
Bob Hope Bldg., #200
Los Angeles, CA 90038

DEBORAH BARYLSKI CASTING
Walt Disney Studios
500 S. Buena Vista St.
Production Building, 3rd fl.
Burbank, CA 91521

FRAN BASCOM
Studio Plaza
3400 Riverside Dr., #765
Burbank, CA 91505

CHERYL BAYER CASTING
ABC Productions
2020 Ave. of the Stars, 5th fl.
Los Angeles, CA 90067

ANNETTE BENSON
Kushner Locke
11601 Wilshire Blvd., 21st fl.
Los Angeles, CA 90025

CHEMIN BERNARD CASTING
4435 West Slauson Ave., #146
Los Angeles, CA 90043

JUEL BESTROP
Sony Pictures
10202 West Washington Blvd., Poitier
Bldg., #1108
Culver City, CA 90232

SHARON BIALY
P.O. Box 570308
Tarzana, CA 91356

BILLIK/JACOBY CASTING
Walt Disney Studios
500 South Buena Vista St.
Trailer 32
Burbank, CA 91521

CARISSA BLIX
Media Casting
6963 Douglas Blvd., #294
Granite Bay, CA 95746

EUGENE BLYTHE, VP OF CASTING
Walt Disney/Touchstone Television
500 South Buena Vista St.
Team Disney Bldg., #417E
Burbank, CA 91521

JUDITH BOULEY
536 Pearl St.
Monterey, CA 93940

MEGAN BRANMAN
4029 Lankershim Blvd.
Universal City, CA 91608

BUCK/EDELMAN CASTING
4045 Radford Ave., Suite B
Studio City, CA 91604

PERRY BULLINGTON
MacDonald–Bullngton Casting
3030 Andrita St., Suite A
Los Angeles, CA 90028

REUBEN CANNON AND ASSOCIATES
1640 South Sepulveda Blvd., #218
Los Angeles, CA 90025

FERNE CASSEL
20th Century Fox
10201 West Pico Blvd.
Los Angeles, CA 90035

LUCY CAVALLO, VP OF TALENT
Stephen J. Cannell Productions
7083 Hollywood Blvd., 3rd fl.
Los Angeles, CA 90028

DENISE CHAMIAN CASTING
Aaron Spelling Productions
5700 Wilshire Blvd., #575
Los Angeles, CA 90036

ELLEN CHENOWETH
Werthemer Armstrong & Hirsc
1888 Century Park East, Suite 1888
Los Angeles, CA 90067

BARBARA CLAMAN, INC.
8281 Melrose Ave., #300
Los Angeles, CA 90046

LORI COBE
3599 Cahuenga Blvd. West, 3rd fl.
Los Angeles, CA 90068

ANDREA COHEN
Warner Studios
4000 Warner Blvd., Bldg. 5, #27
Burbank, CA 91522

RUTH CONFORTE
5300 Laurel Canyon Blvd., #168
North Hollywood, CA 91607

ALLISON COWITT
Mike Fenton & Associates
14724 Ventura Blvd., Suite 510
Sherman Oaks, CA 91403

BILLY DAMOTA CASTING
P.O. Box 4635
Glendale, CA 91222

ANITA DANN
270 North Canon Dr., #1147
Beverly Hills, CA 90210

ERIC DAWSON
Ulrich/Dawson Casting
5750 Wilshire Blvd., Suite 250
Los Angeles CA 90036

DIANE DIMEO AND ASSOCIATES
12754 Sarah St.
Studio City, CA 91604

PAM DIXON
P.O. Box 672
Beverly Hills, CA 90213

DONNA DOCKSTADER
Universal Studios
100 Universal City Plaza, Bldg. 463,
#110
Universal City, CA 91608

SUSAN EDELMAN
Buck/Edelman Casting
4045 Radford Ave., Suite B
Studio City, CA 91604

DONNA EKHOLDT, MANAGER OF CASTING
NBC
3000 West Alameda Ave., #231
Burbank, CA 91523

PENNY ELLERS CASTING
5700 Wilshire Blvd., #116
Los Angeles, CA 90028

MIKE FENTON AND ASSOCIATES
14724 Ventura Blvd., #510
Sherman Oaks, CA 91043

STEVEN FERTIG
8271 Melrose Ave., #208
West Hollywood, CA 90046

FINN CASTING
Warner Studios
4000 Warner Blvd.
Producers Bldg. 1, #103
Burbank, CA 91522

DAVID GIELLA
3151 Cahuenga Blvd. West, Suite 210
Los Angeles, CA 90068

JAN GLASER
Concorde Pictures
11600 San Vicente Blvd., 2nd fl.
Los Angeles, CA 90049

LAURA GLEASON
Berman/Gleason Casting Ltd.
12400 Ventura Blvd., Suite 312
Studio City, CA 91604

SUSAN GLICKSMAN
5433 Beethoven St.
Los Angeles, CA 90066

PETER GOLDEN
St. Clare Productions
Universal Studios
Bldg. 506, Suite A
Universal City, CA 91608

GOODMAN/EDELMAN CASTING
10100 Santa Monica Blvd., #700
Los Angeles, CA 90067

JEFF GREENBERG AND ASSOCIATES
Paramount Studios
5555 Melrose Ave.
Marx Brothers Bldg., #102
Los Angeles, CA 90038

HARRIET GREENSPAN
9242 Beverly Blvd.
Beverly Hills, CA 90210

IRIS GROSSMAN, VP OF CASTING
TNT
1888 Century Park East, 14th fl.
Los Angeles, CA 90067

SHEILA GUTHRIE
Paramount TV
5555 Melrose Place
Marx Bros. Bldg., #102
Los Angeles, CA 90038

TED HANN
Warner Bros. Television
300 Television Plaza
Bldg. 140, 1st fl.
Burbank, CA 91505

BOB HARBIN, VP OF TALENT AND CASTING
Fox Broadcasting Company
10201 West Pico Blvd.
Executive Bldg. 88, #325
Los Angeles, CA 90035

CATHY HENDERSON CASTING
13517 Ventura Blvd., Suite 2
Sherman Oaks, CA 91423

MARC HIRSCHFELD
Liberman Hirschfeld Casting
5979 West 3rd St., Suite 204
Los Angeles, CA 90036

JANET HIRSHENSON
The Casting Company
7461 Beverly Blvd., PH
Los Angeles, CA 90036

ALAN C. HOCHBERG
4063 Radford Ave., #103
Studio City, CA 91604

DONNA ISAACSON, VP, FEATURE CASTING
20th Century Fox
10201 West Pico Blvd.
Bldg. 12, #225
Los Angeles, CA 90035

JUSTINE JACOBY
Billik/Jacoby Casting
8642 Melrose Ave., Suite 2
Los Angeles, CA 90069

JANE JENKINS
The Casting Company
7461 Beverly Blvd., PH
Los Angeles, CA 90036

CARO JONES CASTING
P.O. Box 3329
Los Angeles, CA 90078

ELLIE KANNER
Warner Bros. Television
300 Television Plaza
Bldg. 140, 1st fl.
Burbank, CA 91505

KAPLAN/WINTHROP CASTING
P.O. Box 261160
Encino, CA 91426-1160

MICHAEL A. KATCHER
CBS Entertainment
7800 Beverly Blvd., #284
Los Angeles, CA 90036

EILEEN KNIGHT CASTING
12009 Guerin St.
Studio City, CA 91604

JOANNE KOEHLER
Warner Bros. Television
300 Television Plaza, Bldg. 140
Burbank, CA 91505

SHANA LANDSBURG
The Landsburg Building
11811 West Olympic Blvd.
Los Angeles, CA 90064

ELIZABETH LARROQUETTE
Port St. Films, Inc.
4000 Warner Blvd.
Producers Bldg. 1, #102
Burbank, CA 91522

GERALDINE LEDER
Warner Bros. Television
300 Television Plaza, Bldg. 140, #139
Burbank, CA 91505

KATHLEEN LETTERIE, HEAD OF CASTING
Warner Bros. Television
3701 West Oak St., Bldg. 34R, #161
Burbank, CA 91505

JOHN LEVEY
Warner Bros. Television
300 Television Plaza, Bldg. 140, #138
Burbank, CA 91505

HEIDI LEVITT
Television Center
1020 North Cole Ave., 2nd fl.
Los Angeles, CA 90038

MEG LIBERMAN
5979 West 3rd St., Suite 204
Los Angeles, CA 90036

ROBIN LIPPIN AND ASSOICATES
NBC Productions
330 Bob Hope Dr., Suite C-110
Burbank, CA 91523

MOLLY LOPATA
12725 Ventura Blvd., Suite 1
Studio City, CA 91604

JUNIE LOWRY JOHNSON CASTING
Paramount Studios
5555 Melrose Ave.
Von Sternberg, Suite 104
Los Angeles, CA 90038

MACDONALD/BULLINGTON CASTING
3030 Andrita St., Suite A
Los Angeles, CA 90065

DEBI MANWILLER
Pagano/Manwiller Casting
10201 W. Pico Blvd., Trailer 767
Los Angeles, CA 90035

MARGIOTTA CASTING
8265 Sunset Blvd., #200
Los Angeles, CA 90046

IRENE MARIANO, VP OF CASTING
Warner Bros. Television
300 Television Plaza, Bldg. 140, #134A
Burbank, CA 91505

MINDY MARIN
Casting Artists, Inc.
609 Broadway
Santa Monica, CA 90401

VALERIE MCCAFFREY, VP OF FEATURE
CASTING
New Line Cinema
116 N. Robertson Blvd., 6th fl.
Los Angeles, CA 90048

VIVIAN MCRAE
P.O. Box 1351
Burbank, CA 91507

TOM MCSWEENEY
6040 Van Noord Ave.
Sherman Oaks, CA 91401

JEFF MESHEL, DIRECTOR OF CASTING
NBC
3000 West Alameda Ave., #231
Burbank, CA 91523

ELLEN MEYER
Meyer & Oberst Casting
301 N. Canon Dr., #300
Beverly Hills, CA 90210

LYNN D. MEYERS
P.O. Box 3277
N. Hollywood, CA 91609

BARBARA MILLER, SENIOR VP OF TALENT &
CASTING
Warner Bros. Television
300 Television Plaza, Bldg. 140, 1st fl.
Burbank, CA 91505

BOB MORONES
KCET
4401 Sunset Blvd.
Los Angeles, CA 90027

HELEN MOSSLER, VP OF TALENT
Paramount Studios
5555 Melrose Ave., Bludhorn Bldg., #128
Los Angeles, CA 90038

ROGER MUSSENDEN
Manager of Feature Casting
20th Century Fox Studios
10201 West Pico Blvd., Bldg. 12, #225
Los Angeles, CA 90035

ROBIN STOLTZ NASSIF, DIRECTOR OF
CASTING
ABC
2040 Ave. of the Stars, 5th fl.
Los Angeles, CA 90067

NANCY NAYOR, VP FEATURE FILM CASTING
MCA/Universal
100 Universal Plaza, Bldg. 500, 1st fl.
Universal City, CA 91608

BRUCE NEWBERG
c/o Edward Rada
5670 Wilshire Blvd, Suite 1450
Los Angeles, CA 90036

GARY OBERST
Meyer & Oberst Casting
300 North Canon Dr., #300
Beverly Hills, CA 90210

LORI OPENDEN, SENIOR VP OF TALENT &
CASTING
NBC
3000 West Alameda Ave., #231
Burbank, CA 91523

FERN ORENSTEIN
5433 Beethoven St.
Los Angeles, CA 90066

JEFF OSHEN AND ASSOCIATES
Paramount Studios
5555 Melrose Ave., Gower Mill Bldg.,
#117
Los Angeles, CA 90038

JESSICA OVERWISE
17250 Sunset Blvd.
Pacific Palisades, CA 90272

PAGANO/MANWILLER CASTING
20th Century Fox Studios
10201 West Pico Blvd., Trailer 767
Los Angeles, CA 90035

MARVIN PAIGE
P.O. Box 69964
West Hollywood, CA 90069

LINDA PHILLIPS PALO
Raleigh Studios
650 North Bronson Ave., Bronson
Bldg., #144
Los Angeles, CA 90004

JOHN PAPSIDERA
Casting Artists, Inc.
609 Broadway St.
Santa Monica, CA 90401

DAN PARADA
Montgomery/Parada Casting
1020 N. Cole Ave., Suite 4267
Hollywood, CA 90038

CAMI PATTON
Witt–Thomas Productions
1438 N. Gower St., Bldg 35, Rm. 577
Los Angeles, CA 90028

DONALD PAUL PEMRICK
3520 Hayden Ave.
Culver City, CA 90232

JOHANNA RAY CASTING
1022 Palm Ave., #2
West Hollywood, CA 90069

ROBI REED AND ASSOCIATES
8170 Beverly Blvd., #202
Los Angeles, CA 90048

BARBARA REMSEN AND ASSOCIATES
Raleigh Studios
650 North Bronson Ave., #124
Los Angeles, CA 90004

STUART M. ROSEN
7631 Lexington Ave.
West Hollywood, CA 90046

DONNA ROSENSTEIN, VP OF TALENT AND
CASTING
ABC
2040 Ave. of the Stars, 5th fl.
Los Angeles, CA 90067

MARCIA ROSS CASTING
500 South Buena Vista, Casting Bldg.,
#10
Burbank, CA 91521

DAVID RUBIN CASTING
8721 Sunset Blvd., #208
Los Angeles, CA 90069

DEBRA RUBINSTEIN CASTING
Museum Square
5757 Wilshire Blvd., #670
Los Angeles, CA 90036

MARK SAKS
Warner Bros. Television
300 South Television Plaza, Bldg. 140,
1st fl.
Burbank, CA 91505

SUSAN SCUDDER
6565 Sunset Blvd., Suite 306
Hollywood, CA 90028

TONY SEPULVEDA, DIRECTOR OF CASTING
Warner Bros. Television
300 Television Plaza, Bldg. 140, 1st fl.
Burbank, CA 91505

DAN SHANER
Wilshire Court Productions
1840 Century Park East, Suite 400
Los Angeles, CA 90067

BARBARA SHANNON
1537 Rosecrans, Suite G
San Diego, CA 92106

MELISSA SKOFF
11684 Ventura Blvd., #5141
Studio City, CA 91604

SLATER/BROOKSBANK CASTING
MGM
2500 Broadway
Santa Monica, CA 90404

STANLEY SOBLE
Center Theatre Group
601 West Temple St.
Los Angeles, CA 90012

PAMELA SPARKS
Chelsea
3859 Lankershim Blvd.
Studio City, CA 91604

DAWN STEINBERG
Big Ticket Television
5700 Wilshire Blvd., #478
Los Angeles, CA 90036

RON STEPHENSON
MCA/Universal Studios
4029 Lankershim Blvd., Bldg. 463,
Rm. 100
Universal City, CA 91608

SALLY STINER CASTING
12228 Venice Blvd.
Los Angeles, CA 90066

RANDY STONE, VP TALENT AND CASTING
20th Century Fox Television
10201 West Pico Blvd., Bldg. 54, #6
Los Angeles, CA 90035

STRATTON/ROBERTS
Television Center
6311 Romaine St., #7219
Los Angeles, CA 90038

MONICA SWANN CASTING
12009 Guerin St.
Studio City, CA 91604

TAYLOR/GORDON CASTING
P.O. Box 461198
Los Angeles, CA 90046

MARK TESCHNER
General Hospital,
ABC Prospect
4151 Prospect Ave., Stage 54
Los Angeles, CA 90027

ULRICH/DAWSON CASTING
6421 Coldwater Canyon
North Hollywood, CA 91606

KAREN VICE
12001 Ventura Place, #203
Studio City, CA 91604

DAVA WAITE
Universal Television
100 Universal City Plaza, Bldg. 463,
#104
Universal City, CA 91608

SAMUEL WARREN JR.
Warren & Associates International
Casting Services
2244 4th Ave., Suite D
San Diego, CA 92101

NICK WILKINSON, DIRECTOR OF CASTING
ABC
2040 Ave. of the Stars, 5th fl.
Los Angeles, CA 90067

KIM WILLIAMS
HBO
2049 Century Park East, 42nd fl.
Los Angeles, CA 90067

GERI WINDSOR–FISCHER
11333 Moorpark St.
P.O. Box 402
Studio City, CA 91602

ANNE WINTHROP
P.O. Box 261160
Encino, CA 91426

DIANNE YOUNG
15001 Calvert St.
Van Nuys, CA 91411

RHONDA YOUNG
10350 Santa Monica Blvd.
Los Angeles, CA 90025

GARY ZUCKERBROD
CBS Television City
7800 Beverly Blvd., #284
Los Angeles, CA 90036

*The following independent casting
directors are best reached at:*

THE CASTING SOCIETY OF AMERICA
6565 Sunset Blvd., Suite 306
Los Angeles, CA 90028

Julie Alter
Donna Anderson
Maureen A. Arata
Simon Ayer
Pamela Basker
Lisa Beach
Susan Bluestein
Jacklynn Briskey
Jackie Burch
Irene Cagen
Anne Capizzi
Alice Cassidy
Fern Champion
Brian Chavanne
Barbara Cohen
Glenn Daniels
Leslee Dennis
Dick Dinman
Dorian Dunas
Nan Dutton
Nancy Foy
Carrie Frazier
Melinda Gartzman
Shani Ginsberg
Christopher Gorman
Michael Greer
Milt Hamerman
Natalie Hart
Judith Holstra
Vicki Huff
Beth Hymson-Ayer
Steven Jacobs
Nancy Klopper
Allison Kohler
Wendy Kurtzman
Jason La Padura
Sally Lear
Elisabeth Leustig
Carol Lewis
Terry Liebling
Tracy Lilienfield
Leslie Litt

Lisa London
Amanda Mackey
Francine Maisler
Jackie Margey
Liz Marx
Valorie Massalas
Rick Millikan
Lisa Mionie
Patricia Mock
Meryl O'Loughlin
Mark Paladini
Joey Paul
Holly Powell
Pamela Rack
Robyn Ray
Karen Rea
Joe Reich
Gretchen Rennell
Shari Rhodes
Vicki Rosenberg
Eleanor Ross
Renee Rousselot
Cathy Sandrich
Ellen Lubin Sanitsky
Jean Scoccimarro
Julie Kaplan Selzer
Bill Shepard
Jennifer Shull
Margery Simkin
Sharon Soble
Stanzi Stokes
Joel Thurm
Mark Tillman
Joy Todd
Nikki Valko
Jose Villaverde
April Webster
Rosemary Welden
Susan Wieder
Ronnie Yeskel
Debra Zane

CHICAGO

JANE ALDERMAN CASTING
2105 N. Southport, Suite 202
Chicago, IL 60614
(312) 549-6464

JANE BRODY CASTING
20 W. Hubbard
Chicago, IL 60610
(312) 527-0665

HEITZ CASTING, INC.
920 N. Franklin, #205
Chicago, IL 60610
(312) 664-0601

HOLZER & RIDGE CASTING
700 S. Des Plaines
Chicago, IL 60607
(312) 922-9860
Registration information lines:
Women, (312) 922-4043
Men, (312) 922-4042

LYNN LEVINSON
3536 N. Pinegrove
Chicago, IL 60657
(312) 327-6384

CHERIE MANN & ASSOCIATES
1540 N. LaSalle, #1004
Chicago, IL 60610
(312) 751-2927

BETH RABEDEAU CASTING
225 W. Ohio, Suite 400
Chicago, IL 60610
(312) 222-0181

JEFFREY LYLE SEGAL
1525 W. Homer St., 3rd fl.
Chicago, IL 60622
(312) 509-2943

Personal Managers

The following managers are members of the National Conference of Personal Managers (NCOPM), with offices on both the East and West coasts. The name of the owner/manager is listed first, followed by the company name. Associate members are shown below the phone number. The list of categories that follows serves as a guideline to the different fields of entertainment in which a member is engaged. In some cases, a specific explanation can be found next to a number. To find managers who deal in comedy acts, for example, look for the number 5 under each listing.

If a personal manager claims to belong to the NCOPM, you can call the organization's headquarters to double-check. Be advised, though, that managers who are not members of the NCOPM may be very qualified. It's best to get recommendations and ask for references. Gerard W. Purcell, President, heads the NCOPM, 964 Second Ave., New York, NY 10022; phone (212) 421-2670.

1. Actors/actresses.
2. Directors, producers, writers.
3. Children, teenagers.
4. Newscasters, sports personalities.
5. Variety and/or comedy acts.
6. Music performers, composers, recordings, concerts, lounge, rock 'n' roll.
7. Miscellaneous fields not mentioned above (artists, photographers, etc.).

EAST COAST CHAPTER

Joseph Rapp, Executive Director, heads the East Coast Chapter of the NCOPM, 1650 Broadway, Suite 705, New York, NY 10019; phone (212) 265-3366.

ROGER AILES
Roger Ailes Communications
440 Park Ave. So.
New York, NY 10016
(212) 685-8400
Judy Laterza
(2,4)

AMY AMBROSINO
1027 Shippan Ave.
Stamford, CT 06902
(203) 964-0170
(1,3,5)

MR. DEE ANTHONY
P.O. Box 3509
Westport, CT 06880
(6,7)

SETH APPEL
20 E. 35th St., Suite 2E
New York, NY 10016
(212) 725-9746
(1)

BUD AYERS
Fastbreak Management, Inc.
70 Clay Hill Rd.
Stamford, CT 06905
(203) 329-7335
(1,5,6)

HARVEY BELLOVIN
410 E. 64th St.
New York, NY 10021
(212) 752-5181
(1,2,6)

JOANNE BERKMAN
Bennu Talent Management, Inc.
626 McLean Ave.
Yonkers, NY 10705
(914) 964-1828
Ron Uva
(1,6)

BOBBY BERNARD
40 Central Park So.
New York, NY 10019
(212) 688-1065
(2,5,6)

CLINTON FORD BILLUPS, JR.
78 Taylor Rd., P.O. Box 273
Riverton, CT 06065
(203) 738-3801
Wanda J. Rogers
(5)

PHIL BOUGHTON
211 S. Federal Highway, D9
Boynton Beach, FL 33435
(407) 736-8060
(1,2)

MS. DREW BURKE
Modern Artists Management Associates
150 Fifth Ave., Suite 72B
New York, NY 10011
(201) 962-0263
(1,3,4)

MICHAEL J. BURRIS
Burris Management Group
6120-10 Powers Ave., Suite 164
Jacksonville, FL 32217
(904) 730-9516
(6)

ANTONIO CAMACHO
Top Draw Entertainment
108-22 Queens Blvd., Suite 1
Forest Hills, NY 11375
(718) 896-4001
(5)

RONALD M. CAMPBELL
4381 Hudson Dr., Suite 109
Stow, OH 44224
(216) 688-6778
(6)

DAVID CAMPBELL
Campbell/Martin Associates
75 Spring St., 6th fl.
New York, NY 10012
(212) 343-1923
(1,2)

JOYCE CHASE
2 Fifth Ave.
New York, NY 10011
(212) 473-1234
(1,2)

SUSAN CRAIG
Craig Group
1018 Wild Road Dr.
Lutz, FL 33549
(813) 948-8096
(1,6)

THOMAS A. CURRIE
553 Third Ave., Suite 34
New York, NY 10016-3555
(212) 481-8728
(1, directors)

LORI DANZIGER
Persona Management
40 E. 9th St.
New York, NY 10003
(212) 674-7078
(3)

MS. K. CHARISSE DICKS
Podesoir International Management
211 W. 56th St., Suite 3L
New York, NY 10019
(212) 767-0520
(1,3,5,6)

MS. WINTER DONALDSON
Winter Donaldson Management
33 Cedar Lane
Ossining, NY 10562
(914) 941-6063
(1,3)

MICHELE DONAY
Michele Donay Talent Management
236 E. 74th St.
New York, NY 10021
(212) 769-0924
(1,3)

JOHN ESSAY
P.O. Box 755, Times Square Station
New York, NY 10036
(212) 581-0396
(1)

JOEL A. FELTMAN
Think Tank Talent
389 Fifth Ave., Suite 1010
New York, NY 10016
(914) 237-5834
Grace White Lohr
(1,4)

JONATHAN FIRST
Sound Entertainment Inc.
729 Seventh Ave., 14th fl.
New York, NY 10019
(212) 221-0600
(1,6)

ALAN FOSHKO
305 W. 52nd St.
New York, NY 10019
(212) 757-6085
(1)

MS. JEAN T. FOX
Fox-Albert Management Enterprises,
Inc.
308 W. 48th St.
New York, NY 10036
(212) 262-4300
Denise Dunayer Simon
(1,3)

DICK FOX
Fox Entertainment Company, Inc.
1650 Broadway
New York, NY 10019
(212) 582-9072
(1,5,6)

ESTELLE FUSCO
Discovery Talent Management, Ltd.
72 Moriches Rd.
Lake Grove, NY 11755
(212) 877-6670
(1,3)

MS. TOBE GIBSON
Young Talent, Inc.
301 E. 62nd St., Suite 2C
New York, NY 10021
(212) 308-0930
(1,3,6)

MARILYN GLASSER
MG Management
233 W. 77th St., Suite 3E
New York, NY 10024
(212) 496-0550
(1)

MS. AGGIE GOLD
Fresh Faces Management, Inc.
2911 Carnation Ave.
Baldwin, NY 11510
(516) 223-0034
(3)

MR. SID GOLD
Goldstar Talent Management
161 W. 54th St.
New York, NY 10019
(212) 315-4429
(3: infants)

DICK GRASS
GMS Management
585 Ellsworth St., Suite 2G
Bridgeport, CT 06605
(203) 334-9285
Danny Scarpone
(2,5,6,7)

LLOYD GREENFIELD
Greenfield Associates
1140 Ave. of the Americas, 18th fl.
New York, NY 10036
(212) 245-8130
(5,6)

SETH R. GREENKY
Green Key Management
251 W. 89th St., Suite 4A
New York, NY 10024
(212) 874-7373
(1,2,5,6,7)

CAROLINE HIRSCH
Media and Management
1626 Broadway
New York, NY 10019
(212) 956-0101
Joe Falzarano
(5)

MARC HOFFMAN
119 Langham St.
Brooklyn, NY 11235
(718) 332-7147
(1,6)

JOHN N. JENNINGS
881 10th Ave., Suite 1A
New York, NY 10019
(212) 581-0377
(1,3,5,6)

CATHY KANNER
Kanner/Thor Entertainment
125 W. 72nd St., Suite 3R
New York, NY 10023
(212) 787-1179
Tina Thor
(1)

LAURIE KANNER
Kanner Talent Management
200 Central Park So.
New York, NY 10019
(212) 397-3766
(1)

JONATHAN C. KINLOCH
Kinloch Entertainment Inc.
3500 Oak Lawn, Suite 400
Dallas, TX 75219
(214) 528-3788
(6)

LLOYD KOLMER
Lloyd Kolmer Enterprises
65 W. 55th St.
New York, NY 10019
(212) 582-4735

JENNIFER LAMBERT
1600 Broadway, Suite 1001
New York, NY 10019
(212) 315-0665
(1,3,5,6)

MARIANNE LEONE
Terrific Talent Associates
419 Park Avenue So., Suite 1009
New York, NY 10016
(212) 689-2800
(1,3,6)

JOSEPH LODATO
264 W. 35th St., Suite 10
New York, NY 10001
(212) 967-3320
(5,6: records)

RICK MARTIN
Rick Martin Productions
125 Fieldpoint Rd.
Greenwich, CT 06830
(203) 661-1615
(1,5,6: record production)

ARLINE MCGOVERN
Goodwin & McGovern Theatrical
Management
Mine Layton Ave.
Hicksville, NY 11801
(516) 932-5310
(1,3)

DANIEL MCGOVERN
Lakeland Enterprises
8 Franklin Ave.
New Hyde, New York 11040
(516) 327-0205
*(1,3, physically challenged, hearing and
visually impaired performers)*

MS. SANDI MERLE
101 W. 57th St.,
New York, NY 10019
(212) 489-1578
(5,6)

DAVID MILLER
David Miller Management
306 W. 50th St.
New York, NY 10022
(212) 980-4180
(1)

LOIS N. MILLER
Star Talent Management
1109 Union Blvd., 2nd fl.
Allentown, PA 18103
(610) 770-1200
(1,3)

JEFF MITCHELL
J. Mitchell Management
440 Park Ave. So., 11th fl.
New York, NY 10016
(212) 679-3550
(1,3)

FRED J. MONTILLA, JR.
F.J.M. Productions, Inc.
7305 W. Sample Rd., Suite 1
Coral Springs, FL 33063
(305) 753-8591
(6)

BARBARA MOORE
Moore Entertainment Group
11 Possum Trail
Upper Saddle River, NJ 07458
(201) 327-3698
(1,2,3,6)

REGINALD A. MURRAY
RAM Entertainment
400 Cozine Ave., Suite 7C
Brooklyn, NY 11207
(718) 257-8014
(1,6)

DOREEN NAKAMURA
Dee-Mura Enterprises, Inc.
269 W. Shore Dr.
Massapequa, NY 11758
(516) 795-1616

ROSELLA OLSON
Rosella Olson Management
319 W. 105th St., Suite 1F
New York, NY 10025
(212) 864-0336
(1,5,6)

CATHY PARKER
Cathy Parker Management, Inc.
P.O. Box 716
Voorhees Township, NJ 08043
(609) 354-2020
(1,3)

MARVIN PEARL
Pearl Management
1650 Broadway, Suite 508
New York, NY 10019
(212) 399-7224
(1)

GERARD W. PURCELL
Gerard W. Purcell Associates
964 2nd Ave., New York, NY 10022
(212) 421-2670
Faith Ball
(2,5,6: TV, records)

VIC RAMOS
Vic Ramos Management
49 W. 9th St., 5B
New York, NY 10011
(212) 473-2610
(1)

HOWARD RAPP
Charles Rapp Enterprises, Inc.
1650 Broadway, Suite 609
New York, NY 10019
(212) 247-6646
(1,2,4,5)

JOSEPH RAPP
Joseph Rapp Enterprises
1650 Broadway, Suite 705
New York, NY 10019
(212) 265-3366
(5,6: TV, records)

KAREN RHODES-CALISTI
Class Act Entertainment
102 South St.
Jeannette, PA 15644
(412) 523-3590
(5)

EDIE ROBB
Edie Robb Talent Works, Inc.
301 W. 53rd St., Suite 4K
New York, NY 10019
(212) 245-3250
(1,3)

LINDA ROHE
Coastal Entertainment Productions
32-31 35th St.
Astoria, NY 11106
(718) 728-8581
(5)

JACK ROLLINS
130 W. 57th St.
New York, NY 10019
(212) 582-1940
(2,5)

PHILIP ROSE
137 W. 78th St., Apt. 1 Garden
New York, NY 10024
(212) 877-5538
(1,2)

JOAN M. ROSENBERG
Talent & Comedy Management
145B Allen Blvd.
Farmingdale, NY 11735
(516) 249-9896

RICHARD S. ROSENWALD
300 W. 55th St., Suite 14Y
New York, NY 10019
(212) 245-4515
(1)

PETER N. SALERNO
317 Temple Place
Westfield, NJ 07090
(908) 232-8766
(1)

SUZANNE SCHACHTER
Suzelle Enterprises
116 Central Park So., Suite 12B
New York, NY 10019
(212) 397-2047
(1,3)

EDIE F. SCHUR
Edie F. Schur, Inc.
176 E. 71st St.
New York, NY 10021
(212) 734-5100
(1,3,4,7)

CHERYL A. SCOTT
Cheryl Scott Management
25 Breezy Hill Rd.
Collinsville, CT 06022
(203) 693-0891
(6: rock)

JACK SEGAL
Jack Segal Enterprises
10 Park Ave.
West Orange, NJ 07052
(201) 731-8801
(5)

SID SEIDENBERG
1414 Avenue of the Americas
New York, NY 10019
(212) 421-2021
(6)

ARTHUR SHAFMAN
Shafman International Ltd.
P.O. Box 352
Pawling, NY 12564
(914) 855-3005
(1,5,6)

MARTIN SIEGEL
Scott Eden Creative Management
P.O. Box 186
Millwood, NY 10546
(914) 941-8684
(1,3)

JOAN SILVERMAN
Multi-Ethnic
415 E. 52nd St., Suite 6DA
New York, NY 10022
(212) 832-2668
(1,2)

HELENE SOKOL
Cuzzins Management
250 W. 57th St., Suite 2601
New York, NY 10107
(212) 765-6559
Victoria Frankmano
(1,3)

MR. RADAMES SOTO
Blue Pearl, Inc.
1600 Broadway, Suite 306
New York, NY 10019
(212) 974-1735
(1,2,5)

CHRISTOPHER SPIERER
Christopher Group Productions
1775 Broadway, 7th fl.
New York, NY 10019
(718) 601-1951
(1,6)

BURT STRATFORD
221 W. 57th St.
New York, NY 10019
(212) 757-2211
(1,2,5)

JEFF SUSSMAN
50 W. 34th St., Suite #15
New York, NY 10001
(212) 268-2940
(2,5)

JACQUELINE TELLALIAN
Vesta Talent Services
500 2nd Ave., 16C
New York, NY 10016
(212) 685-7151
(1)

LARRY TUNNY
Larry Tunny Enterprises, Inc.
30 Lincoln Plaza
New York, NY 10023
(212) 582-2023
(6)

CHARLENE TURNEY
484 W. 43rd St., Suite 11S
New York, NY 10036
(212) 564-3536
(1,2)

FRANK E. UNDERWOOD, SR.
1547 Westover Ave.
Petersburg, VA 23805
(804) 861-5691
(1)

ALEX VALDEZ
793 Lexington Ave.
New York, NY 10021
(212) 688-6054
(1)

SALVATORE VASI
114 Lexington Ave.
New York, NY 10016
(212) 532-6843
(1,5,6)

MS. AYESHA Z. WILSON
Omizelli Management
P.O. Box 1802
New York, NY 10025
(212) 222-3806
(1,5)

FRANK M. ZAZZA
Zazza Talent Management
Astoria Studios
34-12 36th St.
Astoria, NY 11106
(718) 729-9288
(1,2)

MARILYN ZITNER
Global Sports & Entertainment
300 Park Ave. So., 3rd fl.
New York, NY 10010
(212) 979-9797
(1,2,3,6)

WEST COAST CHAPTER

*Stanley Evans, Executive Director, heads
the West Coast Chapter of the NCOPM,
10231 Riverside Dr., Suite 303, Toluca
Lake, CA 91602; phone (818) 762-NCPM.*

TOMMY AMATO
Tap, Inc.
825 Twin Pines Rd.
Reno, NV 89509
(702) 826-5899
(5,6)

CANDEE BARSHOP
P.O. Box 606
Palm Desert, CA 92261-0606
(619) 341-1565
(1)

TINO BARZIE
Tin-Bar Amusement Corp.
10590 Wilshire Blvd.
Los Angeles, CA 90024
(310) 474-4763
(2,5,6,7)

SAM BAUMAYS
8016 Willow Glen Rd.
Los Angeles, CA 90046
(310) 202-3473
(1,5)

PAUL CANTOR
Paul Cantor Enterprises, Ltd.
33042 Ocean Ridge
Dana Point, CA 92629
(714) 240-4400
(6)

BILL CIVITELLA
Persona Management
1070 Terrace Hill Circle
Westlake Village, CA 91362
(818) 865-8188
(1,3)

ANTHONY CRESSWELL
2508 Strongs Dr.
Venice, CA 90291
(310) 306-2001
(1,5)

HILLARD ELKINS
Hillard Elkins Entertainment Corp.
8306 Wilshire Blvd., Suite 438
Beverly Hills, CA 90211
(310) 285-0700
(1,2,4,5,6)

STANLEY EVANS
Evans Management
10231 Riverside Dr., Suite 303
Toluca Lake, CA 91602
(818) 766-0114
(1,2,4,5,6)

THEODORE GEKIS
Braverman, Gekis, Bloom Management
6399 Wilshire Blvd., Suite 901
Los Angeles, CA 90048
(213) 782-4900
Michael Braverman, Barry Bloom
(1,2,3,4)

DAVID GLADSTONE
Off 'n' Running Management
300 Manhattan Beach Blvd., Suite 4
Manhattan Beach, CA 90266
(310) 798-2501
(1,5)

MICHAEL GLYNN
Mixed Media Entertainment Corp.
10153½ Riverside Dr.
Toluca Lake, CA 91602
(800) 647-3404
(1,5,7)

HOWARD HINDERSTEIN
Howard Hinderstein Productions
c/o Mark Goodson
5750 Wilshire Blvd., Suite 475
Los Angeles, CA 90036
(213) 965-6500
(1,2,5)

ANDREA JONES
5102 Tujunga Ave., Apt. 16
North Hollywood, CA 91601
(818) 762-2008
(1,3)

JERRY KIRSCH
Terrific Talent Associates, Inc.
The Grand
4735 Sepulveda Blvd., Suite 420
Sherman Oaks, CA 91403
(818) 784-6863
(1,3,6)

ABBE LEVITON
Leviton Management
624 Sunset Ave., Apt. 3
Venice, CA 90291
(310) 452-7400
(1,5)

RICHARD LINKE
Richard O. Linke Personal Management
177 Longview Heights
Athens, OH 45701
(614) 593-8700
(1,5)

SANDRA LORD
Creative Management Network, Inc.
P.O. Box 3225
Hollywood, CA 90078
(213) 469-5985
(1,2,3,5,6)

JEFFREY C. LOSEFF
4521 Colfax Ave., Suite 205
North Hollywood, CA 91602
(818) 505-9468

KATHLEEN MANN
22808 Crespi St.
Woodland Hills, CA 91364
(818) 224-2232
(1)

RICHARD MOON
Mooner Entertainment Management
P.O. Box 657
Hollywood, CA 90078
(213) 960-9422
(1)

PATRICK REAVES
Reavestock Management
550 S. Barrington Ave., Suite 1214
Los Angeles, CA 90049
(310) 476-6641
(1,2)

EARL SHANK
520 N. Kings Rd.
West Hollywood, CA 90048
(213) 651-5241
(1,5)

BARBARA J. SILVER
8089 Pinnacle Peak
Las Vegas, NV 89113
(800) 343-0669
(1)

MS. FONDA ST. PAUL
Fonda St. Paul Management
3811 Multiview Dr.
Los Angeles, CA 90068
(213) 876-6161
(1)

M. SCOTT STANDER
Stander Management
13834 Magnolia Blvd.
Sherman Oaks, CA 91423
(818) 990-0292
(1,2,5)

MIMI WEBER
Mimi Weber Management, Ltd.
9738 Arby Dr.
Beverly Hills, CA 90210
(310) 278-8440
(1,7: productions)

National and Regional Union Offices

The following is a list of nationwide offices for Actors' Equity Association, Screen Actors Guild, American Federation of Television and Radio Artists, American Guild of Musical Artists, and American Guild of Variety Artists. If you are making an inquiry about membership, address your letter "To the Attention of Membership Department," in care of (c/o) the office for your region.

ACTORS' EQUITY ASSOCIATION

NATIONAL/EASTERN OFFICE
165 W. 46th St.
New York, NY 10036
(212) 869-8530

CENTRAL OFFICE
203 N. Wabash Ave.
Chicago, IL 60601
(312) 641-0393

DISNEY OFFICE
10369 Orangewood Blvd.
Orlando, FL 32821
(407) 345-8600

SAN FRANCISCO OFFICE
235 Pine St., 11th fl.
San Francisco, CA 94104
(415) 391-3838

WESTERN OFFICE
6430 Sunset Blvd.
Los Angeles, CA 90028
(213) 462-2334

SCREEN ACTORS GUILD

NATIONAL OFFICE
5757 Wilshire Blvd.
Los Angeles, CA 90036-3600
(213) 954-1600

ATLANTA
455 E. Paces Ferry Rd., #334
Atlanta, GA 30305
(404) 239-0131

BOSTON
11 Beacon St., #515
Boston, MA 02108
(617) 742-2688

CHICAGO
75 E. Wacker Dr., 14th fl.
Chicago, IL 60601
(312) 372-8081

CLEVELAND
1030 Euclid Ave., #429
Cleveland, OH 44115
(216) 579-9305

DALLAS
6060 N. Central Expressway
Suite 302, LB 604
Dallas, TX 75206
(214) 363-8300

DENVER
(Regional—covers Colorado, Nevada, New Mexico, and Utah)
950 S. Cherry St., #502
Denver, CO 80222
(303) 757-6226

DETROIT
28690 Southfield Rd.
Lathrup Village, MI 48076
(313) 559-9540

HONOLULU
949 Kapiolani Blvd., #105
Honolulu, HI 96814
(808) 538-6122

HOUSTON
2650 Fountainview, #326
Houston, TX 77057
(713) 972-1806

MIAMI
(Regional—covers Alabama, Arkansas, Florida, Louisiana, Mississippi, North Carolina, South Carolina, West Virginia, Virginia, Puerto Rico, and the Caribbean)
7300 N. Kendall Dr., Suite 620
Miami, FL 33156
(305) 670-7677

MINNEAPOLIS/ST. PAUL
708 N. 1st St., #343A
Minneapolis, MN 55401
(612) 371-9120

NASHVILLE
1108 17th Ave. South
Nashville, TN 37212
(615) 327-2958

NEW YORK
1515 Broadway, 44th fl.
New York, NY 10036
(212) 944-1030

PHILADELPHIA
230 S. Broad St., 10th fl.
Philadelphia, PA 19102
(215) 545-3150

PHOENIX
1616 E. Indian School Rd., #330
Phoenix, AZ 85016
(602) 265-2712

ST. LOUIS
906 Olive St., #1006
St. Louis, MO 63101
(314) 231-8410

SAN DIEGO
7827 Convoy Court #400
San Diego, CA 92111
(619) 278-7695

SAN FRANCISCO
235 Pine St., 11th fl.
San Francisco, CA 94104
(415) 391-7510

SEATTLE
608 Valley St., #200
Seattle, WA 98109
(206) 282-2506

WASHINGTON, D.C.
The Highland House
5480 Wisconsin Ave., #201
Chevy Chase, MD 20815
(301) 657-2560

AMERICAN FEDERATION OF TELEVISION AND RADIO ARTISTS

NATIONAL OFFICE
260 Madison Ave.
New York, NY 10016
(212) 532-0800

ATLANTA
455 E. Paces Ferry Rd., #334
Atlanta, GA 30305
(404) 239-0131
(800) 544-4799

BOSTON
11 Beacon St., #512
Boston, MA 02108
(617) 742-2688

CINCINNATI
(Regional—covers Columbus, Dayton,
Indianapolis, Louisville, West Virginia)
128 E. 6th St., #802
Cincinnati, OH 45202
(513) 579-8668

CHICAGO
75 E. Wacker Drive, 14th fl.
Chicago, IL 60601
(312) 372-8081

CLEVELAND
1030 Euclid Ave., #429
Cleveland, OH 44115-1504
(216) 781-2255

DALLAS—FORT WORTH
6060 N. Central Expressway, #302
L.B. 604
Dallas, TX 75206
(214) 363-8300

DENVER
950 S. Cherry St., #502
Denver, CO 80222
(303) 757-6226

DETROIT
28690 Southfield Rd.
Lathrup Village, MI 48076
(313) 559-9540

FRESNO
P.O. Box 11961
Fresno, CA 93776
(209) 222-7065

HONOLULU
949 Kapiolani Blvd., #105
Honolulu, HI 96814
(808) 538-6122

HOUSTON
2650 Fountainview, #325
Houston, TX 77057
(713) 972-1806

KANSAS CITY
4000 Baltimore, 2nd fl.
P.O. Box 32167
Kansas City, MO 64111
(816) 753-4557

LOS ANGELES
6922 Hollywood Blvd., 8th fl.
Los Angeles, CA 90028-6128
(213) 461-8111

MIAMI
20401 N.W. Second Ave., #102
Miami, FL 33169
(305) 652-4824

NASHVILLE
P.O. Box 121087
1108 17th Ave. S.
Nashville, TN 37212
(615) 327-2944

NEW ORLEANS
247 S. Canal St., #108
New Orleans, LA 70119
(504) 822-6568

NEW YORK
260 Madison Ave., 7th fl.
New York, NY 10016
(212) 532-0800

OMAHA
3000 Farnam, #3 East
Omaha, NE 68131
(402) 346-8384

ORLANDO
Major Building
5728 Major Blvd., #264
Orlando, FL 32819
(407) 354-2230
(800) 330-AFTRA

PHILADELPHIA
230 S. Broad St., 10th fl.
Philadelphia, PA 19102
(215) 732-0507

PHOENIX
1616 E. Indian School Rd., #330
Phoenix, AZ 85016
(602) 265-2712

PITTSBURGH
625 Stanwix St., Penthouse
Pittsburgh, PA 15222
(412) 281-6767

PORTLAND
516 S.E. Morrison, #M3
Portland, OR 97214
(503) 238-6914

ROCHESTER
1600 Crossroads Office Building
Rochester, NY 14614
(716) 232-3730

SACRAMENTO–STOCKTON
836 Garnet St.
West Sacramento, CA 95691
(916) 372-1966

SAN DIEGO
7827 Convoy Ct., #400
San Diego, CA 92111
(619) 278-7695

SAN FRANCISCO
235 Pine St., 11th fl.
San Franciso, CA 94104
(415) 391-7510

ST. LOUIS
906 Olive St., #1006
St. Louis, MO 63101
(314) 231-8410

SCHENECTADY
170 Ray Ave.
Schenectady, NY 12304
(518) 381-4836

SEATTLE
P.O. Box 9688
601 Valley St., #200
Seattle, WA 98109
(206) 282-2506

STAMFORD
100 Prospect St.
Stamford, CT 06901
(203) 327-1400

MINNEAPOLIS (TWIN CITIES REGION)
Itasca Bldg., Suite 343A
708 N. First St.
Minneapolis, MN 55401
(612) 371-9120

WASHINGTON, D.C.–BALTIMORE
4340 East West Hwy., Suite 204
Bethesda, MD 20814
(301) 657-2560

AMERICAN GUILD OF MUSICAL ARTISTS

NATIONAL OFFICE
1727 Broadway
New York, NY 10019-5284
(212) 266-3687

AMERICAN GUILD OF VARIETY ARTISTS

NEW YORK OFFICE
184 Fifth Ave., 6th fl.
New York, NY 10010
(212) 675-1003

CALIFORNIA OFFICE
4741 Laurel Canyon Blvd.
North Hollywood, CA 91607
(818) 508-9984

League of Resident Theatres

The following theatres operate under Equity's LORT (League of Resident Theatres) contract. They are listed alphabetically according to state, then by city within each state, and then by theatre within each city. The letter that follows the name of each theatre (A, B, B+, C, D, or Experimental) indicates the category in which that theatre operates. These categories are based on the certified actual maximum weekly box office gross of each theatre. The breakdown is as follows: D = $17,999.99 and below; C = $18,000–$32,999.99; B = $33,000–$54,999.99; B+ = $55,000 and above. There are no box office gross figures for A theatres.

In some instances, theatre companies have two or more theatres; therefore, each theatre is categorized, which is why you might read two or more letters next to a company's name.

These are not the only Equity regional theatres. The 50 states are filled with Equity theatres that operate under Small Professional Theatre contracts (SPT) and Letters of Agreement (LOA). An all-inclusive list of those theatres would be too extensive to include here.

ALABAMA

ALABAMA SHAKESPEARE FESTIVAL (C) (D)
1 Festival Dr.
Montgomery, AL 36117
(205) 271-5300
Kent Thompson, artistic director
Kevin K. Maifeld, managing director

ARIZONA

ARIZONA THEATRE COMPANY (C)
P.O. Box 1631
Tucson, AZ 85702
(602) 884-8210
David Ira Goldstein, artistic director
Robert Alpaugh, managing director

CALIFORNIA

BERKELEY REPERTORY THEATRE (B)
2025 Addison St.
Berkeley, CA 94704
(510) 204-8901
Sharon Ott, artistic director
Susan Medak, managing director

CALIFORNIA SHAKESPEARE FESTIVAL (D)
P.O. Box 969
Berkeley, CA 94701
(510) 548-3422
Marcia O'Dea

SOUTH COAST REPERTORY THEATRE (B) (D)
P.O. Box 2197
655 Town Center Dr.
Costa Mesa, CA 92628-2197
(714) 957-2602
David Emmes, producing artistic director
Martin Benson, artistic director

LA JOLLA PLAYHOUSE (B) (C)
P.O. Box 12039
La Jolla, CA 92039
(619) 555-1070
Michael Grief, artistic director
Terrence Dwyer, managing director

MARK TAPER FORUM (A) (B)
135 North Grand Ave.
Los Angeles, CA 90012
(213) 972-0700
Gordon Davidson, artistic director
Charles Dillingham, managing director

PASADENA PLAYHOUSE (B+)
39 South El Molino Ave.
Pasadena, CA 91101
(818) 792-8672
Lars Hansen

OLD GLOBE THEATRE (B+) (B) (C)
P.O. Box 2171
San Diego, CA 92112-2171
(619) 231-1941
Jack O'Brien, artistic director
Tom Hall, managing director

AMERICAN CONSERVATORY THEATER (A)
30 Grant Ave., 6th fl.
San Francisco, CA 94108-5800
(415) 834-3200
Carey Perloff, artistic director
Thomas W. Flynn, administrative
director

SAN JOSE REPERTORY COMPANY (C)
P.O. Box 2399
San Jose, CA 95109-2399
(408) 291-2266
Timothy Near, artistic director
Alexandra U. Boisvert, managing
director

COLORADO

DENVER CENTER THEATRE COMPANY (C) (D)
1050 13th St.
Denver, CO 80204
(303) 893-4000
Donovan Marley, artistic director
J. Christopher Wineman, executive
director

CONNECTICUT

GOODSPEED OPERA HOUSE (B) (D)
P.O. Box A
East Haddam, CT 06423
(203) 873-8664
Michael P. Price, executive director
Sue Frost, associate producer

HARTFORD STAGE COMPANY (B)
50 Church St.
Hartford, CT 06103
(203) 525-5601
Mark Lamos, artistic director
Stephen J. Albert, managing director

LONG WHARF THEATRE (B) (C)
222 Sargent Dr.
New Haven, CT 06511
(203) 787-4284
Arvin Brown, artistic director
M. Edgar Rosenblum, executive director

YALE REPERTORY THEATRE (C)
P.O. Box 208244 Yale Station
222 York St.
New Haven, CT 06520-8244
(203) 432-1515
Stan Wojewodski Jr., artistic director
Victoria Nolan, managing director

EUGENE O'NEILL MEMORIAL THEATER
CENTER (D)
National Playwrights Conference
305 Great Neck Road
Waterford, CT 06385
(203) 443-5378
Lloyd Richards, artistic director
George C. White, president

DISTRICT OF COLUMBIA

ARENA STAGE (B+) (D)
6th & Maine Ave. S.W.
Washington, DC 20024
(202) 554-9066
Douglas C. Wager, artistic director
Stephen Richard, executive director

THE SHAKESPEARE THEATRE (C) (D)
301 E. Capitol St. S.E.
Washington, DC 20003
(202) 547-3230
Michael Kahn, artistic director

FLORIDA

CALDWELL THEATRE COMPANY (C)
P.O. Box 277
Boca Raton, FL 33429-0277
(407) 241-7432
Michael Hall, artistic director

COCONUT GROVE PLAYHOUSE (B) (D)
P.O. Box 616
Miami, FL 33133
(305) 442-2662
Arnold Mittelman, Bruce Leslie

ASOLO THEATRE COMPANY (C)
Asolo Center for the Performing Arts
5555 N. Tamiami Trail
Sarasota, FL 34243
(813) 351-9010
Howard Millman, artistic director

GEORGIA

ALLIANCE THEATRE COMPANY (B) (D)
Robert W. Woodruff Arts Center
1280 Peachtree St. N.E.
Atlanta, GA 30309
(404) 733-4650
Kenneth Leon, artistic director
Edith H. Love, managing director

ILLINOIS

GOODMAN THEATRE COMPANY (B+) (D)
200 S. Columbus Dr.
Chicago, IL 60603
(312) 443-3811
Robert Falls, artistic director
Roche Schulfer, executive director

THE NORTHLIGHT THEATRE (D)
600 Davis St., 2nd fl.
Evanston, IL 60201
(708) 869-7732
Russell Vandenbroucke, artistic director
Richard Friedman, managing director

INDIANA

INDIANA REPERTORY THEATRE (C) (D)
140 W. Washington St.
Indianapolis, IN 46204-3465
(317) 635-5277
Libby Appel, artistic director

KENTUCKY

ACTORS THEATRE OF LOUISVILLE (B) (D)
316-320 W. Main St.
Louisville, KY 40202-4218
(502) 584-1265
Jon Jory, producing director
Alexander Speer, executive director

MAINE

PORTLAND STAGE COMPANY (D)
P.O. Box 1458
Portland, ME 04104
(207) 774-1043
Greg Leaming, artistic director
William Chance, managing director

MARYLAND

CENTER STAGE (B) (C)
700 North Calvert St.
Baltimore, MD 21202-3686
(410) 685-3200
Irene Lewis, artistic director
Peter W. Culman, managing director

MASSACHUSETTS

HUNTINGTON THEATRE COMPANY (B)
264 Huntington Ave.
Boston, MA 02115-4606
(617) 266-7900
Peter Altman, producing director
Michael Maso, managing director

AMERICAN REPERTORY THEATRE (B)
Loeb Drama Center
64 Brattle St.
Cambridge, MA 02138
(617) 495-2668
Robert Brustein, artistic director
Robert J. Orchard, managing director

MERRIMACK REPERTORY THEATRE (D)
P.O. Box 228
Lowell, MA 01853
(508) 454-6324
David G. Kent, producing artistic
director
Chuck Still, managing director

STAGEWEST (C)
1 Columbus Center
Springfield, MA 01103
(413) 781-4470
Albert Ihde, artistic director
Kate Maguire, managing director

BERKSHIRE THEATRE FESTIVAL (C)
P.O. Box 797
Stockbridge, MA 01262
(413) 298-5536
Arthur Storch, artistic director
Cynthia Wassell, managing director

MICHIGAN

MEADOW BROOK THEATRE (B)
Oakland University
Rochester, MI 48309-4401
(313) 370-3310
Gregg Bloomfield, managing director

MINNESOTA

THE GUTHRIE THEATER (A) (D)
725 Vineland Place
Minneapolis, MN 55403
(612) 347-1100
Joe Dowling, artistic director
Edward A. Martenson, executive
director

MISSOURI

MISSOURI REPERTORY THEATRE (B)
4949 Cherry St.
Kansas City, MO 64110
(816) 235-2727
George Keathley, artistic director
James D. Costin, executive director

THE REPERTORY THEATRE OF ST. LOUIS (C)
(D)
P.O. Box 191730
130 Edgar Rd.
St. Louis, MO 63119
(314) 968-7340
Steven Woolf, artistic director
Mark D. Bernstein, managing director

NEW JERSEY

CROSSROADS THEATRE COMPANY (D)
7 Livingston Ave.
New Brunswick, NJ 08901
(908) 249-5581
Ricardo Khan, artistic director

GEORGE ST. PLAYHOUSE (C)
9 Livingston Ave.
New Brunswick, NJ 08901
(908) 846-2895
Gregory S. Hurst, producing artistic
director
Diane Claussen, managing director

MCCARTER THEATRE CENTER FOR THE
PERFORMING ARTS (B+) (D)
91 University Place
Princeton, NJ 08540
(609) 683-9100
Emily Mann, artistic director
Jeffrey Woodward, managing director

NEW YORK

CAPITAL REPERTORY COMPANY (D)
P.O. Box 399
Albany, NY 12201-0399
(518) 462-4531
Maggie Mancinelli-Cahill, artistic
director

STUDIO ARENA THEATRE (B)
710 Main St.
Buffalo, NY 14202-1990
(716) 856-8025
Gavin Cameron-Webb, artistic director
Raymond Bonnard, producing director

THE ACTING COMPANY (C) (D)
P.O. Box 898, Times Square Station
New York, NY 10108
(212) 564-3510
Margot Harley, producing director

CIRCLE IN THE SQUARE (A) (EXP.)
1633 Broadway
New York, NY 10019
(212) 307-2700
Theodore Mann, Josephine Abady, co-
artistic directors

LINCOLN CENTER THEATER (A) (C)
150 W. 65th St.
New York, NY 10023
(212) 362-7600
André Bishop, artistic director
Bernard Gersten, executive producer

NATIONAL ACTORS THEATRE (A)
c/o Niko Associates
234 W. 44th St., Suite 1003
New York, NY 10036
(212) 382-3410
Tony Randall, artistic director
Manny Kladitis, executive producer

NEW YORK SHAKESPEARE FESTIVAL (B)
Joseph Papp Public Theater
425 Lafayette St.
New York, NY 10003
(212) 598-7100
George C. Wolfe, producer

ROUNDABOUT THEATRE COMPANY (B)
1530 Broadway
New York, NY 10036
(212) 719-9393
Todd Haimes, artistic director

GEVA THEATRE (B)
75 Woodbury Blvd.
Rochester, NY 14607
(716) 232-1366
Timothy J. Shields, managing director

SYRACUSE STAGE (C)
820 East Genesee St.
Syracuse, NY 13210-1508
(315) 443-4008
Tazewell Thompson, artistic director
James A. Clark, producing director

NORTH CAROLINA

PLAYMAKERS REPERTORY COMPANY (D)
CB #3235 Graham Memorial Bldg.
052A
Chapel Hill, NC 27599-3235
(919) 962-1122
Milly S. Barranger, producing director
David Hammond, associate producing
director

NORTH CAROLINA SHAKESPEARE FESTIVAL (D)
P.O. Box 6066
High Point, NC 27262
(919) 841-2273
Lou Rackoff, Thomas Gaffney

OHIO

CINCINNATI PLAYHOUSE IN THE PARK (B) (D)
P.O. Box 6537
Cincinnati, OH 45206-0537
(513) 345-2242
Edward Stern, producing artistic director
Buzz Ward, executive director

THE CLEVELAND PLAY HOUSE (C)
P.O. Box 1989
Cleveland, OH 44106-0189
(216) 795-7010
Peter Hackett, artistic director
Dean R. Gladden, managing director

GREAT LAKES THEATER FESTIVAL (B)
1501 Euclid Ave., Suite 423
Cleveland, OH 44115-2108
(216) 241-5490
Gerald Freedman, artistic director
Anne B. DesRosiers, managing director

OREGON

OREGON SHAKESPEARE FESTIVAL (B)
P.O. Box 158
Ashland, OR 97520
(503) 482-2111

PORTLAND CENTER STAGE (B)
P.O. Box 9008
Portland, OR 97207
(503) 274-6581
Elizabeth Huddle, producing artistic director
Martha Richards, administrative director

PENNSYLVANIA

PENNSYLVANIA STAGE COMPANY (D)
J.I. Rodale Theatre
837 Linden St.
Allentown, PA 18101
(610) 434-6110
Charles Richter, artistic director
Ellen Baker Baltz, managing director

THE PEOPLE'S LIGHT AND THEATRE COMPANY (D)
39 Conestoga Rd.
Malvern, PA 19355-1798
(610) 647-1900
Abigail Adams, Stephen Novelli, co-artistic directors

PHILADELPHIA FESTIVAL THEATRE FOR NEW PLAYS (D)
c/o Annenberg Center
3680 Walnut St.
Philadelphia, PA 19104
(215) 898-5828
Carol Rocamora, founding artistic director
Stephen Goff, managing director

PHILADELPHIA THEATRE COMPANY
21 S. 5th St.
The Bourse Building
Philadelphia, PA 19106
(215) 592-8333
Sara Garonzik, producing artistic director
Ada Coppock, general manager

THE WALNUT ST. THEATRE (A) (D)
825 Walnut St.
Philadelphia, PA 19107
(215) 574-3550
Bernard Havard, executive director
Ken Wesler, managing director

PITTSBURGH PUBLIC THEATER (B)
Allegheny Sq.
Pittsburgh, PA 15212-5349
(412) 323-8200
Edward Gilbert, artistic director

RHODE ISLAND

TRINITY REPERTORY COMPANY (B) (C)
201 Washington St.
Providence, RI 02903
(401) 521-1100
Oskar Eustis, artistic director
Patricia Egan, managing director

TENNESSEE

CLARENCE BROWN THEATRE COMPANY (D)
206 McClung Tower
Knoxville, TN 37996-4800
(615) 974-6011
Thomas P. Cooke, producing director
Margaret Ferguson, general manager

TENNESSEE REPERTORY THEATRE (C)
427 Chestnut St.
Nashville, TN 37203
(615) 244-4878
Mac Pirkle, artistic director
Brian J. Laczko, managing director

TEXAS

DALLAS THEATER CENTER (C)
3636 Turtle Creek Blvd.
Dallas, TX 75219-5598
(214) 526-8210
Richard Hamburger, artistic director
Robert Yesselman, managing director

ALLEY THEATRE (B) (C)
615 Texas Ave.
Houston, TX 77002
(713) 228-9341
Gregory Boyd, artistic director
Paul Tetreault, managing director

UTAH

PIONEER THEATRE COMPANY (B)
Pioneer Memorial Theatre
University of Utah
Salt Lake City, UT 84112
(801) 581-6356
Charles Morey, artistic director
Christopher Lino, managing director

VIRGINIA

BARTER THEATRE (D)
P.O. Box 867
Abingdon, VA 24210-0867
(703) 628-2281
Richard Rose, producing artistic
director

VIRGINIA STAGE COMPANY (C)
P.O. Box 3770
Norfolk, VA 23514
(804) 627-6988
Charlie Hensley, artistic director
Doug Perry, managing director

THEATREVIRGINIA (C) (D)
2800 Grove Ave.
Richmond, VA 23221
(804) 367-0840
George Black, producing artistic
director
R.L. Rowsey, associate artistic director

WASHINGTON

A CONTEMPORARY THEATRE (C)
P.O. Box 19400
Seattle, WA 98109
(206) 285-3220
Phil Schermer, producing director
Susan Trapnell Moritz, managing director

INTIMAN THEATRE COMPANY (C)
P.O. Box 19760
Seattle, WA 98109
(206) 626-0775
Warner Shook, artistic director
Laura Penn, managing director

SEATTLE REPERTORY THEATRE (B+) (D)
155 Mercer St.
Seattle, WA 98109
(206) 443-2210
Daniel Sullivan, artistic director
Benjamin Moore, managing director

WISCONSIN

MILWAUKEE REPERTORY THEATER (A) (C)
(D)
108 E. Wells St.
Milwaukee, WI 53202
(414) 224-1761
Joseph Hanreddy, artistic director
Dan Fallon, managing director

Dinner Theatres

This list of dinner theatres nationwide is arranged alphabetically by state. An asterisk (*) denotes theatres which operate under an Actors' Equity Dinner Theatre contract. The designation ADTI or NDTA indicates membership in one of two national dinner theatre organizations: the American Dinner Theatre Institute (ADTI) is almost exclusively Equity; the National Dinner Theatre Association (NDTA) is almost exclusively non-Equity.

Equity Dinner Theatre contract weekly minimum salaries are categorized by tier levels, determined by seating capacity. Tier 1 is 0–199 seats; Tier 2, 200–329 seats; Tier 3, 330–449 seats; Tier 4, 450–649 seats; and Tier 5, 650–1,200 seats.

The ADTI address is P.O. Box 7057, Akron, OH 44306, phone (216) 724-8605. The NDTA is at 525 Marriott Dr., Clarksville, IN 47130; phone (812) 288-2632.

ALASKA

ALASKA CABIN NITE DINNER THEATRE
ARA Denali Park Hotels
825 W. 8th Ave., Suite 220
Anchorage, AK 99501
(907) 279-2653
(NDTA)

ARIZONA

GASLIGHT THEATRE
7010 E. Broadway
Tucson, AZ 85710
(602) 886-9428

ARKANSAS

MURRAY'S DINNER PLAYHOUSE
6323 Asher Ave.
Little Rock, AR 72204
(501) 562-3131
(NDTA)

CALIFORNIA

CANDLELIGHT PAVILION DINNER THEATRE
555 W. Foothill Blvd.
Claremont, CA 91711
(909) 626-1254
(NDTA)

CURTAIN CALL DINNER THEATRE
690 El Camino Real
Tustin, CA 92680
(714) 838-1540

GARBEAU'S DINNER THEATRE
12401 Folsom Blvd.
Rancho Cordova, CA 95742-6413
(916) 985-6361
(NDTA)

LAWRENCE WELK VILLAGE THEATRE*
8860 Lawrence Welk Dr.
Escondido, CA 92026
(619) 749-3000
(Equity Tier 2)

ROGER ROCKA'S MUSIC HALL
1226 N. Wishon Ave.
Fresno, CA 93728
(209) 266-9493

STARS THEATRE RESTAURANT
324 Bernard
Bakersfield, CA 93305
(805) 325-6100
(NDTA)

COLORADO

BOULDER'S DINNER THEATRE
5501 Arapahoe Ave.
Boulder, CO 80303-1391
(303) 449-6000
(NDTA)

CAROUSEL DINNER THEATRE
3509 Mason St.
Fort Collins, CO 80525
(303) 225-2555
(NDTA)

COUNTRY DINNER PLAYHOUSE*
6875 S. Clinton St.
Englewood, CO 80112
(303) 799-0112
(Equity Tier 4; NDTA)

HERITAGE SQUARE MUSIC HALL
18301 W. Colfax D103
Golden, CO 80401
(303) 279-7800

DELAWARE

THREE LITTLE BAKERS COUNTRY CLUB &
DINNER THEATRE
3540 Foxcroft Dr.
Pike Creek Valley
Wilmington, DE 19808
(302) 368-1694
(NDTA)

FLORIDA

ALHAMBRA DINNER THEATRE*
12000 Beach Blvd.
Jacksonville, FL 32246
(904) 642-9307
(Equity Tier 3; NDTA; ADTI)

BROADWAY PALM DINNER THEATRE
1380 Colonial Blvd.
Fort Myers, FL 33907-1023
(NDTA)

GOLDEN APPLE DINNER THEATRE*
25 N. Pineapple Ave.
Sarasota, FL 34236
(813) 366-2646
(Equity Tier 2; ADTI)

JUPITER THEATRE*
1001 E. Indiantown Rd.
Jupiter, FL 33477
(407) 747-5261
(Equity Tier 3; NDTA; ADTI)

MARK TWO DINNER THEATRE*
3376 Edgewater Dr.
Orlando, FL 32804
(407) 843-6275
(Equity Tier 2; NDTA; ADTI)

NAPLES DINNER THEATRE
1025 Piper Blvd.
Naples, FL 33942
(813) 597-6031
(NDTA)

ROYAL PALM DINNER THEATRE*
Royal Palm Plaza
303 S.E. Mizner Blvd.
Boca Raton, FL 33432
(407) 392-3455
(Equity Tier 2; ADTI)

SHOWBOAT DINNER THEATRE*
3405 Ulmerton Rd.
St. Petersburg, FL 34622
(813) 573-3777
(Equity Tier 3; ADTI)

ILLINOIS

BARN II
Box 310, Conklin Ct.
Goodfield, IL 61742
(309) 965-2545

CANDLELIGHT DINNER PLAYHOUSE*
5620 S. Harlem Ave.
Summit, IL 60501
(708) 496-3000
(Equity Tier 3 and 4; ADTI)

CIRCA '21 DINNER PLAYHOUSE
1828 Third Ave., Box 3784
Rock Island, IL 61201
(309) 786-2667
(NDTA)

CLOCK TOWER DINNER THEATRES
P.O. Box 5285
7801 E. State St.
Rockford, IL 61125-0285
(NDTA)

DRURY LANE OAKBROOK THEATRE*
100 Drury Lane
Oakbrook Terrace, IL 60181
(708) 530-8300
(Equity Tier 5; ADTI)

DRURY LANE SOUTH*
2500 W. 95th St.
Evergreen Park, IL 60642
(708) 422-0404
(Equity Tier 4; ADTI)

FORUM DINNER THEATRE*
5620 S. Harlem Ave.
Summit, IL 60501
(708) 496-3000
(Equity Tier 3; ADTI)

MARRIOTT'S LINCOLNSHIRE THEATRE*
10 Marriott Dr.
Lincolnshire, IL 60069
(708) 634-0204
(Equity Tier 5; ADTI)

PHEASANT RUN DINNER THEATRE
P.O. Box 64, 401 E. Main St.
St. Charles, IL 60174
(708) 584-6342

SUNSHINE DINNER PLAYHOUSE
115 W. Kirby Ave.
Champaign, IL 61820
(217) 359-4503
(NDTA)

ZELLMER'S MAIN STREET DINNER THEATRE
45 N. Main St., P.O. Box 37
Farmington, IL 61531
(309) 245-2554
(NDTA)

INDIANA

BEEF & BOARDS DINNER THEATRE*
9301 N. Michigan Rd.
Indianapolis, IN 46268
(317) 872-9664
(Equity Tier 3; NDTA; ADTI)

DERBY DINNER PLAYHOUSE
525 Marriott Dr.
Clarksville, IN 47129
(812) 288-2632
(NDTA)

GOOD TIMES THEATRE
Rt. 1, Box 180B
Bryant, IN 47326
(219) 997-6822
(NDTA)

IOWA

INGERSOLL DINNER THEATRE
3711 Ingersoll Ave.
Des Moines, IA 50312
(515) 274-4686
(NDTA)

KANSAS

CROWN UPTOWN DINNER THEATRE
3207 E. Douglas
Wichita, KS 67218
(316) 681-1566
(NDTA)

MARYLAND

ACT TWO DINNER THEATRE
8014 Pulaski Hwy.
Baltimore, MD 21237
(410) 686-1126

BURN BRAE DINNER THEATRE
3811 Blackburn Lane
Burtonsville, MD 20866
(301) 384-5800

OREGON RIDGE DINNER THEATRE
13403 Beaver Dam Rd.
Cockysville, MD 21030
(410) 771-8427

TOBY'S DINNER THEATRE OF COLUMBIA
P.O. Box 1003
Columbia, MD 21044
(410) 730-8311
(NDTA)

TOWSON DINNER THEATRE
100 E. Chesapeake
Towson, MD 21286
(410) 321-6595

MASSACHUSETTS

MEDIEVAL MANOR THEATRE RESTAURANT
246 E. Berkeley St.
Boston, MA 02118
(617) 423-4900

MYSTERY CAFE DINNER THEATRE
11 Green St.
Boston, MA 02130
(617) 524-CAFE

PLAYHOUSE DINNER THEATRE
194 Main St.
Amesburg, MA 01913
(508) 388-9059
(NDTA)

MICHIGAN

CORNWELL'S DINNER THEATRE
P.O. Box 556
Marshall, MI 49068
(616) 781-7933
(NDTA)

PRITCHARD PRODUCTIONS
P.O. Box 693
Marshall, MI 49068
(616) 781-7933
(NDTA)

MINNESOTA

CHANHASSEN DINNER THEATRE*
501 W. 78th St.
Chanhassen, MN 55317
(612) 934-1500
(Equity Tier 1, 2 and 4; ADTI)

MISSOURI

AMERICAN HEARTLAND THEATRE*
2450 Grand Ave., Suite 314
Kansas City, MO 64108
(816) 842-9900
(Equity Tier 3)

NEW THEATRE RESTAURANT*
9229 Foster
Kansas City, MO 66212
(913) 649-0103
(ADTI)

NEBRASKA

FIREHOUSE DINNER THEATRE*
514 S. 11th St.
Omaha, NE 68102
(402) 346-6009

NEW YORK

CURTAIN CALL DINNER THEATRE
189 Wolf Rd.
Albany, NY 12205
(518) 877-7529
(NDTA)

LAKE GEORGE DINNER THEATRE*
P.O. Box 266
Lake George, NY 12845
(518) 668-2198
(Equity Tier 1)

WESTCHESTER BROADWAY THEATRE*
1 Broadway Plaza
Elmsford, NY 10523
(914) 592-2268
(Equity Tier 3; ADTI)

NORTH CAROLINA

BARN DINNER THEATRE
120 Stagecoach Trail
Greensboro, NC 27409
(910) 292-2211

OHIO

CAROUSEL DINNER THEATRE*
1275 E. Waterloo Rd.
Akron, OH 44306
(216) 724-9855
(Equity Tier 5; ADTI; NDTA)

MIAMI VALLEY DINNER THEATRE
765 W. Central Ave.
Springboro, OH 45066
(513) 746-3114
(NDTA)

PLAYHOUSE SQUARE CENTER*
1501 Euclid Ave., Suite 810
Cleveland, OH 44115-2197
(216) 771-4444
(Equity Tier 3)

SPIRIT DINNER PLAYHOUSE
657 Sunsbury Dr. East
Worthington, OH 43085
(614) 846-2361
(NDTA)

OREGON

SYLVIA'S DINNER THEATRE
5115 Northeast Sandy Blvd.
Portland, OR 97213
(503) 288-6828

PENNSYLVANIA

CONLEY INN SHOWROOM OF IRWIN
Route 30, Conley La.
Irwin, PA 15642
(800) 683-1255

THE DAVID GROUP
3083 Altoona Rd.
Bethlehem, PA 18017
(610) 868-0056
(NDTA)

DUTCH APPLE DINNER THEATRE
510 Centerville Rd.
Lancaster, PA 17601
(717) 898-1900
(NDTA)

PEDDLER'S VILLAGE MURDER MYSTERIES
Cock 'n' Bull Restaurant
Peddler's Village, Box 218
Lahaska, PA 18931
(215) 794-4000

RIVERFRONT DINNER THEATRE
Delaware Ave. at Poplar St.
Philadelphia, PA 19123
(215) 925-7000

RIVERSIDE DINNER THEATRE
One Fountain Ave.
Cambridge Springs, PA 16403
(814) 398-4645
(NDTA)

ROCKWELL GRAND CANDLELIGHT THEATRE
32 S. Turbot Ave.
Milton, PA 17847
(717) 742-2511
(NDTA)

SHAWNEE PLAYHOUSE
P.O. Box 159
Shawnee-on-Delaware, PA 18356
(717) 421-5093

TENNESSEE

CHAFFIN'S BARN DINNER THEATRE
8204 Highway 100
Nashville, TN 37221
(615) 646-9977
(ADTI assoc. member; NDTA)

VIRGINIA

BARKSDALE DINNER THEATRE
P.O. Box 7
Hanover, VA 23069
(804) 559-4804

SWIFT CREEK MILL PLAYHOUSE
P.O. Box 41
Colonial Heights, VA 23834
(804) 748-5203

WEST END DINNER THEATRE
4615 Duke St.
Alexandria, VA 22304
(703) 370-2500
(ADTI assoc. member; NDTA)

WASHINGTON

AUBURN AVENUE DINNER THEATRE &
OPERA HOUSE
10 Auburn Ave. N.
Auburn, WA 98002
(206) 833-0620
(NDTA)

WISCONSIN

FANNY HILL INN & DINNER THEATRE
3919 Crescent Ave.
Eau Claire, WI 54703
(715) 836-8184

FIRESIDE RESTAURANT & PLAYHOUSE
1131 Janesville Ave.
P.O. Box 7
Fort Atkinson, WI 53538
(414) 563-9505
(NDTA)

MOLLY'S SHOWPLACE
1541 Wisconsin Dells Parkway
P.O. Box 473
Lake Delton, WI 53940
(608) 254-6222
(NDTA)

NORTHERN LIGHTS PLAYHOUSE
P.O. Box 256
Hazelhurst, WI 54531
(715) 356-7173
(NDTA)

Off- and Off-Off-Broadway Theatre Companies

The following is a list of mailing addresses for Off- and Off-Off-Broadway theatre companies in New York City. (For some, the performance space is at the same address.) Included are both Equity and non-Equity groups. Some of the Equity companies produce under Actors' Equity Showcase or Tier Codes, while others may produce under an Equity contract. Although this list is extensive, it is not all-inclusive; as some theatres close, new ventures start up.

AAI PRODUCTIONS
JAF P.O. Box 7370
New York, NY 10116-4630
(212) 802-5373
Melanie Sutherland, artistic director

THE ABOUTFACE THEATRE COMPANY
Nat Horne Theatre
442 W. 42nd St.
New York, NY 10036
(212) 268-9638
Sean Burke, artistic director
Allison Jones, managing director

THE ACTORS COLLECTIVE
145 E. 27th St., Suite 4K
New York, NY 10016
Warren Manzi, artistic director
Catherine Russell, managing director

ACTORS' COMPANY THEATRE
43 E. 10th St., Suite 6K
New York, NY 10003
(212) 645-8228
Maia Danziger, Scott Alan Evans,
Cynthia Harris, co-artistic directors

THE ACTORS THEATRE WORKSHOP
145 W. 28th St., 3rd fl.
New York, NY 10001
(212) 947-1386
Thurman E. Scott, artistic director and
founder
Janet P. Scott, general manager

ADOBE THEATRE COMPANY
21 E. 22nd St., 2F
New York, NY 10010
(212) 477-3661
Jeremy Dobrish, artistic director
Christopher Roberts, producing
director

AFRICA ARTS THEATRE COMPANY
660 Riverside Dr., #2J
New York, NY 10031
(212) 926-9203
Adusah Boakye, artistic director

AFRIKAN WOMEN'S REPERTORY
600 E. 137th St., 13G
Bronx, NY 10454

ALCHEMY COURTHOUSE THEATER
COMPANY
P.O. Box 2561, Times Square Station
New York, NY 10108
(212) 841-0894
Stephen O'Rourke, managing director
Louise Freistadt, managing director

ALICE'S FOURTH FLOOR
432 W. 42nd St.
New York, NY 10036
(212) 967-0400
Susann Brinkley, artistic director

AMAS MUSICAL THEATRE INC. & ROSETTA
LENOIRE MUSICAL THEATRE ACADEMY
450 W. 42nd St., Suite 2J
New York, NY 10036
(212) 563-2565
Rosetta LeNoire, artistic director and
founder
Donna Trinkoff, producing director

AMERICAN ENSEMBLE COMPANY
6 Burns St., #417
Forest Hills, NY 11375
(718) 544-8074
Robert Dominguez, managing director

AMERICAN GLOBE THEATRE
145 W. 46 St., 3rd fl.
New York, NY 10036
(212) 869-9809
John Basil, artistic director
Jacqueline Lowry, producing director
Elizabeth Keefe, general manager

AMERICAN INDIAN COMMUNITY HOUSE
THEATRE SPACE
404 Lafayette St., 2nd fl.
New York, NY 10003
(212) 598-0100
Jim Cyrus, performing arts director

AMERICAN JEWISH THEATRE
307 W. 26th St.
New York, NY 10001
(212) 633-9797
Stanley Brechner, artistic director

AMERICAN PLACE THEATRE
111 W. 46th St.
New York, NY 10036
(212) 840-2960
Wynn Handman, artistic director
Susannah Halston, executive director

AMERICAN RENAISSANCE THEATRE OF
DRAMATIC ARTS
10 W. 15th St., #325
New York, NY 10011
(212) 924-6862
Rich Stone, artistic director
Darren Farrington, business manager

AMERICAN THEATRE OF ACTORS
314 W. 54th St.
New York, NY 10019
(212) 581-3044
James Jennings, artistic director.

ANCHOR THEATRE COMPANY
354 E. 66th St., #6F
New York, NY 10021
(212) 249-2230
John McDonough, artistic director

ART & WORK ENSEMBLE
P.O. Box 20332, Greeley Square Station
New York, NY 10001-0007
(212) 227-5814
Derek Todd, artistic director
Alison Lani Broda, managing director

ARTISTS IN SEARCH OF..., INC.
206 W. 99th St., #2C
New York, NY 10025
(212) 663-6459
Kim Johnson, artistic director
Pamela Sabrin, managing director

ATLANTIC THEATER COMPANY
336 W. 20th St.
New York, NY 10011
(212) 645-8015
Neil Pepe, artistic director
Joshua Lehrer, managing director

AZZIZZ THEATRE
58 Fourth Place, #1
Brooklyn, NY 11231
(718) 722-7491
Robert James Bellamy, artistic director

THE BARROW GROUP
P.O. Box 5112, Times Square Station
New York, NY 10185
(212) 522-1421
Seth Barrish, artistic director

THE BASIC THEATRE
Box 434, Radio City Station
New York, NY 10101
(212) 397-1511
Fax: (212) 243-1402
Jared Hammond, artistic director
Pamela Mobilia, executive director

BELMONT ITALIAN AMERICAN PLAYHOUSE
2385 Arthur Ave.
Bronx, NY 10458
(718) 364-4700
Dante Alberti, artistic director
Marco Greco, executive director

BLACK SPECTRUM THEATRE COMPANY, INC.
119th Ave. and Merrick Blvd.
Jamaica, NY 11434
(718) 723-1800
Carl Clay, executive producer

BLUE HERON THEATRE
645 West End Ave., #7B
New York, NY 10025
(212) 787-0422
Ardelle Striker, producing director

BOND STREET THEATRE COALITION
2 Bond St.
New York, NY 10012
(212) 254-4614
Joanna M. Sherman, artistic director
Michael McGuigan, managing director

BROADWAY TOMORROW
191 Claremont Ave., Suite 53
New York, NY 10027
(212) 864-4736
Elyse Curtis, artistic director

THE BULL FAMILY ORCHESTRA,
an Inter-Arts Theater Company
One Union Square West, Room 712
New York, NY 10003
(212) 647-9229
Katie Bull, artistic director
Leslie Kincaid, associate artistic director

CHAIN LIGHTNING THEATRE
51 Spring St., Suite 12
New York, NY 10012
(212) 219-2085
Claire Higgins, producer
Todd Pieper, artistic director
Kricker James, managing director

CHICAGO CITY LIMITS
1105 First Ave.
New York, NY 10021
(212) 888-5233
Paul Zuckerman, artistic director
Ges Selmont, producer

CIRCLE REPERTORY COMPANY
632 Broadway
New York, NY 10012-2614
(212) 505-6010
Austin Pendleton, artistic director

CLASSIC STAGE COMPANY
136 E. 13th St.
New York, NY 10003
(212) 477-5808
David Esbjornson, artistic director
Patricia Taylor, managing director

CONEY ISLAND, USA
Boardwalk & W. 12th St.
Coney Island, NY 11224
(718) 372-5159
Dick D. Zigun, artistic director

CUCARACHA THEATRE
500 Greenwich St., Suite 302
New York, NY 10013
(212) 966-8596
Richard Caliban, artistic director
Mary McBride, managing director

DANCE THEATER WORKSHOP
219 W. 19th St.
New York, NY 10011
(212) 691-6500
David White, executive
director/producer

D'ARC
721 Broadway, 9th fl.
New York, NY 10003
(212) 998-1700
Campbell Dalglish, director

DARK HORSE THEATER GROUP
230 West End Ave., #2A
New York, NY 10023
(212) 721-9456
Cindy Sandmann, artistic director

DICAPO OPERA THEATRE
220 E. 54 St., #11J
New York, NY 10022
(212) 288-9438
Diane Martindale, artistic director
Michael Capasso, general director

THE DIRECTORS COMPANY
Theatre 603
311 W. 43rd St. #206
New York, NY 10036
(212) 246-5877
Michael Parva, Victoria Chesshire,
artistic directors

DUO THEATRE
Box 1200, Cooper Station
New York, NY 10276
(212) 598-4320
Michaelangelo Alasa, executive/artistic
director

ECONOMY TIRES THEATER
Bessie Schonberg Theater
219 W. 19th St.
New York, NY 10011
(212) 691-6500
David R. White, executive
director/producer

EDWINSCOTT PRODUCTIONS
839 West End Ave., Apt. 1C
New York, NY 10025
(212) 749-9598
Scott Miller, Ralph Mitchell, artistic
directors

EMERGING ARTISTS THEATRE
426 W. 22nd St., #3
New York, NY 10011
(212) 627-5792
Paul Adams, artistic director
Donna Moreau-Cupp, producing director

EN GARDE ARTS
225 Rector Pl., Suite 3A
New York, NY 10280
(212) 941-9793
Anne Hamburger, executive producer
Carol Bixler, managing
director/associate producer

ENCOMPASS MUSIC THEATRE
484 W. 43rd St., Suite 20H
New York, NY 10036
(212) 594-7880
Nancy Rhodes, artistic director

ENSEMBLE STUDIO THEATRE
549 W. 52nd St.
New York, NY 10019
(212) 247-4982
Curt Dempster, artistic director
Jacqueline Anne Siegel, managing
director

ESSENTIAL STAGES
112 W. 72 St., 12A
New York, NY 10023
(212) 721-5409
Ann Harvey, artistic director
Kay Rothman, producing director

FALSTAFF PRESENTS
2790 Broadway, Suite 1B
New York, NY 10025
(212) 866-7542
Michael Winter, producer
Rachel Colbert, managing director

FREESTYLE REPERTORY THEATRE
120 W. 86th St., Suite 1A
New York, NY 10024
(212) 642-8202
Laura Livingston, artistic director
Michael Durkin, executive director

THE GALLERY PLAYERS OF PARK SLOPE
199 14th St.
Brooklyn, NY 11215
(718) 832-0617
Dominic Cuskern, president

GERTRUDE STEIN REPERTORY THEATRE
c/o HERE
145 Ave. of the Americas
New York, NY 10013
(212) 647-9684
Cheryl Faver, artistic director
John Reaves, co-director

GILGAMESH THEATRE GROUP
425 W. 46th St., #3A
New York, NY 10036
(212) 581-8956
Suzanne von Eck, artistic director

THE GLINES, INC.
240 W. 44th St.
New York, NY 10036
(212) 354-8899
John Glines, artistic director

GORILLA REPERTORY THEATRE COMPANY, INC.
P.O. Box 551, Cooper Station
New York, NY 10276
(212) 330-8086
Christopher Sanderson, director and president
William Wilkie, production manager
Diane Magnuson, producing director

GREENWICH HOUSE THEATRE COMPANY
27 Barrow St.
New York, NY 10014
(212) 633-8360
Joseph M. Farina, artistic director

THE GREENWICH STREET THEATRE
286 Spring St., 2nd fl.
New York, NY 10013
(212) 255-3940
Ludovica Villar-Hauser, artistic director
Jana Lee Brockman, manager

GROVE STREET PLAYHOUSE
39 Grove St.
New York, NY 10014
(212) 841-0259; (212) 741-6436
Marilyn Majeski, artistic director

H.A.D.L.E.Y. PLAYERS
207 W. 133rd St.
New York, NY 10030
(212) 368-9314
Gertrude Jeannette, artistic director

HAWK & HANDSAW THEATRE CO.
690 Greenwich St., Suite 5A
New York, NY 10014
(212) 741-1737
Dina Hampton, artistic director

THE HEIGHTS PLAYERS
26 Willow Place
Brooklyn, NY 11201
(718) 237-2752
Ed Healy, president

HOME
c/o HERE
145 Ave. of the Americas
New York, NY 10013
(212) 647-0202
Randy Rollison, artistic director

INNER FIRES COMPANY
214 Meads Mountain Rd., #6
Woodstock, NY 12498
(914) 679-5543
Glenn Weiss, artistic director

INTAR HISPANIC AMERICAN ARTS CENTER
420 W. 42nd St.
New York, NY 10036
(212) 695-6134
Max Ferra, artistic director
David Minton, managing director

IRISH ARTS CENTER
553 W. 51st St.
New York, NY 10019
(212) 757-3318
Nye Heron, artistic director
Marianne Delaney, executive director

IRISH REPERTORY THEATRE
163 W. 17th St.
New York, NY 10011
(212) 255-0270
Charlotte Moore, artistic director
Ciaran O'Reilly, producing director

IRONDALE ENSEMBLE PROJECT
P.O. Box 1314, Old Chelsea Station
New York, NY 10011-1314
(212) 633-1292
Jim Niesen, artistic director
Terry Greiss, executive director

JEAN COCTEAU REPERTORY
Bouwerie Lane Theatre
330 Bowery
New York, NY 10012
(212) 677-0060
Robert Hupp, Scott Shattuck, artistic
directors

JEWISH REPERTORY THEATRE
c/o 92nd Street YM/YWHA
1395 Lexington Ave.
New York, NY 10128
(212) 415-5550
Ran Avni, artistic director

KINGS COUNTY SHAKESPEARE COMPANY
155 Henry St., #8B
Brooklyn, NY 11201
(718) 596-9685
Deborah Wright Houston, Liz Shipman,
artistic directors

LA MAMA E.T.C.
74-A E. 4th St.
New York, NY 10003
(212) 254-6468
Ellen Stewart, artistic director
Meryl Vladimer, associate director

LAMB'S THEATRE COMPANY
130 W. 44th St.
New York, NY 10036
(212) 997-0210
(212) 997-1780
Carolyn Rossi Copeland, producing
artistic director
Nancy Nagel Gibbs, general manager

THE LESBIAN THEATER PROJECT
77 Perry St., #2B
New York, NY 10014
(212) 243-5770
Hope Forstenzer, artistic director

LIGHTNING STRIKES THEATRE COMPANY
55 Mercer St.
New York, NY 10013
(212) 713-5334
D. Candis Paule, artistic director

LINCOLN CENTER THEATER
Mitzi E. Newhouse Theater
150 W. 65th St.
New York, NY 10023
(212) 362-7600
André Bishop, artistic director
Bernard Gersten, executive producer

LIVE EYES THEATER COMPANY
220 Madison Ave., Apt. 9H
New York, NY 10019
(212) 779-0524
Ian Kahn, artistic director

THE LIVING THEATRE
800 West End Ave., #5A
New York, NY 10025
(212) 865-3957
Judith Malina, artistic director
Hanon Reznikov, executive director

LOVE CREEK PRODUCTIONS
Nat Horne Theatre
440 W. 42nd St.
New York, NY 10036
Philip Galbraith, artistic director

MABOU MINES
150 First Ave.
New York, NY 10009
(212) 473-0559
Collective artistic leadership

MANHATTAN TAP
Attn: Heather Cornell
2350 Broadway, #1010
New York, NY 10024
(212) 787-7181
or contact: Ann Stuart (212) 674-1572

MANHATTAN THEATRE CLUB
453 W. 16th St., 2nd fl.
New York, NY 10011
(212) 645-5590
Lynne Meadow, artistic director
Barry Grove, managing director

MCC THEATER
120 W. 28th St., 2nd fl.
New York, NY 10001
(212) 727-7722
Robert LuPone, Bernard Telsey,
executive directors

MEASURED BREATHS THEATRE COMPANY
193 Spring St., #3R
New York, NY 10012
(212) 334-8402
Robert Press, artistic director

MEDICINE SHOW THEATRE ENSEMBLE
Box 20240
New York, NY 10025
(212) 262-4216
Barbara Vann, artistic director

METROPOLITAN PLAYHOUSE
460 W. 49th St., #5
New York, NY 10019-7240
(212) 757-4452
David Zarko, artistic director

MINT THEATER COMPANY
311 W. 43rd St., 5th fl.
New York, NY 10036
(212) 315-9434
Jonathan Bank, artistic director

MIRANDA THEATRE COMPANY
259 W. 30th St.
New York, NY 10003
(212) 268-9829
Valentina Fratti, artistic director
Catherine Triant Buxton, executive
director

MUSIC THEATRE GROUP
(Sept.–May)
29 Bethune St.
New York, NY 10014
(212) 924-3108
(June–August)
P.O. Box 641
Stockbridge, MA 01262
(413) 298-5504
Lyn Austin, producing director
Diane Wondisford, general director

MUSICAL THEATRE WORKS
440 Lafayette St.
New York, NY 10003
(212) 677-0040
Anthony J. Stimac, executive director

MUTT REP
446 W. 50th St., Suite 1W
New York, NY 10019
Don Wilson Glenn, artistic director

NADA
167 Ludlow St.
New York, NY 10002
(212) 420-1466
Aaron Beall, executive director
Laura Zambrano, technical director

NATIONAL ASIAN–AMERICAN THEATRE CO.
37 St. Mark's Place
New York, NY 10003
(212) 505-3003
Mia Katigbak, artistic director
Richard Eng, executive director

NATIONAL BLACK THEATRE
2033 Fifth Ave.
New York, NY 10035
(212) 722-3800
Barbara Ann Teer, chief executive
Tunde Samuel, producer/director

NATIONAL SHAKESPEARE COMPANY
414 W. 51st St.
New York, NY 10019
(212) 265-1340
Gregory Lombardo, artistic director
Thomas Trudgeon, managing director

NEGRO ENSEMBLE COMPANY
1600 Broadway, Suite 500
New York, NY 10019
(212) 582-5860
Douglas Turner Ward, artistic director
Susan Watson Turner, producing director

NEUROTIC THEATRICAL COMPANY
465 W. 23rd St., #2C
New York, NY 10011
(212) 242-3657
Steve Diefenderfer, administrative
director

NEW FEDERAL THEATRE
466 Grand St.
New York, NY 10002
(212) 598-0400
Woodie King, Jr., producing director
Pat White, company manager

NEW GEORGES
550 W. 43rd St.
New York, NY 10036
(212) 967-2718
Susan Bernfield, artistic director

NEW PERSPECTIVES THEATRE COMPANY
750 Eighth Ave., #601
New York, NY 10036
(212) 730-2030
Melody Brooks, artistic director
Greg Weiss, managing director

NEW YORK DEAF THEATRE
305 Seventh Ave., 11th fl.
New York, NY 10001-6008
(212) 924-9491
Tony Allicino, general manager

NEW YORK GILBERT & SULLIVAN PLAYERS
251 W. 91st St., 4C
New York, NY 10024
(212) 769-1000
Albert Bergeret, artistic director

NEW YORK ITALIAN THEATRE COMPANY, INC.
119 W. 23rd St., Room 305
New York, NY 10011
(212) 929-6392
Piero Dusa, artistic director

NEW YORK SHAKESPEARE FESTIVAL
Joseph Papp Public Theater
425 Lafayette St.
New York, NY 10003
(212) 598-7100
George C. Wolfe, producer

NEW YORK THEATRE WORKSHOP
220 W. 42nd St., 18th fl.
New York, NY 10036
(212) 780-9037
James C. Nicola, artistic director
Nancy Kassak Diekmann, managing
director

NEW YORK YOUTH THEATER
P.O. Box 2153, Times Square Station
New York, NY 10108-2153
(212) 315-1737
Lawrence Axmith, artistic director

THE NO-PANTS THEATRE COMPANY
Synchronicity Space
55 Mercer St.
New York, NY 10013
(212) 673-3852
Dominic Orlando, artistic director
Karin Bowersock, producing director

NUYORICAN POETS CAFE
236 E. 3rd St.
New York, NY 10019
(212) 465-3167
Rome Neal, artistic theatre director
Miguel Algarin, producer

OASIS THEATRE COMPANY
Play Ground Theatre
230 E. 9th St.
New York, NY 10003
(212) 673-3706
Brenda Lynn Bynum, artistic director

OFF WEST BROADWAY THEATER
The Lamb's Little Theatre
130 W. 44th St.
New York, NY 10036
(212) 768-9117
Barbara Wesner, artistic director

OHIO THEATRE PROJECT
66 Wooster St.
New York, NY 10012
(212) 966-4844
Robert Lyons, artistic director

ON STAGE PRODUCTIONS
50 W. 97th St., #8H
New York, NY 10025
(212) 666-1716
Lee Frank, artistic director

ONE DREAM
232 West Broadway
New York, NY 10013
(212) 274-1450
David Ferdinand, artistic director
Laine Valentino, managing director

ONTOLOGICAL-HYSTERIC THEATER
260 W. Broadway
New York, NY 10013
(212) 941-8911
Richard Foreman, artistic director

ONYX THEATRE COMPANY
P.O. Box 1659, Cooper Station
New York, NY 10276-1659
(212) 427-1880
Michelle Banks, artistic director

OUTREACH THEATRE, INC./THEATRE OF
DREAMS
1219 77th St.
Brooklyn, NY 11228
(718) 680-3319
Bob Paton, artistic director

PAN ASIAN REPERTORY THEATRE
47 Great Jones St.
New York, NY 10012
(212) 505-5655
Tisa Chang, artistic/producing director
Russell Murphy, general manager

PANDEMONIUM STAGE COMPANY
The Hamlet of Bank Street Theatre
155 Bank St.
New York, NY 10014
(212) 989-6445
Mayra Ferrer, artistic director

THE PAPER BAG PLAYERS
185 E. Broadway
New York, NY 10002
(212) 362-0431
Judith Martin, artistic director

PEARL THEATRE COMPANY
80 St. Mark's Place
New York, NY 10003
(212) 598-9802
Shepard Sobel, artistic director
Parris Relkin, managing director

PECULIAR WORKS PROJECT
595 Broadway
New York, NY 10012
(212) 947-5207, ext. 100
Barry Rowell, Ralph Lewis, Catherine
Porter, producing partners

PING CHONG & COMPANY
47 Great Jones St.
New York, NY 10012
(212) 529-1557
Ping Chong, artistic director
Bruce Allardice, managing director

PINK, INC.
62 Grand St., #3
New York, NY 10013
(212) 941-1949
Debra Roth, artistic director

PLAYQUEST THEATER COMPANY
4 E. 28th St.
New York, NY 10016
(212) 779-0170
Peter Rogan, artistic director
Zorka Kovacevich, executive producer

PLAYWRIGHTS/ACTORS CONTEMPORARY
THEATER
c/o Juel Wiese
105 W. 13th St., #5G
New York, NY 10011
(212) 242-5888
Nancy Wallace Henderson, artistic
director
Juel Wiese, managing director

THE PLAYWRIGHTS' COLLECTIVE
74 Varick St., #207
New York, NY 10013-1914
(212) 334-9594
Collective artistic leadership

PLAYWRIGHTS HORIZONS
416 W. 42nd St.
New York, NY 10036
(212) 564-1235
Don Scardino, artistic director

PREGONES THEATRE
700 Grand Concourse, 2nd fl.
Bronx, NY 10451
(718) 585-1202
Rosalba Rolon, executive director

PRIMARY STAGES COMPANY
584 Ninth Ave.
New York, NY 10036
(212) 333-7471
Casey Childs, artistic director
Gina Gionfriddo, general manager

PUERTO RICAN TRAVELING THEATRE
141 W. 94th St.
New York, NY 10025
(212) 354-1293
Miriam Colon Valle, artistic director
Geoff Shlaes, managing director

PULSE ENSEMBLE THEATRE
432 W. 42nd St.
New York, NY 10036
(212) 695-1596
Alexa Kelly, artistic director

THE PYRAMID THEATRE ARTS FOUNDATION
159 W. 53rd St., Suite 21F
New York, NY 10019
(212) 541-8293
Nico Hartos, artistic director

QUAIGH THEATRE
205 W. 89th St.
New York, NY 10024
(212) 787-0862

QUEENS THEATRE IN THE PARK
P.O. Box 520069
Flushing, NY 11352
(718) 760-0064
Jeffrey Rosenstock, director
Bob Foreman, general manager

QWIRK PRODUCTIONS
201 W. 70th St., 15L
New York, NY 10023
(212) 595-5673
Laurence Addeo, associate producer

RAKKA-THAMM!!! THEATER COMPANY
P.O. Box 1078, Cooper Station,
New York, NY 10276-1078
(212) 603-9987
John Wuchte, artistic director
Lorraine Stobbe, executive director

RED EARTH ENSEMBLE
55 Mercer St.
New York, NY 10013
Richard Lichte, artistic director

REPERTORIO ESPAÑOL
Gramercy Arts Theatre
138 E. 27th St.
New York, NY 10016
(212) 889-2850
René Buch, artistic director
Gilberto Zaldivar, producer
Robert Weber Federico, associate
producer

RIANT THEATRE
161 Hudson St., 4th fl.
New York, NY 10013
(212) 925-8353
Van Dirk Fisher, artistic director

RIDICULOUS THEATRICAL COMPANY
(212) 989-6524
Everett Quinton, artistic director

RIVER ENSEMBLE
215 W. 92nd St., Suite 10F
New York, NY 10019
(212) 957-7297 10025
Martin Krasnoff, artistic director

ROOTS & BRANCHES THEATRE
c/o JASA
40 W. 68th St.
New York, NY 10023
(212) 501-1042
Arthur Strimling, artistic director

ROYAL BUCKINGHAM THEATRE COMPANY
P.O. Box 7527, FDR Station
New York, NY 10150
(212) 447-5564
Alexandra Jones, artistic
director/producer

RYAN REPERTORY COMPANY
Harry Warren Theatre
2445 Bath Ave.
Brooklyn, NY 11214
(718) 996-4800
John Sannuto, artistic director
Barbara Parisi, executive director

SALAMANDER REPERTORY THEATRE
400 W. 43rd St., #20H
New York, NY 10036
Joel Leffert, artistic director

SALT & PEPPER MIME COMPANY
218 W. 64 St.
New York, NY 10023
(212) 262-4989
Scottie Davis, director

SECOND MESSENGER THEATRE COMPANY
270 W. 91st St.
New York, NY 10024
(212) 724-5231
Cindy Mullen, artistic director
Cindy Nelson, business manager

SECOND STAGE THEATRE
P.O. Box 1807, Ansonia Station
New York, NY 10023
(212) 787-8302
Carole Rothman, artistic director
Suzanne Davidson, producing director
Carol Fishman, associate producer

SHADOW BOX THEATRE
325 West End Ave., #12B
New York, NY 10023
(212) 724-0677
Sandra Robbins, artistic
director/founder
Marlyn Baum, managing director

SHAKESPEARE PROJECT
310 E. 6th St., #25
New York, NY 10003
Scott Cargle, artistic director

SIDEWALKS THEATRE
40 W. 27th St., 3rd. fl.
New York, NY 10001
(212) 481-3077
Gary Beck, artistic director

SIGNATURE THEATRE COMPANY
422 W. 42nd St., 2nd fl.
New York, NY 10036
(212) 967-1913
James Houghton, artistic director
Thomas C. Proehl, managing director

SOHO REP
524 W. 57th St., Bldg. 533-1
New York, NY 10019
(212) 977-5955
Julian Webber, artistic director

SOME ASSEMBLY REQUIRED
P.O. Box 331
New York, NY 10009
(212) 875-7550
Molly Brown, director

SOUNDANCE
385 Broadway, 4th fl.
New York, NY 10013
(212) 941-6457
Sandra Stratton-Gonzalez, executive
director

SOUPSTONE PROJECT
309 E. 5th St., #19
New York, NY 10003-8828
(212) 473-7584
Neile Weissman, director

SOURCEWORKS THEATRE INC.
332 Bleecker St., #K15
New York, NY 10014
(212) 330-6990
Mark Cannistrano, artistic director

SPECTRUM STAGE
c/o Georgia Buchanan
12 Liberty Place, #D2
Weehawken, NJ 07087
(212) 567-7274
Georgia Buchanan, artistic director

SPIDERWOMAN THEATER WORKSHOP, INC.
77 Seventh Ave., #8S
New York, NY 10011
(212) 691-1970
Muriel Miguel, artistic director
Lisa Mayo, president

STAGE LEFT
P.O. Box 3251
New York, NY 10185
(212) 522-5104
Pat Vanderbeck, artistic director
Kirk Woodward, managing director

STORMY WEATHER PRODUCTIONS
P.O. Box 1449, Grand Central Station
New York, NY 10163
(212) 969-0748
Beverly Smith-Dawson, artistic producer

SURVIVOR PRODUCTIONS
10 W. 65th St., #2L
New York, NY 10023
(212) 877-2988
Leslie Sara Carroll, artistic director

SYNCHRONICITY THEATRE GROUP
55 Mercer St.
New York, NY 10013
(212) 925-5240
Peter Sylvester, artistic director

TADA!
120 W. 28th St., 2nd fl.
New York, NY 10001
(212) 627-1732
Janine Nina Trevens, artistic director
Tobe Sevush, managing director

TEN TEN PLAYERS
1010 Park Ave.
New York, NY 10028
(212) 879-7669
Lynn Marie Macy, Judith Jarosz, co-
artistic directors

THALIA SPANISH THEATRE
41-17 Greenpoint Ave.
Sunnyside, NY 11104
(718) 729-3880
Silvia Brito, artistic/executive director
Kathryn Giaimo, administrative director
Heriberto Gonzalez, development
coordinator

THEATER FOR THE NEW CITY
155 First Ave.
New York, NY 10003
(212) 254-1109
Crystal Field, executive director

THEATER 22
54 W. 22nd St.
New York, NY 10010
(212) 243-2805
Sidney Armus, artistic director

THEATRE ARTS PRODUCTIONS
425 E. 63rd St.
New York, NY 10021-7828
(212) 759-8418
Florence Hayle, director

THEATRE FOR A NEW AUDIENCE
154 Christopher St., #3D
New York, NY 10014-2839
(212) 229-2819
Jeffrey Horowitz, artistic/producing
director
Michael Solomon, general manager

THEATRE OFF PARK
224 Waverly Place, 2nd fl.
New York, NY 10014
(212) 627-2556
Albert Harris, artistic director

THEATRE ON 3
10 W. 18th St.
New York, NY 10011
(212) 255-2282
Ida Carusio, artistic director

THE THEATRE–STUDIO
750 Eighth Ave., Suite 200
New York, NY 10036
(212) 719-0500
A.M. Raychel, artistic director

THEATREWORKS/USA
890 Broadway, 7th fl.
New York, NY 10003
(212) 677-5959
Jay Harnick, artistic director

13TH STREET THEATRE REPERTORY
COMPANY
50 W. 13th St.
New York, NY 10011
(212) 675-6677
Edith O'Hara, artistic director
Bernard Falor, general manager
Robert Kreis, associate artistic director

TINY MYTHIC THEATRE COMPANY
c/o HERE
145 Ave. of the Americas
New York, NY 10013
(212) 647-0202
Tim Mayner, Kristen Marting, co-
artistic directors

TOM CAT COHEN PRODUCTIONS
162 E. 80 St., Suite 4B
New York, NY 10021
(212) 988-8042
Aphrodite Clamar, producer

TURNIP FESTIVAL COMPANY
P.O. Box 455, Times Square Station
New York, NY 10108-0455
(212) 768-4016
Joseph Massa, artistic director
Gloria Falzer, managing director

T.W.E.E.D. (THEATREWORKS:
EMERGING/EXPERIMENTAL DIRECTIONS)
332 Bleecker St., Box G36
New York, NY 10014
(212) 777-0536
Kevin Malony, artistic director

29TH STREET REPERTORY THEATER, INC.
212 W. 29th St.
New York, NY 10001
(212) 465-0575
Tim Corcoran, artistic director

TWINFISH PRODUCTIONS, INC.
27-20 27th St., #2
Astoria, NY 11102
(212) 875-7785
Rachel-Louise Rubin, artistic director

UBU REPERTORY THEATER
15 W. 28th St.
New York, NY 10001
(212) 679-7540
Franáoise Kourilsky, artistic director

VILLAR–HAUSER THEATRE CO.
286 Spring St., 202B
New York, NY 10013
(212) 255-3940
Ludovica Villar-Hauser, executive
director

THE VINEYARD THEATRE
108 E. 15th St.
New York, NY 10003
(212) 353-3366
Doug Aibel, artistic director

VOICE & VISION
P.O. Box 021529
Brooklyn, NY 11202
(212) 502-1151
Marya Mazor & Jean Wagner, artistic
directors

VORTEX THEATER COMPANY
164 Eleventh Ave.
New York, NY 10011
(212) 206-1764
Robert Coles, artistic director
Anthony John Lizzul, assistant to
artistic director

WATERMARK THEATER
202 Ave. of the Americas, #2C
New York, NY 10013
(212) 966-9290
Nela Wagman, artistic director

WESTBETH THEATRE CENTER
151 Bank St.
New York, NY 10014
(212) 691-2272
Arnold Engelman, producing director

WESTSIDE REPERTORY THEATRE
252 W. 81st St.
New York, NY 10024
(212) 874-7290
David Zyla, artistic director
Elizabeth K. Mahon, managing director

WET DOG REPERTORY
The Hamlet of Bank Street Theatre

155 Bank St.
New York, NY 10014
(212) 989-6445

THE WILLOW CABIN THEATRE COMPANY
226 W. 47th St., 2nd fl.
New York, NY 10036
(212) 921-9040
Edward Berkeley, artistic director

WINGS THEATRE COMPANY
154 Christopher St.
New York, NY 10014
(212) 627-2960
Jeff Corrick, artistic director
Michael Hillyer, associate director

WOMEN'S PROJECT & PRODUCTIONS
10 Columbus Circle, Suite 2270
New York, NY 10019
(212) 765-1906
Julia Miles, artistic director
Samuel J. Bellinger, general manager

THE WOOSTER GROUP
The Performing Garage
33 Wooster St.
New York, NY 10013
(212) 966-3651

WORKING STAGES
316 W. 93rd St.
New York, NY 10025
(212) 866-5759
Terry Adrian, artistic director

WPA THEATRE
519 W. 23rd St.
New York, NY 10011
(212) 206-0523
Kyle Renick, artistic director
Lori Sherman, managing director

THE XOREGOS PERFORMING COMPANY
496 Ninth Ave., #4A
New York, NY 10018
(212) 239-8405
Shela Xoregos, producing director

YORK THEATRE COMPANY
2 E. 90th St.
New York, NY 10128
(212) 935-5820
Janet Hayes Walker, producing director

YORKVILLE REPERTORY COMPANY
Theatre at Zion Saint Mark's Church
339 E. 84th St.
New York, NY
(212) 737-7289

YOUNG PLAYWRIGHTS, INC.
Young Playwrights Festival
321 W. 44th St., Suite 906
New York, NY 10036
(212) 307-1140
Sheri M. Goldhirsch, artistic director
Brett W. Reynolds, managing director

THE YUEH LUNG SHADOW THEATRE
33-47 91st St.
Jackson Heights, NY 11372
(718) 803-9029
Margarita Borissova, executive director

Los Angeles 99-Seat Theatres

The following theatres in the Los Angeles area have been approved by Actors' Equity Association. Members of Equity or its sister unions may perform in these theatres under the Los Angeles 99-Seat Theatre Plan only.

ACTORS ALLEY
P.O. Box 8500
Van Nuys, CA 91409-8500

ACTOR'S COMPANY
1100 West Clark Ave.
Burbank, CA 91510
(818) 848-9858

ACTOR'S GANG THEATRE
6201 Santa Monica Blvd.
West Hollywood, CA 90038
(213) 465-0566

ADAM HILL THEATRE
8517 Santa Monica Blvd.
West Hollywood, CA 90069
(310) 854-3988

ALLIANCE REPERTORY THEATRE
3204 West Magnolia Blvd.
Burbank, CA 91505
(818) 566-7935

AMERICAN NEW THEATRE
1540 North Cahuenga Blvd.
Hollywood, CA 90028
(213) 960-1604

AMERICAN RENEGADE THEATRE
11305 Magnolia Blvd.
North Hollywood, CA 91601
(818) 763-4430

ANGEL'S THEATRE
2106 Hyperion Ave.
Los Angeles, CA 90027
(213) 666-6789

ATTIC THEATRE
6562½ Santa Monica Blvd.
Los Angeles, CA 90038
(213) 462-9720

BEVERLY HILLS PLAYHOUSE
254 South Robertson Blvd.
Beverly Hills, CA 90211
(310) 855-1556

BILINGUAL FOUNDATION OF THE ARTS
421 North Ave. 19
Los Angeles, CA 90031
(213) 225-4044

CALIFORNIA COTTAGE THEATRE
5220 Sylmar Ave.
Van Nuys, CA 91401
(818) 990-5773

CAST THEATRE
804 North El Centro Ave.
Los Angeles, CA 90038
(213) 462-0265
(213) 462-9872

CELEBRATION THEATRE
7051 Santa Monica Blvd.
Hollywood, CA 90028
(213) 464-0411
Mailing address:
4470-107 Sunset Blvd., #353
Los Angeles, CA 90027

CHANDLER STUDIO
12443 Chandler Blvd.
North Hollywood, CA 91607

COAST PLAYHOUSE
8325 Santa Monica Blvd.
West Hollywood, CA 90069
(310) 650-8507
(310) 654-9657

CROSSLEY THEATRE
1760 North Gower St.
Hollywood, CA 90028
(213) 462-8460

DEAF WEST
660 North Heliotrope Dr.
Los Angeles, CA 90004
(213) 660-0877

GROUP REPERTORY THEATRE
10900 Burbank Blvd.
North Hollywood, CA 91601
(818) 760-9368

HARMAN THEATRE
522 North La Brea Ave.
Hollywood, CA 90036
(213) 931-8130

HUDSON THEATRE/HUDSON BACKSTAGE
6539 Santa Monica Blvd.
Hollywood, CA 90038
(213) 856-4249

INTERNATIONAL CITY THEATRE
4901 East Carson St.
Long Beach, CA 90808
(310) 420-4275
(310) 420-4128

KNIGHTSBRIDGE THEATRE
35 South Raymond Ave.
Pasadena, CA 91105
(818) 440-0821

MELROSE THEATRE
733 North Seward
Hollywood, CA 90038
(213) 465-1885

MET THEATRE
1089 North Oxford Ave.
Los Angeles, CA 90029
(213) 957-1741
(213) 957-1831

MOVING ARTS
1822 Hyperion Ave.
Los Angeles, CA 90027
(213) 665-8961

A NOISE WITHIN
234 South Brand Ave.
Glendale, CA 91202
(818) 753-7750

NOSOTROS
1314 North Wilton Place
Hollywood, CA 90028
(213) 465-4167

ODYSSEY THEATRE ENSEMBLE
2056 South Sepulveda Blvd.
Los Angeles, CA 90025
(310) 477-2055

OFF RAMP THEATRE
1053 North Cahuenga Blvd.
Hollywood, CA 90028
Mailing address:
6394 Ivarene Ave.
Hollywood, CA 90068
(213) 469-4343
(213) 465-8059

OPEN FIST
1625 North La Brea Ave.
Hollywood, CA 90028
(213) 281-8325

PACIFIC RESIDENT THEATRE ENSEMBLE
8780 Venice Blvd.
Los Angeles, CA 90230
Mailing address:
P.O. Box 26A77
Los Angeles, CA 90026
(310) 484-9757

PLAYBOX THEATRE
1955 Cahuenga Blvd.
Hollywood, CA 90028
(213) 469-9434

ROAD THEATRE
14141 Covello St., 9D
Van Nuys, CA 91367
(818) 785-6175

SECOND STAGE
6500 Santa Monica Blvd.
Hollywood, CA 90038
(213) 465-6029

STAGES THEATRE CENTER
1540 North McCadden Place
Hollywood, CA 90028
(213) 465-1010
(213) 463-5356

STUDIO THEATRE PLAYHOUSE/THE COLONY
1944 Riverside Dr.
Los Angeles, CA 90039
(213) 665-3011
(213) 667-9851

TAMARIND THEATRE
5919 Franklin Ave.
Hollywood, CA 90028
(213) 465-7980

THEATRE 40
Beverly Hills High School
241 Moreno Dr.
Beverly Hills, CA 90212
Mailing address:
P.O. Box 5401
Beverly Hills, CA 90210
(310) 277-4221

THEATRE EAST
12655 Ventura Blvd.
Studio City, CA 91604
(818) 760-4160

THEATRE GEO
1229 North Highland Ave.
Hollywood, CA 90038
(213) 462-3348

THEATRE/THEATER
1713 North Cahuenga Blvd.
Hollywood, CA 90028
(213) 871-0210
(213) 850-6941

TRACY ROBERTS THEATRE
141 South Robertson Blvd.
West Hollywood, CA 90048
(310) 271-2730

TWO ROADS THEATRE
4383 Tujunga Ave.
Studio City, CA 91604
(818) 766-9381

VENTURA COURT THEATRE
12417 Ventura Court
Studio City, CA 91604
(818) 763-3856

VICTORY THEATRE
3324 Victory Blvd.
Burbank, CA 91505
(818) 843-9253
(818) 841-4404

WEST COAST ENSEMBLE
6240 Hollywood Blvd.
Hollywood, CA 90028
(213) 871-1052
(213) 871-8673

Chicago Theatres

This list of selected Chicago-area theatres was compiled primarily by the League of Chicago Theatres, 67 E. Madison Ave., Suite 2116, Chicago, IL 60603. Business phone numbers are listed, along with names of key artistic and administrative personnel.

AMERICAN BLUES THEATRE
1909 W. Byron
Chicago, IL 60604
(312) 929-1031
Kate Buddeke, Carmen Roman
Nonprofit, Equity

APPLE TREE THEATRE
595 Elm Place, #210
Highland Park, IL 60035
(708) 432-4335
Eileen Boevers, Alan Salzenstein
Nonprofit, Equity

ATHENAEUM THEATRE CO.
P.O. Box 578026
Chicago, IL 60657
(312) 525-0195
Debbie Pekin, Jim Struthers
Nonprofit, non-Equity

AVENUE THEATRE
4223 N. Lincoln Ave.
Chicago, IL 60618
(312) 404-1780
Doug Binkley
Nonprofit, non-Equity

BAILIWICK REPERTORY
1229 W. Belmont
Chicago, IL 60657
(312) 883-1090
Cecilie Keenan, David Zak
Nonprofit, Equity

BLACK ENSEMBLE THEATRE
4520 N. Beacon
Chicago, IL 60640
(312) 769-5516
Calandra Gandy
Nonprofit, Equity

BLUE RIDER THEATRE
1822 S. Halsted
Chicago, IL 60608
(312) 733-4668
Tim Fiori, Donna Blue Lachman
Nonprofit, non-Equity

BUFFALO THEATRE ENSEMBLE
Arts Center, College of DuPage
22nd St. and Lambert Rd.
Glen Ellyn, IL 60137
(708) 858-2800, ext. 2100
Craig Berger
Nonprofit, Equity

CENTER THEATER
1346 W. Devon
Chicago, IL 60660
(312) 508-0200
Dan LaMorte, Robin Stanton
Nonprofit, Equity

CHICAGO ACTORS ENSEMBLE
P.O. Box 409216
Chicago, IL 60640
(312) 275-4463
Hilary MacAustin
Nonprofit, non-Equity

CHICAGO THEATRE COMPANY
500 E. 67th St.
Chicago, IL 60637
(312) 493-0901
Douglas Mann
Nonprofit, Equity

CITY LIT THEATER COMPANY
410 S. Michigan, #813A
Chicago, IL 60605
(312) 913-9446
Mark Richard, Mary Hatch
Nonprofit, non-Equity

CLOUD 42
3354 N. Paulina, #206F
Chicago, IL 60657
(312) 477-4446
Patrick Trettenero, Nathan Rankin
Nonprofit, non-Equity

COMEDYSPORTZ
2148 N. Halsted, #3R
Chicago, IL 60614
(312) 549-8080
Jill Shely, David Gaudet
Commercial, non-Equity

COURT THEATRE
5535 S. Ellis
Chicago, IL 60637
(312) 702-7005
Charles Newell, Sandy Karuschak
Nonprofit, Equity

DREISKE PERFORMANCE COMPANY
1517 W. Fullerton
Chicago, IL 60614
(312) 281-9075
Nicole Dreiske
Nonprofit, non-Equity

ECLIPSE THEATRE COMPANY
2074 N. Leavitt
Chicago, IL 60647
(312) 862-7415
Robert Mohler, Kenn Puttbach
Nonprofit, Equity

EQUITY LIBRARY THEATRE
345 W. Dickens
Chicago, IL 60614
(312) 743-0266
Darwin Apel, Leah Roshal
Nonprofit, Equity

ETA CREATIVE ARTS FOUNDATION
7558 S. Chicago Ave.
Chicago, IL 60619
(312) 752-3955
Abena Joan Brown, Runako Jahi
Nonprofit, non-Equity

FAMOUS DOOR THEATRE COMPANY
3212 N. Broadway
Chicago, IL 60657
(312) 404-8283
Marc Grapey, Dan Rivkin
Nonprofit, non-Equity

FOOTSTEPS THEATRE COMPANY
5230 N. Clark
Chicago, IL 60640
(312) 465-8323
Jean Adamak, Dale Heinen
Nonprofit, non-Equity

GOODMAN THEATRE
200 S. Columbus
Chicago, IL 60603
(312) 443-3811
Roche Schulfer, Robert Falls
Nonprofit, Equity

GRIFFIN THEATRE COMPANY
5404 N. Clark
Chicago, IL 60640
(312) 769-2228
Richard Barlena, William Massolia
Nonprofit, non-Equity

HYSTOPOLIS PUPPET THEATRE
c/o Rosary College
7900 W. Division
River Forest, IL 60305
(312) 787-7387
Michael Schwabe, Larry Basgall, Jim
Rossow
Nonprofit, non-Equity

ILLINOIS THEATRE CENTER
400A Lakewood Blvd.
Park Forest, IL 60466
(708) 481-3510
Etel Billig, Steve Billig
Nonprofit, Equity

THE IMPROV INSTITUTE
2319 W. Belmont
Chicago, IL 60618
(312) 929-2323
Patricia Musker, Jack Bronis
Nonprofit, non-Equity

INTERPLAY
135 S. Cuyler (mail only)
Oak Park, IL 60302
(708) 848-3245
David Perkovich, Donald Miller
Nonprofit, Equity

IVANHOE THEATER
180 E. Pearson, #4602
Chicago, IL 60611
(312) 642-2342
Douglas Bragan
Commercial, Equity

LATINO CHICAGO
1625 N. Damen
Chicago, IL 60647
(312) 486-5151
Juan Ramirez, Nilda Hernandez
Nonprofit, Equity

LIFELINE THEATRE
6912 N. Glenwood
Chicago, IL 60626
(312) 761-0667
Meryl Friedman, Scott Olson
Nonprofit, non-Equity

LIGHT OPERA WORKS
927 Noyes St.
Evanston, IL 60201
(708) 869-6300
Bridget McDonough, Tim Pleiman
Nonprofit, non-Equity

LIVE BAIT THEATRICAL COMPANY
3914 N. Clark St.
Chicago, IL 60613
(312) 871-3191
Sharon Evans, John Ragir
Nonprofit, non-Equity

LOOKINGGLASS THEATRE COMPANY
3309 N. Seminary
Chicago, IL 60657
(312) 477-9257
Laura Eason, David Catlin
Nonprofit, non-Equity

MUSIC/THEATRE WORKSHOP
5647 N. Ashland
Chicago, IL 60660
(312) 561-7100
Elbrey Harrell, Meade Padidofsky
Nonprofit, Equity, TYA

NATIONAL JEWISH THEATER
Horwich/Kaplan JCC
5050 W. Church St.
Skokie, IL 60077
(708) 675-2200
Lisa Bany-Winters, Susan Padveen
Nonprofit, Equity

NEW REGAL THEATER
1645 E. 79th St.
Chicago, IL 60649
(312) 721-9301
Wilma Washington
Nonprofit, Equity

NEXT THEATRE COMPANY
927 Noyes St.
Evanston, IL 60201
(708) 475-6763
Steve Pickering, Peter Rybolt
Nonprofit, non-Equity

NORTHLIGHT THEATRE
600 Davis St.
Evanston, IL 60201
(708) 869-7732
Russell Vandenbroucke, Richard
Friedman
Nonprofit, Equity, LORT

OAK PARK FESTIVAL THEATRE
P.O. Box 4114
Oak Park, IL 60303
(708) 524-2050
Tom Mula
Nonprofit, Equity

ORGANIC THEATER COMPANY
3319 N. Clark St. 4V
Chicago, IL 60657
(312) 327-2427
Paul Frellick
Nonprofit, Equity, non-Equity

PALOOKAVILLE
5835 W. Grace
Chicago, IL 60634
(312) 833-0449
Warren Sampson, Bonnie Lucas
Nonprofit, non-Equity

PARALLAX THEATRE
2009 W. North Ave.
Chicago, IL 60647
(312) 489-0205
Henrietta B. Pearsall, Scott Holstein
Non-profit, non-Equity

PEGASUS PLAYERS
O'Rourke Center for Performing Arts
1145 W. Wilson
Chicago, IL 60640
(312) 878-9761
Arlene Crewdson, Paul Klaeyson
Nonprofit, non-Equity

PERFORMING ARTS CHICAGO
410 S. Michigan, Suite 911
Chicago, IL 60605
(312) 663-1628
Carol Fox
Nonprofit, Equity

PERKINS PRODUCTIONS, INC.
1633 N. Halsted, Suite 400
Chicago, IL 60614
(312) 944-5626
Bob Perkins, Jim Jensen
Commercial, Equity

PIVEN THEATRE WORKSHOP
927 Noyes
Evanston, IL 60201
(708) 866-6597
Joyce Piven, Caroline Schless
Nonprofit, non-Equity

PROFILES PERFORMANCE ENSEMBLE
4206 N. Hermitage, 1st fl.
Chicago, IL 60613
(312) 404-8341
Cynthia Jahraus, Joe Jahraus
Nonprofit, non-Equity

RAVEN THEATRE COMPANY
6931 N. Clark St.
Chicago, IL 60626
(312) 338-2177
Michael Menendian, JoAnn
Montemurro
Nonprofit, non-Equity

REMAINS THEATRE
863 N. Dearborn
Chicago, IL 60610
(312) 335-9595
Neel Keller
Nonprofit, Equity

ROADWORKS PRODUCTIONS
1532 N. Milwaukee, Suite 208
Chicago, IL 60622
(312) 489-7623
Abby Epstein, Karen Turk
Nonprofit, non-Equity

SAINT SEBASTIAN PLAYERS
c/o St. Bonaventure
1641 W. Diversey
Chicago, IL 60614
Terri Dsida, Jill Chukerman
Nonprofit, non-Equity

SECOND CITY
1616 N. Wells St.
Chicago, IL 60614
(312) 664-4032
Joyce Sloane, Kelly Leonard
Commercial, Equity

SHAKESPEARE REPERTORY
820 N. Orleans, Suite 340
Chicago, IL 60610
(312) 642-8394
Barbara Gaines, Criss Henderson
Nonprofit, Equity

SHATTERED GLOBE THEATRE
2856 N. Halsted
Chicago, IL 60657
(312) 404-1237
Brian Pudil, Joseph Porbrich
Nonprofit, non-Equity

SPLINTER GROUP
1937 W. Division
Chicago, IL 60622
Matt O'Brien
Nonprofit, non-Equity

STAGE LEFT THEATRE
3408 N. Sheffield Ave.
Chicago, IL 60657
(312) 883-8830
Mike Troccoli, Sandra Verthein
Nonprofit, non-Equity

STEPPENWOLF THEATRE COMPANY
1650 N. Halsted
Chicago, IL 60614
(312) 335-1888
Stephen Eich
Nonprofit, Equity

STRAWDOG THEATRE COMPANY
3829 N. Broadway
Chicago, IL 60613
(312) 528-9889
Richard Shavzin, Steve Savage
Nonprofit, non-Equity

TALISMAN THEATRE
1847 W. Carroll
Chicago, IL 60612
(312) 235-7763
Mark Hardiman
Nonprofit, non-Equity

TEATRO VISTA
3712 N. Broadway, Suite 213
Chicago, IL 60613
(312) 878-8773
Henry Godinez, Tami Workentin-Ness
Nonprofit, Equity

THEATRE BUILDING/NEW TUNERS THEATRE
1225 W. Belmont
Chicago, IL 60657
(312) 929-7367
Ruth Higgins, Joan Mazzonelli
Nonprofit, non-Equity

THEATRE II COMPANY
St. Xavier College, McGuire Hall
3700 W. 103rd St.
Chicago, IL 60655
(312) 298-3561
JoAnne Fleming, Stephen Micotto
Nonprofit, non-Equity

TORSO THEATRE
2827 N. Broadway, 2nd fl.
Chicago, IL 60657
(312) 549-3330
Billy Bermingham
Nonprofit, non-Equity

TOUCHSTONE THEATRE
2851 N. Halsted
Chicago, IL 60657
(312) 477-5779
Ina Marlowe, Tamra Powell
Nonprofit, non-Equity

TRINITY SQUARE ENSEMBLE
927 Noyes, #224
Evanston, IL 60201
(708) 328-0330
Kathleen Martin
Nonprofit, non-Equity

VICTORY GARDENS THEATER
2257 N. Lincoln Ave.
Chicago, IL 60614
(312) 549-5788
Dennis Zacek, John Walker
Nonprofit, Equity

WISDOM BRIDGE THEATRE
332 S. Michigan
Chicago, IL 60604
(312) 341-2550
Jeffrey Ortmann, Terry McCabe
Nonprofit, Equity

WOODSTOCK OPERA HOUSE
121 Van Buren
Woodstock, IL 60098
(815) 338-4212
John Scharres
Nonprofit, non-Equity

WRITERS' THEATRE—CHICAGO
1101 W. Pratt, Suite 3E
Chicago, IL 60626
(312) 338-7166
Michael Halberstam, Betty Askow
Nonprofit, Equity

ZEBRA CROSSING THEATRE
4223 N. Lincoln
Chicago, IL 60618
(312) 248-6401
Marlene Zuccaro, Bob Buck
Nonprofit, non-Equity

Acting Schools and Teachers

The following are sources of training in stage, commercial, and film acting in New York City, Los Angeles, Chicago, and London. Other class categories are also included. Although this list is extensive, it is not all-inclusive. (Where no address is given, it means that classes are held in a location that could change.)

NEW YORK CITY AND ENVIRONS

STAGE

THE ACTING STUDIO, INC.
29 E. 19th St., 4th fl.
New York, NY 10003
(212) 228-2700

ACTORS ADVENT LTD.
212 W. 29th St.
New York, NY 10001
(212) 627-0854
Contact: Esther Brandice, director

ACTOR'S ARENA 370 W. 30TH ST., #4E
New York, NY 10001
(212) 268-4177
Contact: Cee Ali

THE ACTORS INSTITUTE
48 W. 21st St., 4th fl.
New York, NY 10010
(212) 924-8888

ACTORS MOVEMENT STUDIO
5 W. 31st St., 6th fl.
New York, NY 10001
(212) 736-3309

ACTORS TRAINING INSTITUTE
P.O. Box 2096
91 Monmouth St.
Red Bank, NJ 07701

ACTORS WORKSHOP
205 W. Houston St.
New York, NY
(212) 724-9441
Contact: Lewis Van Bergen

STELLA ADLER CONSERVATORY OF ACTING
419 Lafayette St., 6th fl.
New York, NY 10003
(212) 260-0525
Fax: (212) 260-8944

ELAINE AIKEN ACTORS CONSERVATORY
750 Eighth Ave.
New York, NY 10036
(212) 764-0543
Contact: Lily Lodge, associate director

AMARANTH STUDIO
164 Lake St.
Englewood, NJ 07631
(212) 360-7006
Contact: Pamela Childs, director

AMERICAN ACADEMY OF DRAMATIC ARTS
120 Madison Ave.
New York, NY 10016
(212) 686-9244

AMERICAN DANCE & DRAMA STUDIO
188-22 Union Tpke.
Flushing, NY 11366
(718) 479-8522

AMERICAN GLOBE THEATRE CONSERVATORY
145 W. 46th St.
New York, NY 10036
(212) 869-9809

THE AMERICAN MIME THEATRE
61 Fourth Ave.
New York, NY 10003
(212) 777-1710

AMERICAN MUSICAL AND DRAMATIC ACADEMY
2109 Broadway
New York, NY 10023
(212) 787-5300

ATLANTIC THEATER COMPANY ACTING SCHOOL
Practical Aesthetics Workshop
336 W. 20th St.
New York, NY 10011
(212) 645-8015

RON AUGUST
516 E. 83rd St.
New York, NY 10028
(212) 861-4528

MARJORIE BALLENTINE STUDIO
115 MacDougal St.
New York, NY 10012
(212) 780-9520

MICHAEL BARBARY
(212) 245-3084

JOYCE BARKER SCHOOL FOR ACTORS
Guild Rehearsal Studios
Hotel Ansonia
2109 Broadway, #977
New York, NY 10023
(212) 873-6208

THE BARROW GROUP SCHOOL
P.O. Box 5112
New York, NY 10185
(212) 522-1421

BB PRODUCTIONS
325 W. 45th St., Suite 512
New York, NY 10036
(212) 246-6005

JO ANNA BECKSON
636 Broadway, Studio 708
New York, NY 10012
(212) 353-0114
(212) 586-6300

JIM BONNEY STUDIO
Theatre Row Studios
412 W. 42nd St.
New York, NY 10036
(212) 713-5277

DELOSS BROWN
444 Central Park West, #5A
New York, NY 10025
(212) 865-1127

ELIZABETH BROWNING
(212) 541-7600
Classes in Manhattan

DAVID BRUNETTI
71 W. 71st St.
New York, NY 10023
(212) 580-3292

WALTRUDIS BUCK
155 W. 68th St.
New York, NY 10023
(212) 787-3104
Fax: (212) 787-2830

CASTLE LANE
(718) 369-1121
Classes in Manhattan

THE CENTAUR STAGE
(212) 724-2800
Contact: Gillien Goll, artistic director
Classes in Manhattan

CHEKHOV THEATRE ENSEMBLE
(718) 832-3630
Classes in Manhattan

CIRCLE IN THE SQUARE THEATRE SCHOOL
1633 Broadway
New York, NY 10019-6795
(212) 307-2732

CIRCLE REPERTORY SCHOOL OF THEATRE
632 Broadway, 6th fl.
New York, NY 10012
(212) 505-6010

DAVID COHEN
(212) 592-4118
Classes in Manhattan

COLLABORATIVE ARTS PROJECT 21
One Union Square West, Suite 907
New York, NY 10003
(212) 807-0202

THE COLUMN THEATRE & STUDIO
48 W. 21st St., 8th fl.
New York, NY 10010
(212) 229-0020

MARNIE COOPER SCHOOL OF ACTING
155 E. 23rd St., Suite 101
New York, NY 10010
(212) 477-1818

THE CREATIVE ACTOR'S WORKSHOP
451 W. 43rd St.
New York, NY 10036
(212) 245-1237
Contact: Jeffrey Zeiner

ROBERT DAGNY
Box 852, FDR Station
New York, NY 10150-0852
(212) 371-8258

THE DIRECTORS COMPANY
311 W. 43rd St., Suite 206
New York, NY 10036
(212) 246-5877

THE PIERO DUSA ACTING STUDIO
Duality Playhouse
119 W. 23rd St., #305
New York, NY 10011
(212) 929-6392

PAUL EISEMAN
305 E. 40th St., #4H
New York, NY 10016
(212) 953-6926

ENSEMBLE STUDIO THEATRE INSTITUTE
549 W. 52nd St.
New York, NY 10019
(212) 581-9409

WILLIAM ESPER STUDIO
250 Third Ave.
New York, NY 10010
(212) 673-6713

THE 42ND STREET COLLECTIVE
412 W. 42nd St.
New York, NY 10036
(212) 967-1481

GENE FRANKEL THEATRE WORKSHOP
24 Bond St.
New York, NY 10012
(212) 777-1767
Catherine Gaffigan
(212) 586-6300

THE GATELY/POOLE ACTING STUDIO, INC.
543 W. 43rd St., Suite 8079
New York, NY 10036
(212) 517-1677

JOSEPH GIARDINA
235 E. 22nd St., PH-C
New York, NY 10010
(212) 725-2015

DAVID GIDEON/THE ACTING CLASS, INC.
111 Barrow St.
New York, NY 10014
(212) 645-1025

PHILIP GUSHEE STUDIO
636 Broadway, Room 708
New York, NY 10012
(212) 353-0114

HB STUDIO
120 Bank St.
New York, NY 10014
(212) 675-2370

HISPANIC ORGANIZATION OF LATIN ACTORS
(HOLA)
250 W. 65th St.
New York, NY 10023
(212) 595-8286

MARY HOLLOWELL
191 Devoe St., 2R
New York, NY 11211
(212) 229-8297

MICHAEL HOWARD STUDIO
152 W. 25th St.
New York, NY 10001
(212) 645-1525

CHARLES KAKATSAKIS
202 W. 80th St., #1W
New York, NY 10024
(212) 362-5757

JULIA L. KEEFER
408 E. 78th St., #3B
New York, NY 10021
(212) 734-1083

RAPHAEL KELLY SHAKESPEARE STUDIO
168 E. 89th St.
New York, NY 10028
(212) 289-1392

ED KOVENS
The Professional Workshop
20 Dongan Pl., #311
New York, NY 10040
(212) 567-6761

CATHLEEN LESLIE
(212) 371-1652

THE ERIC LOEB STUDIO
(212) 243-5331

BERNICE LORE/EXPRESSIONS
350 W. 55th St., #3F
New York, NY 10019
(212) 586-8604

THE BOB LUKE ACTING STUDIO
349 W. 44th St.
New York, NY 10036
(212) 245-2831

MAGGIE MAES
Actors' Loft
944 Eighth Ave., 2nd fl.
New York, NY 10019
(212) 397-0904

JUDY MAGEE
401 E. 89th St.
New York, NY 10128
(212) 722-5694

PATRICIA McGINNIS
344 W. 89th St.
New York, NY 10024
(212) 362-3374

MARGO McKEE'S SOUNDSTAGE, INC.
630 Ninth Ave.
New York, NY 10036
(212) 757-5436

STEPHEN MICHAELS
114 E. 7th St., Apt. 4
New York, NY 10009
(212) 473-8854

THE MINT THEATER ACTOR TRAINING
PROGRAM
311 W. 43rd St., 5th fl.
New York, NY 10036
(212) 315-9434

ROBERT X. MODICA
881 Seventh Ave., Room 809
New York, NY 10025
(212) 245-2089

JOY MORRIS
New York, NY 10019
(212) 397-8795

LUCY MOSES SCHOOL
Elaine Kaufman Cultural Center
129 W. 67th St.
New York, NY 10028
(212) 362-8060

DOUG MOSTON DRAMA PROJECT
440 Lafayette St.
New York, NY 10003
(212) 674-1166

MUSICAL THEATRE WORKS CONSERVATORY
440 Lafayette St.
New York, NY 10003
(212) 677-0040

NATIONAL SHAKESPEARE CONSERVATORY
440 Lafayette St.
New York, NY 10003
(212) 260-8660
(800) 472-6667

NATIONAL THEATRE WORKSHOP OF THE
HANDICAPPED
354 Broome St., Suite 5F
New York, NY 10013
(212) 941-9511

NEIGHBORHOOD PLAYHOUSE SCHOOL OF
'THE THEATRE
340 E. 54th St.
New York, NY 10022
(212) 688-3770

RUTH NERKEN
11 E. 4th St.
New York, NY
(212) 362-5277

NEW ACTORS WORKSHOP
259 W. 30th St., 2nd fl.
New York, NY 10001
(212) 947-1310

NEW CONSERVATORY THEATRE WORKSHOP
334 Bowery
New York, NY 10012
(212) 777-1855

NEW YORK PERFORMANCE WORKS
85 West Broadway, 2nd fl.
New York, NY 10004
(212) 566-1500

ONE ON ONE PRODUCTIONS
126 W. 23rd St.
New York, NY 10011
(212) 691-6000

ROBERT PATTERSON STUDIO
170 W. 74th St.
New York, NY 10023
(212) 840-1234

DAVID PERRY
881 Seventh Ave., Studio 808
New York, NY 10019
(212) 866-8929

TODD PETERS
345 W. 85th St.
New York, NY 10024
(212) 873-5836

AVRA PETRIDES' TRAINING FOR ACTORS
101 W. 78th St., Suite 21
New York, NY 10024
(212) 877-3155

VINCENT PHILLIP MONOLOGUE, VOICE,
AND SPEECH SCHOOL
339 W. 48th St.
New York, NY 10036
(212) 246-3558

PLAYQUEST THEATER COMPANY
4 E. 28th St.
New York, NY 10016
(212) 779-0170

CAROL FOX PRESCOTT
221 W. 82nd St.
New York, NY 10024
(212) 877-2780

MARILYN RALL
201 W. 70th St., 20K
New York, NY 10023
(718) 434-6405

JUDITH ROSENBLATT
Actor's Theatre Workshop
145 W. 28th St.
New York, NY 10001
(212) 260-2295

ROUNDABOUT THEATRE CONSERVATORY &
ENSEMBLE
The Criterion Center
1530 Broadway
New York, NY 10036
(212) 719-9393

ALEC RUBIN
(212) 724-7508

FLOYD RUMOHR
84 Windsor Place
Brooklyn, NY 11215
(718) 832-5943

T. SCHREIBER STUDIO
83 E. 4th St.
New York, NY 10003
(212) 420-1249

MICHAEL SCHULMAN WORKSHOP
28 E. 10th St.
New York, NY 10003
(212) 777-3055

JACQUELINE SEGAL
88 Lexington Ave., PH G
New York, NY 10016
(212) 683-9428

78TH STREET THEATRE LAB
236 W. 78th St.
New York, NY 10024
Contact: Mark Zeller (212) 362-1736
Dana Zeller-Alexis (212) 724-4862

SUZANNE SHEPHERD
(212) 873-5324

BETSY SHEVEY
(212) 787-8943

SANDE SHURIN ACTING STUDIO N.Y.
335 W. 38th St.
New York, NY 10018
(212) 563-2298

ROGER HENDRICKS SIMON STUDIO
540 Seminary Row, #32
New York, NY 10027
(212) 932-9604

SUSAN SLAVIN ACTORS & SINGERS
ACADEMY
Carnegie Hall
154 W. 57th St.
New York, NY 10019
(212) 582-0321

BARBARA SPIEGEL THEATRE WORKSHOPS
534 Madison Ave.
New York, NY 10022
(212) 688-0945

ALICE SPIVAK
c/o AIA/Three of Us Studios
39 W. 19th St.
New York, NY 10011
(212) 924-0561

LEE STRASBERG THEATRE INSTITUTE
115 E. 15th St.
New York, NY 10003
(212) 533-5500

STEPHEN STRIMPELL
201 W. 70th St., 20K
New York, NY 10023
(212) 873-7311

THEATRE NEXT DOOR
101-06 Queens Blvd., 2nd fl.
Forest Hills, NY 11375
(718) 830-0265
(718) 459-1928
Contact: Jim Cowen

CAROLINE THOMAS' TOTAL THEATRE LAB
118 W. 79th St., Suite 12A
New York, NY 10024
(212) 799-4224

PATRICIA WING TOBIAS
305 E. 86th St., #5PW
New York, NY 10028
(212) 289-4322

ELIZA VENTURA
150 W. 74th St., Suite 2C
New York, NY 10023
(212) 362-2686

VOICEWORKS: THE LYNN SINGER GROUP
201 W. 16th St.
New York, NY 10011
(212) 242-3297

BILL WENDT
115 MacDougal St.
New York, NY 10012
(212) 925-0036

WALT WITCOVER
40 W. 22nd St.
New York, NY 10010
(212) 691-4367

TED ZURKOWSKI
Musical Theatre Works
440 Lafayette St.
New York, NY 10003
(212) 866-7280

COMEDY/IMPROVISATION

CHICAGO CITY LIMITS IMPROVISATIONAL
THEATRE
1105 First Ave.
New York, NY 10021
(212) 888-5233

FREESTYLE REPERTORY THEATRE
120 W. 86th St., #1A
New York, NY 10024
(212) 642-8202

GOTHAM CITY IMPROV
450 W. 42nd St., Suite 2A
New York, NY 10036
(212) 714-1477

MICHAEL HORN IMPROVISATIONAL SCHOOL
OF ACTING
115 MacDougal St.
70 University Place, #1
New York, NY 10003
(212) 505-8068

SOME ASSEMBLY REQUIRED
P.O. Box 331
New York, NY 10009
(212) 875-7550
Classes in Manhattan

TOM SOTER WINGNUT COMEDY STUDIO
1264 Amsterdam Ave., #3B
New York, NY 10027
(212) 316-4916
Classes in Manhattan

THE STAND-UP COMEDY EXPERIENCE
1600 Broadway
New York, NY 10019
(212) 247-5555

ON-CAMERA
(FILM, TV, COMMERCIAL)

ACTING FOR CAMERA
The Film Center Building
630 Ninth Ave., Suite 702
New York, NY 10036
(212) 247-2011
Contact: Maria Greco, Tony Greco

ACTING MANAGEMENT INC.
140 W. 22nd St., 4th fl.
New York, NY 10011
(212) 989-8709

AIA/THREE OF US STUDIOS
39 W. 19th St., 12th fl.
New York, NY 10010
(212) 645-0030

MADELYN J. BURNS STUDIO
121 W. 27th St., Suite 503
New York, NY 10001
(212) 627-8880

BOB COLLIER'S TV STUDIOS & CASTING
SERVICE
124 W. 18th St., 2nd fl.
New York, NY 10011
(212) 929-4737

NINA DOVA ON-CAMERA COMMERCIAL
TRAINING
280 Riverside Dr., Apt. 10B
New York, NY 10025
(212) 222-7651

GWYN GILLISS COMMUNICATIONS
666 Fifth Ave., Suite 323
New York, NY 10103
(212) 595-9001

CATHERINE MARKS WORKSHOP
250 E. 73rd St.
New York, NY 10021
(212) 737-5911

CHRISTOPHER MERTZ
364 W. 18th St., #3A
New York, NY 10011
(212) 255-4810

NEW YORK FILM ACADEMY
100 E. 17th St.
New York, NY 10003
(212) 674-4300

ON CAMERA AND OFF/LARRY CONROY
42 W. 13th St., #4D
New York, NY 10011
(212) 741-1444

SCOTT POWERS PRODUCTIONS
150 Fifth Ave., Suite 623
New York, NY 10011
(212) 242-4700

JEFFREY D. STOCKER FILM ACTING STUDIO
90 Lexington Ave., Suite 1H
(212) 684-3094

MICHAEL STORCK FILM ACTING
P.O. Box 657
New York, NY 10101
(212) 982-9091

TVI ACTORS CENTER & STUDIO
165 W. 46th St., Suite 509
New York, NY 10036
(212) 302-1900

VIDEO ASSOCIATES STUDIO
311 W. 43rd St., Suite 601
New York, NY 10036
(212) 397-0018
Contact: Kim Todd, Gordon Rigsby

WEIST–BARRON ACTING FOR
TELEVISION/FILM/THEATRE
35 W. 45th St., 6th fl.
New York, NY 10036
(212) 840-7025

**MONOLOGUE/AUDITION/PRIVATE
COACHING**

GLENN ALTERMAN'S WRITING &
PERFORMING YOUR OWN MONOLOGUES
(212) 967-8930

JUDITH BARCROFT
(212) 362-3978

ELINOR BASESCU STUDIO
529 W. 42nd St., #8D
New York, NY 10036
(212) 868-1278

HELEN HANFT
(212) 682-6984
Classes in Manhattan

PRUDENCE HOLMES
255 W. 108th St., #9D
New York, NY 10025
(212) 864-6525

BARBARA KAHN
(212) 840-1234

JACK POGGI, MONOLOGUE COACH
880 W. 181st St., Apt. 4B
New York, NY 10033
(212) 928-6882
(212) 382-3535

DANIEL B. POLLACK
890 West End Ave.
New York, NY 10025
(212) 663-8143

LOIS RAEBECK
31 Joralemon St.
Brooklyn, NY 11201
(718) 624-8145

BARRY SHAPIRO
c/o Herman & Lipson
24 W. 25th St.
New York, NY 10001
(212) 807-7706

JACK WALTZER ACTING WORKSHOPS
5 Minetta St., Apt. 2B
New York, NY 10012
(212) 473-7056
(212) 840-1234

FLORENCE WINSTON
(212) 541-7600
Classes in Manhattan

CATHERINE WOLF
(212) 362-5332

ALAN WYNROTH
61 Morton St.
New York, NY 10014
(212) 675-9267

MELISSA ZULLO
(212) 245-3406
Classes in Manhattan

CHILDREN/TEENS

ACTEEN
c/o Rita Litton, Director
Weist–Barron Studios
35 W. 45th St.
New York, NY 10036
(212) 391-5915

CITY LIGHTS YOUTH THEATRE
City Center
130 W. 56th St.
New York, NY 10019
(212) 262-0200

IMPROVISATIONAL THEATER FOR CHILDREN
(212) 874-5054
Contact: Vivian B. Teich, director

KIDS LOVE ACTING
Weist–Barron Studios
35 W. 45th St.
New York, NY 10036
Inquiries: (212) 874-1081
Studio: (212) 840-7025
Contact: Sharon Richardson

TADA!
120 W. 28th St.
New York, NY 10001
(212) 627-1732

LOS ANGELES
STAGE

HELENE ABRAMS
(310) 285-8172

THE ACTING LAB/BARRY PEARL
(818) 995-1334

ACTION IN ACTING
1918 Magnolia Blvd., #206
Burbank, CA 91506
(818) 563-4142

ACTOR'S ART THEATRE
6128 Wilshire Blvd., #110
Los Angeles, CA 90048
(213) 969-4953
Contact: Jolene Adams

ACTORS CIRCLE THEATRE SCHOOL
7313 Santa Monica Blvd.
West Hollywood, CA 90046
(213) 882-6805
Contact: Jennifer Taylor Scott

ACTORS FORUM THEATRE
10655 Magnolia Blvd.
North Hollywood, CA 91601
(818) 506-0600
Contact: Audrey Marlyn Singer
Programs include musical comedy.

THE ACTORS LAB
(213) 850-8521
Contact: J.D. Lewis

THE ACTORS SHELTER
(310) 838-4114
Contact: Allen Garfield

CATLIN ADAMS ACTING LAB
(213) 851-8811

STELLA ADLER ACADEMY OF ACTING
6773 Hollywood Blvd., 2nd fl.
Hollywood, CA 90028
(213) 465-4446

WILLIAM ALDERSON
3912 Clayton Ave.
Los Angeles, CA 90027
(213) 669-1534

AMERICAN ACADEMY OF DRAMATIC ARTS
2550 Paloma St.
Pasadena, CA 91107
(818) 798-0777

THE AMERICAN CENTER FOR MUSIC
THEATER
6425 Hollywood Blvd.
Hollywood, CA 90028
(213) 871-8083

AMERICAN NATIONAL ACADEMY OF
PERFORMING ARTS
10944 Ventura Blvd.
Studio City, CA 91604
(818) 763-4431
Contact: Francis Lederer

THE AMERICAN REPERTORY COMPANY
The Complex Theatre
(213) 461-9268
Contact: Manu Tupou, artistic director

A NOISE WITHIN
234 Brand Blvd.
Glendale, CA 91204
(818) 546-1449
Classical theatre

ARTISTS & TALENT
12655 Ventura Blvd.
Studio City, CA 91604
(818) 508-8838

JOEL ASHER STUDIO
13448 Albers St.
Sherman Oaks, CA 91401
(818) 785-1551

BALANCE OF ACTING
Lionstar Theatre
12655 Ventura Blvd.
Studio City, CA 91604
(818) 753-1639, ext. 2
Contact: Richard Neil

JERED BARCLAY
(818) 980-5001

ADILAH BARNES
(213) 380-3373

IRA BELGRADE
5850-E W. 3rd St.
Los Angeles, CA 90036
(213) 931-3085

JACKIE BENTON
(310) 393-1410

BARBARA BLISS
(213) 965-8092
Music and musical theatre training

MICHAEL BLOOM
(310) 823-1179

STEPHEN BOOK ACTING WORKSHOP
(213) 467-8083

ROBERT BURGOS
(818) 990-8848

RON BURRUS ACTING CONSERVATORY
Los Feliz Playhouse
4646 Hollywood Blvd.
Hollywood, CA 90027
(213) 953-2823

BILL CAKMIS
(818) 785-1435

ROBERT CALI
(213) 968-2246

MATT CHAIT
The Complex
6476 Santa Monica Blvd.
Los Angeles, CA 90038
(213) 469-5408

CHARLEY'S WORKSHOP
(213) 465-1214

VINCENT CHASE WORKSHOP
7221 Sunset Blvd.
Hollywood, CA 90046
(213) 851-4819

CHURCH OF SCIENTOLOGY CELEBRITY
CENTRE INTERNATIONAL
5930 Franklin Ave.
Hollywood, CA 90028
(213) 960-3100

JEREMIAH COMEY
1648 N. Vine
Hollywood, CA 90028
(213) 469-5302

COMPLETE AUDITION WORKSHOP
(213) 464-5524
Contact: Bill Schneider, David Shine

CHARLES E. CONRAD STUDIO
4110 W. Burbank Blvd.
Burbank, CA 91505
(818) 846-9010

ROBERT CRAIGHEAD
Prime Time Actors Studio
3405 Cahuenga Blvd. West
Los Angeles, CA 90068
(213) 874-4131

GRANT CRAMER'S SCENE STUDY & COLD
READING WORKSHOP
(213) 658-6062

SCOTT CRAWFORD
(213) 663-1664

IVAN CROW, M.F.A.
(310) 587-9093

CAROLE D'ANDREA
5257 Ben Ave.
North Hollywood, CA 91607
(818) 759-9416

BOB DELEGALL ACTOR'S WORKSHOP
P.O. Box 1311
Santa Monica, CA 90406
(310) 281-3343

DELL' ARTE SCHOOL OF PHYSICAL THEATRE
P.O. Box 816
Blue Lake, CA 95525
(707) 668-5663

ANTHONY DINOVI
(310) 392-6482

BRUCE DUCAT
(213) 874-2822

WAYNE DVORAK
Dvorak & Co.
(213) 913-9563

EAST WEST PLAYERS CONSERVATORY
4424 Santa Monica Blvd.
Los Angeles, CA 90029
(213) 666-1929

ROBERT EASTON
(818) 985-2222

ROBIN EISENMAN
(213) 953-7680

ENTERTAINMENT SERVICES INTERNATIONAL
204 S. Beverly Dr., #109
Beverly Hills, CA 90212
(310) 888-1128

FAITH ACTING STUDIOS
3725 Don Felipe Dr.
Los Angeles, CA 90008
(213) 295-4996

OTTO FELIX
11377 W. Olympic, #125
Los Angeles, CA 90025
(310) 470-1939

CHRISTINA FERRA
The Actors Edge Workshop
(310) 652-4399

NINA FOCH STUDIO
(310) 553-5805

BONNIE FORWARD
(310) 399-5544

KATHLEEN FREEMAN ENTERPRISES
11026 Ventura Blvd.
Studio City, CA 91604
(818) 781-5096

FULLERTON ACTING LABORATORY
1619 E. Chapman Ave.
Fullerton, CA 92631
(714) 449-1488

LEO GARCIA
(310) 828-5475

THE GATEWAY THEATRE
3018 Carmel St.
Los Angeles, CA 90065
(818) 247-9544

THE WILL GEER THEATRICUM BOTANICUM
P.O. Box 1222
Topanga, CA 90290
(310) 455-2322
Classical theatre

ELLEN GERSTEIN
(213) 852-0276

MARIA GOBETTI
The Victory Theatre
3326 W. Victory Blvd.
Burbank, CA 91505
(818) 843-9253

ARLENE GOLONKA
Westside Studio
1266 W. Olympic Blvd.
Los Angeles, CA 90015
(310) 281-3130

DON GORDON
(213) 856-2808
Contact: Mark Helm

GERALD GORDON
(818) 994-8684

OFRAY HALL
Haunted Studios
6419 Hollywood Blvd.
Los Angeles, CA 90028
(213) 465-5224
Classical theatre

PAMELA HALL
(818) 996-0505
Music/musical theatre

STANLEY MYRON HANDELMAN
(818) 883-7175

ROBERT HANLEY
Actors Studio
6514 Lankershim Blvd.
North Hollywood, CA
(818) 909-0841

ESTELLE HARMAN ACTORS WORKSHOP, INC.
522 La Brea Ave.
Los Angeles, CA 90046
(213) 931-8137

CHRISTINA HART
Hollywood Court Theater
(213) 464-3018

JACK HELLER
(213) 850-6328

RANDEE HELLER
(818) 901-1066

JUDY HELM
PO Box 2546
Toluca Laka, CA 91610-0546
(818) 848-6887

SHERYL HENDERSON
The Downtown Playhouse
929 E. 2nd St., #105
Los Angeles, CA 90012
(213) 626-6906

DANIEL HENNING
(213) 662-7734, ext. 4

LAURA HENRY STUDIO
626½ Santa Monica Blvd., #207
Santa Monica, CA 90401
(310) 319-1912

ROBERT HERNANDEZ
Showcase Playhouse
6572 Santa Monica Blvd.
Los Angeles, CA 90038
(310) 278-1457

ADAM HILL ACTORS STUDIO
c/o The McCadden Theatre
1157 N. McCadden Place
Hollywood, CA 90028
(213) 466-9774

MICHAEL HOLMES ACTING WORKSHOPS
(818) 786-1045

DIANNE HULL, PRIVATE COACH
(310) 828-0632

LORRIE HULL, PH.D., WORKSHOPS FOR
ADULTS & YOUTH
(310) 828-0632
Classes in Santa Monica and West Los Angeles

INNER CITY CULTURAL CENTER
1605 N. Ivar St.
Los Angeles, CA 90028
(213) 388-3047

INTERNATIONAL CALIFORNIA STUDIO
1111 N. Brand Blvd.
Glendale, CA 91202
(818) 543-1211
Contact: John Macker

TAYLOR JACOBS
10355 Mount Gleason
Sunland, CA 91040
(818) 819-4955

LAURA JAMES
(818) 562-3075

KIMBERLY JENTZEN
Living the Art Institute
P.O. Box 8456
Universal City, CA 91618-0456
(818) 509-1311

ANITA JESSE ACTORS' WORKSHOP
859 Hollywood Way, Suite 251
Burbank, CA 91505-2814
(213) 876-2870

JILL-MORE BROWN PLAYERS
(818) 766-9678

BECKY KEMMERER
(310) 364-2261

TERI KEMPNER
(818) 508-4812

JUDY KERR'S ACTING WORKSHOP
(213) 874-7330

LEIGH KILTON-SMITH
2140 Beech Knoll Road
Los Angeles, CA 90046
(213) 650-4204

DAPHNE ECKLER KIRBY ACTING
WORKSHOPS
(818) 769-9709

JACK KOSSLYN ACTING WORKSHOP
666½ N. Robertson
Los Angeles, CA 90069
(213) 656-1591

L.A. SCENE STEALERS
(310) 302-1166

L.A. SHAKESPEARE COMPANY
15752 Enadia Way
Van Nuys, CA 91406
(818) 989-7221
Classical

ALAN LANGDON
(818) 887-6425

DAVID LEHMAN
(818) 845-1549

BUD LESLIE
(213) 660-5720

M.K. LEWIS WORKSHOPS
1513 6th St.
Santa Monica, CA 90401
(310) 826-8118
(310) 394-2511

JAN LINDER
(818) 996-7464

JOANNE LINVILLE
(213) 656-2040

MICHAEL RAY LLOYD
(818) 592-0778

PETER LOONEY
(213) 257-9741

THE LOS ANGELES REPERTORY CO.
6560 Hollywood Blvd., 2nd fl.
Hollywood, CA 90028
(213) 464-8542

LOS ANGELES WOMEN'S SHAKESPEARE
COMPANY WORKSHOPS
1231 Harvard, #D
Santa Monica, CA 90404
(310) 453-5069

THE LOST STUDIO
130 S. La Brea Ave.
Los Angeles, CA 90036
(213) 933-6944

JONATHAN LURIA
(310) 470-6027

DEBRA MAGIT
(310) 826-2946

ROSIE MALEK-YONAN
(818) 249-8989

NANCY MALONE
9911 W. Pico
Los Angeles, CA 90035
(818) 762-8641

NED MANDERINO
(213) 665-0123

MARTIN ALLEY PLAYERS
10543 Valley Spring Lane
North Hollywood, CA 91602
(818) 760-0339

ALLAN MILLER
(818) 907-6262

MOJO ENSEMBLE
1540 Cahuenga Blvd.
Hollywood, CA 90028
(213) 938-2953

BOB MONROE
American Renegade Theatre
11305 Magnolia
(818) 909-7727

FRAN MONTANO ACTORS WORKOUT
STUDIO
(818) 760-3052

JUDITH DOTY MORSE
(818) 766-5424

MITCHELL NESTOR
(310) 572-7955

SHEREE NORTH
(310) 459-1221

NU WEST PICTURES
15455 Redhill Ave., Bldg. 10, Suite F
Tustin, CA 92680
(714) 258-1922

ODYSSEY THEATRE ENSEMBLE
2055 S. Sepulveda Blvd.
Los Angeles, CA 90025
(310) 477-2055

LAUREL OLLSTEIN
(310) 558-8119

THE ONSTAGE COMPANY
(818) 753-3302

OPEN FIST THEATRE
1625 N. La Brea Ave.
Los Angeles, CA 90028
(213) 882-6912

SUSAN PERETZ STUDIOS
(213) 852-0614

PLAYHOUSE WEST SCHOOL AND REPERTORY
THEATER
4250 Lankershim Blvd.
North Hollywood, CA 91602
(818) 506-6345

PRIMETIME ACTORS STUDIO INC.
3405 Cahuenga Blvd. West
Los Angeles, CA 90068
(213) 874-4131

PROFESSIONAL SCHOOL FOR THE ARTS
1321 Sartori Ave.
Torrance, CA 90501
(310) 328-7664

PRO-SING
(800) 66-VOCAL
Music and musical theatre

RAMONA RHOADES
Take One Studios
(213) 876-2007

MICHAEL RINEY
(213) 964-2286

TRACY ROBERTS ACTORS STUDIO
141 S. Robertson Blvd.
Los Angeles, CA 90048
(310) 271-2730

STUART ROBINSON
(310) 558-4961

RACHEL ROY
(213) 655-4402

JOE SALAZAR
(213) 882-6433

SAN JOSE CIVIC LIGHT OPERA
1717 Technology Dr.
San Jose, CA 95110
(408) 453-7100

PETER SANDS
(818) 759-9928

SANTA MONICA PLAYHOUSE
1211 4th St.
Santa Monica, CA 90401
(310) 394-9779

STU SCHREIBER
(818) 508-4812

AL SECUNDA
(213) 654-8821

RICK SEVY ACTORS STUDIO
7278 Hollywood Blvd.
West Hollywood, CA 90046
(213) 874-7014

SHOWCASE LAB DIRECTED BY MARK
TAYLOR
13020 Otsego St.
Sherman Oaks, CA 91423
(818) 753-6623

GAMMY SINGER'S SCENE STUDY
(213) 460-2453

SOUNDSTAGE STUDIOS
324 S. Beverly Dr., Suite 200
Beverly Hills, CA 90212
(310) 282-0882

SOUTH COAST REPERTORY
655 Town Center Dr.
Costa Mesa, CA 92628-2197
(714) 957-2602, Ext. 210

AARON SPEISER WORKSHOP
2642 Highland Ave.
Santa Monica, CA 90405
(310) 399-4567

GUY STOCKWELL
(818) 761-8240

THE ERIC STONE STUDIO
(213) 460-2580

THE LEE STRASBERG THEATRE INSTITUTE
7936 Santa Monica Blvd.
Los Angeles, CA 90046
(213) 650-7777

STRICTLY THEATRE
(213) 953-4336

TAKE ONE STUDIOS
(213) 876-2007

THEATRE GEO
1229 N. Highland Ave.
Hollywood, CA 90038
(213) 462-3348
Contact: Geo Hartley

THEATRE OF ARTS
4128 Wilshire Blvd.
Los Angeles, CA 90010
(213) 380-0511

TOBIAS COMMUNICATIONS
(800) 995-2096

JOY TODD CASTING CORPORATION
(818) 752-6971

T.O.E. DRAMA WORKSHOP
(818) 344-1618

THE TRAVIS GROUP
12229 Ventura Blvd., Ste. 204
Studio City, CA 91604-2519
(818) 508-4600

ALISON VAIL
(310) 822-9699

THOMAS G. WAITES/NEW YORK THEATER
6468 Santa Monica Blvd.
Hollywood, CA 90038
(213) 462-1973; (310) 478-6399

CAROL WEISS MUSICAL THEATRE
WORKSHOP
(213) 460-6006

DAVID WELLS/SALLY PIPER STUDIO
12500 Riverside Dr., 204
Studio City, CA 91604
(818) 990-0036

CARYN WEST
(818) 785-2392

JUDITH WESTON
Two Lights Acting Studio
3447 Motor Ave.
Los Angeles, CA 90034
(310) 390-1315

VERNA WINTERS STUDIO FOR THE
PERFORMING ARTS
1312 Bonita Ave.
Berkeley, CA 94709
(510) 524-1601

JANET ZARISH/JOHN DE LANCIE
6470 Santa Monica Blvd.
Los Angeles, CA 90038
(310) 330-8892

COMEDY/IMPROVISATION

ACME COMEDY THEATRE
135 N. La Brea Ave.
Los Angeles, CA 90028
(213) 525-0202

GARY AUSTIN WORKSHOPS
(818) 753-9000

JUDY BROWN'S STAND-UP COMEDY
WORKSHOP
Upfront Comedy Club
123 Broadway
Santa Monica, CA 90401
(310) 396-8425

JUDY CARTER'S STAND-UP COMEDY
WORKSHOPS
(310) 915-0555

THE COMEDY COACH
(818) 344-4587
Contact: Steve North

COMEDY HILL
McCadden Theatre
1157 McCadden Place
Hollywood, CA 90046
(213) 467-1745

THE COMEDY STORE
8433 W. Sunset Blvd.
West Hollywood, CA 90046
(213) 460-2426

GREG DEAN'S STAND-UP COMEDY
WORKSHOP
P.O. Box 2929
Hollywood, CA 90078
(310) 285-3799

ANDY GOLDBERG
(213) 658-6945

GOLDEN ENTERTAINMENT & MANAGEMENT
4404 Riverside Dr.
Burbank, CA 91505
(213) 874-9225

THE GROUNDLINGS SCHOOL
7307 Melrose Ave.
Los Angeles, CA 90046
(213) 934-4747

THE ICE HOUSE COMEDY CLINIC COMEDY
WORKSHOPS
(213) 463-1567

THE IMPROV ACADEMY
8162 Melrose Ave.
Los Angeles, CA 90046
(213) 651-2583

L.A. CONNECTION COMEDY THEATRE
13442 Ventura Blvd.
Sherman Oaks, CA 91423
(818) 710-1320

L.A. THEATRESPORTS
Theatre/Theater
1713 Cahuenga Blvd.
Los Angeles, CA 90028
(213) 469-9689

THE HARVEY LEMBECK COMEDY
WORKSHOP
(310) 271-2831

METRO NORTH IMPROV TROUPE
47 N. Grand Oaks Ave.
Pasadena, CA 91107
(818) 793-4752

JOHN MOODY IMPROV WORKSHOP
The Lionstar Theatre
12655 Ventura Blvd.
Studio City, CA
(818) 761-2115

ORANGE COUNTY CRAZIES
IMPROVISATIONAL COMEDY SCHOOL
115 E. Santa Ana Blvd.
Santa Ana, CA 92702
(714) 550-9900

IRA ROSENFELD
(818) 508-4242

THE SPOLIN CENTER
(818) 989-GAME
Contact: Gary Schwartz

ON-CAMERA (FILM, TV, COMMERCIAL)

AMERICAN FILM INSTITUTE
2021 N. Western Ave.
Warner Bldg., Rm. 105
Los Angeles, CA 90027
(213) 856-7690

ANDERSON/MCCOOK/WHITE
(310) 659-6939

PAMELA CAMPUS CASTING & COMMERCIAL
WORKSHOP
(310) 659-5013

FILM ACTING FOR THE
PROFESSIONAL/DAVID KAGEN
(818) 901-8879

FILM INDUSTRY WORKSHOPS, INC.
4047 Radford Ave.
Studio City, CA 91604
(818) 769-4146

MEGAN FOLEY
410 N. La Cienega Ave., #201
Los Angeles, CA 90048
(310) 659-4116

SANDRA FOX FILM ACTING
(818) 991-5931
Classes in Agoura Hills

ORANGE COUNTY COMMERCIAL ACTING
WORKSHOP
222 W. Main St., Suite 201
Tustin, CA 92680
(714) 832-1895

ALEXIA ROBINSON COMMERCIAL ACTING
WORKSHOP
(818) 716-5399

TEPPER/GALLEGOS, INC.
611 N. Larchmont Blvd., 1st fl.
Los Angeles, CA 90004
(213) 469-3577

TVI ACTORS STUDIO
13557 Ventura Blvd., 2nd fl.
Sherman Oaks, CA 91423
(818) 784-6500

VAN MAR ACADEMY OF MOTION PICTURE
& TV ACTING
(213) 650-8823

WEIST–BARRON–HILL ACTING FOR
TELEVISION AND FILM
4300 W. Magnolia Blvd.
Burbank, CA 91505
(818) 846-5595

CHICAGO

STAGE

ACT ONE STUDIOS
640 N. LaSalle, Studio 535
Chicago, IL 60610
(312) 787-9384

ACTORS' CENTER
3047 N. Lincoln Ave., Suite 390
Chicago, IL 60657
(312) 549-3303

THE ACTOR'S CONNECTION
676 N. LaSalle, Suite 418
Chicago, IL 60610
(312) 464-3230

ACTOR'S TRAINING INSTITUTE
3300 N. Lake Shore Dr., Suite 14D
Chicago, IL 60657
(312) 871-0349

ACTOR'S WORKSHOP
1350 N. Wells, Suite A-300
Chicago, IL 60610
(312) 337-6602

CHICAGO ACTORS STUDIO
833 W. Chicago
Chicago, IL 60622
(312) 733-1955

IMPULSE STUDIO
1206 W. Webster Ave.
Chicago, IL 60614
(312) 665-9600

STEVEN IVCICH STUDIO
1836 W. North Ave.
Chicago, IL 60622
(312) 235-9131

PIVEN THEATRE WORKSHOP
927 Noyes
Evanston, IL 60201
(708) 866-6597

RAVEN THEATRE WORKSHOP PROGRAM
6931 N. Clark
Chicago, IL 60626
(312) 338-2177

SARANTOS STUDIOS
2857 N. Halsted
Chicago, IL 60657
(312) 528-7114
(708) 848-1100

SCANLON/SWANBECK
676 N. LaSalle, Suite 418
Chicago, IL 60610
(312) 935-7355

TRAINING CENTER FOR THE WORKING
ACTOR
1346 W. Devon Ave.
Chicago, IL 60660
(312) 508-0200

VICTORY GARDENS THEATRE
2257 N. Lincoln Ave.
Chicago, IL 60614
(312) 549-5788

COMEDY/IMPROVISATION

THE FREE ASSOCIATES
Ivanhoe Theatre
750 W. Wellington
Chicago, IL 60657
(312) 383-1260

IMPROV INSTITUTE
2319 W. Belmont
Chicago, IL 60619
(312) 929-2323

IMPROVOLYMPIC THEATER
3541 Clark
Chicago, IL 60657
(312) 880-0199

PLAYERS WORKSHOP OF THE SECOND CITY
2636 N. Lincoln Ave.
Chicago, IL 60614
(312) 929-6288

SECOND CITY TRAINING CENTER
1616 N. Wells St.
Chicago, IL 60614
(312) 664-9837

MONOLOGUE/AUDITION

THE AUDITION STUDIO
20 W. Hubbard St., Suite 2E
Chicago, IL 60610
(312) 527-4566

THE AUDITION WORKSHOP
5040 N. Marine Dr., Suite 3A
Chicago, IL 60640
(312) 334-4196

LONDON
ACTING SCHOOLS

THE BIRMINGHAM SCHOOL OF SPEECH AND
DRAMA
45 Church Rd.
Edgbaston, Birmingham B15 35W
011-44-121-454-3424

BRITISH AMERICAN DRAMA ACADEMY
136 Hoyt's Hill
Bethel, CT, 06801
(203) 794-1018

CENTRAL SCHOOL OF SPEECH AND DRAMA
The Embassy Theatre
64 Eaton Ave.
London NW3 3HY
011-44-171-722-8183

LONDON ACADEMY OF
MUSIC AND DRAMATIC ART
Tower House
226 Cromwell Road
London SW5 OSR
011-44-171-373-9883

LONDON ACADEMY OF PERFORMING ARTS
2 Effie Rd.
Fulham Broadway,
London SW6 1TB
011-44-171-736-0121

ROYAL ACADEMY OF DRAMATIC ART
62-64 Gower St.
London WC1E 6ED
011-44-171-636-7076

WEBBER DOUGLAS ACADEMY
30 Clareville St.
London SW7 5AP
011-44-171-370-4154

Commercial Print Agencies and Management Firms

The following list of selected East Coast commercial print agencies is supplied courtesy of Scott Powers Productions, Inc. It is not intended as an endorsement but is for informational purposes only. Agents insist that all initial contact be made through the mail.

NEW YORK CITY

ABRAMS ARTISTS & ASSOCIATES LTD.
420 Madison Ave., 14th fl.
New York, NY 10017
(212) 935-8980
Contact: Anna Liza Recto

BOOKERS, INC.
150 Fifth Ave., Suite 834
New York, NY 10011
(212) 645-9706
Contact: Tim Ousey

CUNNINGHAM, ESCOTT, DIPENE & ASSOCIATES
118 E. 25th St., 6th fl.
New York, NY 10010
(212) 477-3838
Contact: Sharon Reich

FUNNYFACE TODAY MODELS
151 E. 31st St., Suite 24J
New York, NY 10016
(212) 686-4343
Contact: Gary Bertalovitz
Jane Blum

THE GARRISON GROUP
151 E. 31st St., Suite 24J
New York, NY 10016
(212) 686-4361
Contact: Gary Bertalovitz
Paula Tackler

ELAINE GORDON MODEL MANAGEMENT, LTD.
1926 Helen Court
Merrick, NY 11566
(212) 936-1001
(516) 623-7736
Contact: Elaine Gordon

LIFESTYLES TALENT MANAGEMENT
900 Broadway, Suite 600
New York, NY 10003
(212) 460-0920
Contact: Michael Gingold
Paul Carmody

MCDONALD/RICHARDS, INC.
156 Fifth Ave., Suite 222
New York, NY 10010
(212) 627-3100
Contact: Debbi Kowall
Maureen Larkin

FIFI OSCARD AGENCY, INC.
24 W. 40th St., 17th fl.
New York, NY 10018
(212) 764-1100
Contact: Tina Cucci

ROGERS & LERMAN
37 E. 28th St., 4th fl.
New York, NY 10016
(212) 889-8233
Contact: Wally Rogers
Peter Lerman

GILLA ROOS, LTD.
16 W. 22nd St., 7th fl.
New York, NY 10010
(212) 727-7820
Contact: David Roos
Janine Minunno
Lauren Green

VAN DER VEER PEOPLE, INC.
400 E. 57th St., Suite 14N
New York, NY 10022
(212) 688-2880
Contact: Sara Zell
Lisa Keys

NEW JERSEY

CHRISTINE MODELS & CASTING
19 Castles Dr.
Wayne, NJ 07470
(201) 696-6950
Contact: Christine Jaeger

MEREDITH MODEL MANAGEMENT
10 Furler St.
Totowa, NJ 07512
(201) 812-0122
Contact: Joyce Meredith
Sharon Norrell

CONNECTICUT

JOHNSTON AGENCY
50 Washington St.
South Norwalk, CT 06854
(203) 838-6188
Contact: Esther Johnston

JOANNA LAWRENCE AGENCY
82 Partrick Rd.
Westport, CT 06880
(203) 226-7239
Contact: Robin Delaney

MARYLAND

CENTRAL CASTING
2229 N. Charles St.
Baltimore, MD 21218
(410) 889-3200
Contact: Beth Schiff
Joni Tackette

TAYLOR ROYALL
2308 South Rd.
Baltimore, MD 21209
(410) 466-5959
Contact: Patty Royall

WASHINGTON, D.C.

CENTRAL CASTING
623 Pennsylvania Ave., S.E.
Washington, DC 20003
(202) 547-6300
Contact: Dagmar Wittmer
Carol Ness

PENNSYLVANIA

EXPRESSIONS MODELING & TALENT
104 Church St.
Philadelphia, PA 19106
(215) 923-4420
Contact: Diana Juliano

GREER LANGE ASSOCIATES, INC.
18 Great Valley Parkway, Suite 180
Malvern, PA 19355
(215) 647-5515
Contact: Greer Lange

REINHARD
2021 Arch St. Suite 400
Philadelphia, PA 19103
(215) 567-2008
Contact: Mary Beth McAndrews

Business Theatre Producers

The following is a list of companies that are signatory with the current agreement of Actors' Equity Association governing employment in business theatre. Some business theatre producers cast through agencies, some from submitted pictures and résumés, and some through casting directors.

ANIFORMS
375 Hudson St.
New York, NY 10014
(212) 714-2550
Gary Seltzer, senior VP, production

BATWIN & ROBIN PRODUCTIONS
151 W. 19th St., 10th fl.
New York, NY 10011
(212) 243-0229
Linda Batwin, president

RAY BLOCH PRODUCTIONS
763 Traberg Ave.
Atlanta, GA 30318
(404) 351-6111
Robert Koors, owner & president

OTHER LOCATION:
RAY BLOCH PRODUCTIONS
16 W. 22nd St.
New York, NY 10010
(212) 366-6565
Franklin Dickson, president

THE CARIBINER GROUP
16 W. 61st St.
New York, NY 10023
(212) 541-3037
Patty Soll, VP in charge of production

MICHAEL CARSON PRODUCTIONS
250 W. 54th St.
New York, NY 10019
(212) 765-2300
Michael Carson, president

NEIL CERBONE ASSOCIATES
137 Riverside Dr., #9E
New York, NY 10024
Mark Tollefson, producer

CORPORATE MAGIC
6221 North O'Connor, #106
Irving, TX 75039
(214) 869-1919
Trish Parks, production coordinator

DRURY DESIGN DYNAMICS
49 W. 27th St.
New York, NY 10001
(212) 213-4600
Michael Metts, talent director

EAST END PRODUCTIONS
768 Brannan St.
San Francisco, CA 94103
(415) 864-4956
Chris Haigh, creative director/executive producer

ENVISION CORPORATION
270 Congress St.
Boston, MA 02210
(617) 482-3444
Andrew Zamore, producer

GOODSIGHT–HERRMANN
7 Macculloch Ave.
Morristown, NJ 07960
(201) 993-8400
Keith Herrmann

HELLER CREATIVE, INC.
14 Foothill St.
Putnam Valley, NY 10579
(914) 528-6328
Buck Heller, president

KBD INNOVATIVE ARTS
5 E. 16th St.
New York, NY 10003
(212) 206-1717

OTHER LOCATION:
KBD INNOVATIVE ARTS
13360 Beach Ave.
Marina del Rey, CA 90292
(310) 578-5452
Dan McPhee, VP of production

MARITZ PERFORMANCE IMPROVEMENT COMPANY
1350 N. Highway Dr.
Fenton, MO 63099
(314) 827-1273
Margaret Brunsman, production coordinator

MCKONE & COMPANY
1900 Westridge
Irving, TX 75038
(214) 550-7433
Ron Biancardi, executive producer

MEGA PRODUCTIONS
420 E. 58th St., #19B
New York, NY 10022
(212) 644-8173
Ken Robbins, executive producer

MJM CREATIVE SERVICES, INC.
255 W. 26th St., 3rd fl.
New York, NY 10001
(212) 924-7070
Bryden Becker

JACK MORTON PRODUCTIONS
680 Lakeshore Dr.
Chicago, IL 60611
(312) 440-9700
William Kahn, VP & general manager

OTHER LOCATIONS:
JACK MORTON PRODUCTIONS
233 Peachtree St., N.E.
Atlanta, GA 30303
(404) 659-2262
Richard Anderson, director of
communication services

JACK MORTON PRODUCTIONS
210 South St.
Boston, MA 02111
(617) 426-6800
Kim Novick, executive producer

JACK MORTON PRODUCTIONS
110 Pine Ave.
Long Beach, CA 90802
(310) 436-6363
Don Kobayashi, general manager

JACK MORTON PRODUCTIONS
300 1st Ave. N., #330
Minneapolis, MN 55401
(612) 338-9000
Steve Anderson, creative director

JACK MORTON PRODUCTIONS
641 Ave. of the Americas
New York, NY 10011
(212) 727-0400
Laura Shuler, VP/general manager

JACK MORTON PRODUCTIONS
31550 W. Big Beaver, Suite 201
Troy, MI 48084
(810) 643-0090
Robert Walker, producer

JACK MORTON PRODUCTIONS
1725 K St., #1400
Washington, DC 20006
(202) 296-9300
Lisa Cordo, producer

PURCELL PRODUCTIONS
484 W. 43rd St., #23M
New York, NY 10036
(212) 279-0795
Don Purcell, president

TWINSUN MUSIC, LTD.
315 Riverside Dr., #16A
New York, NY 10025
(212) 222-3420
Thomas Tierney, president

VISUAL DESIGN GROUP
40 Richards Ave.
Norwalk, CT 06854
(203) 838-3700
Pat Saunders, producer

VISUAL SERVICES, INC.
11135 Knott Ave., Suite C
Cypress, CA 90630
(714) 373-4445
Gary Rivera, executive producer

THE ZINK GROUP
245 W. 19th St.
New York, NY 10011
(212) 929-2949
Bill Buxton, general manager,
productions

Equity Theatre for Young Audiences Companies

The following alphabetically lists TYA companies under Equity contract in the Eastern, Midwestern, and Western United States, followed by an address, phone number, and the name of the artistic and/or producing director. An asterisk (*) indicates companies not currently active on TYA contract.

EASTERN STATES

ALABAMA SHAKESPEARE FESTIVAL
1 Festival Dr.
Montgomery, AL 36117
(334) 271-1640
Contact: Beau Williams

ALHAMBRA DINNER THEATRE
12000 Beach Blvd.
Jacksonville, FL 32246
(904) 642-9307
Contact: Tod Booth

ALLIANCE THEATRE
Robert W. Woodruff Arts Center
1280 Peachtree St. NE
Atlanta, GA 30309
(404) 733-4650
Contact: Edith H. Love

AMERICAN STAGE
P.O. Box 1560
211 3rd St. So.
St. Petersburg, FL 33731
(813) 823-1600
Contact: John Berglund

ARTS GENESIS
310 E. 46th St., Suite 26J
New York, NY 10017
(201) 433-2787
Contact: Roger Shea

ARTS POWER, INC.
P.O. Box 321
Ridgewood, NJ 07451-0321
(201) 652-0100
Contact: Gary Blackman

BLUE HERON THEATRE
645 West End Ave.
New York, NY 10025
(212) 787-0422
Contact: Ardele Striker

BROADWAY ARTS COMPANY
31 W. 56th St.
New York, NY 10019
(212) 245-4680
Contact: Karen Butler

THE BROADWAY PIXIE JUDY TROUPE
8 E. 64th St.
New York, NY 10021
(212) 688-1740
Contact: Judith Abrams

CALEDONIA THEATRE CO.
Totem Pole Playhouse
P.O. Box 603
Fayetteville, PA 17222
(717) 352-2164
Contact: Carl Schurr

CLEVELAND PLAYHOUSE
8500 Euclid Ave.
Cleveland, OH 44106
(216) 795-7010
Contact: Dean Galbdean

CYGNET PRODUCTIONS INC.*
339 E. 10th St., #4E
New York, NY 10009
(212) 473-6678
Contact: Sterling Swann

FANFARE THEATRE ENSEMBLE
100 E. 4th St.
New York, NY 10003
(212) 674-8181
Contact: Joan Shepard

FLATROCK PLAYHOUSE
P.O. Box 310
Flatrock, NC 28731-0310
(704) 693-0731
Contact: Robin Farquhar

FLEETWOOD STAGE COMPANY
701 N. MacQuesten Parkway, Suite 179
Mt. Vernon, NY 10552
(914) 667-3671
Contact: Lewis Arlt

FREEDOM THEATRE
1346 N. Broad St.
Philadelphia, PA 19121
(215) 765-2793
Contact: Walter Dallas

GINGERBREAD PLAYERS & JACK
35-06 88th St.
Jackson Heights, NY 11372
Contact: John Ahearn

KENNEDY CENTER THEATRE FOR YOUNG
PEOPLE
Kennedy Center for the Performing Arts
Washington, DC 20566
(202) 416-8838
Contact: Derek Gordon

LARK THEATRE COMPANY
395 Riverside Dr., #12B
New York, NY 10025
(212) 727-3626
Contact: John C. Eisner

LINCOLN CENTER INSTITUTE
70 Lincoln Center Plaza, 7th fl.
New York, NY 10023
(212) 875-5547
Contact: Andrew Berger

MAXIMILLION PRODUCTIONS
98 Riverside Dr. #7H
New York, NY 10024
(212) 874-3121
Contact: Peggy Traktman, Max
Traktman

NATIONAL COMMUNITY AIDS PARTNERSHIP
Heart Strings
P.O. Box 314
Anniston, AL 36202
(205) 238-8336
Contact: Dena Kirkland

NEW YORK STATE THEATRE INSTITUTE
P.O. Box 28
Troy, NY 12181-0028
(518) 274-3200
Contact: Patricia Snyder

NIGHT KITCHEN
10 E. 53rd St.
New York, NY 10022
(212) 207-7340
Contact: Arthur Yorinks

NORTH SHORE MUSIC THEATRE
Box 62
Beverly, MA 01915
(508) 922-8500
Contact: Jon Kimbell

PITTSBURGH CIVIC LIGHT OPERA
719 Liberty Ave.
Pittsburgh, PA 15222
(412) 281-3973
Contact: Charles Gray

PUBLIC THEATRE OF SOUTH FLORIDA
2301 NE 26th St.
Ft. Lauderdale, FL 33305
(305) 564-6770
Contact: Vince Rhomberg

PUSHCART PLAYERS
197 Bloomfield Ave.
Verona, NJ 07044
(201) 857-1115
Contact: Ruth Fost

SESAME STREET LIVE
VEE Corporation
LaSalle Plaza, Suite 1750
Minneapolis, MN 55402
(612) 375-9670
Contact: Vincent Egan

SHAKESPEARE & COMPANY*
The Mount
2 Plunkett St.
P.O. Box 865
Lenox, MA 01240
(413) 637-1197
Contact: Tina Packer

SHAKESPEARE FOR SCHOOLS*
P.O. Box 1828
Clifton, NJ 07015
(201) 614-9836
Contact: Janet Villas

SLIM GOODBODY CORP.
27 W. 20th St., #1207
New York, NY 10011
(212) 254-3300
Contact: John Burstein

STAGE ONE
Louisville Children's Theatre
425 W. Market St.
Louisville, KY 40202
(502) 589-5946
Contact: Moses Goldberg

STAGEWEST
Springfield Arts Association
One Columbus Center
Springfield, MA 01103-1441
(413) 781-4470
Contact: Eric Hill

STORYBOOK MUSICAL THEATRE
P.O. Box 473
Abington, PA 19001
(215) 659-8550
Contact: Marc Goldberg

STREET THEATRE TOURING COMPANY
228 Fisher Ave., Room 226
White Plains, NY 10606
(914) 761-3307
Contact: Gray Smith

THEATREWORKS/USA
890 Broadway, 7th fl.
New York, NY 10003
(212) 677-5959
Contact: Jay Harnick

TRAVELING PLAYHOUSE
104 Northampton Dr.
White Plains, NY 10603
(914) 946-5289
Contact: Ken Rockefeller

WHEELOCK FAMILY THEATRE
200 The River Way
Boston, MA 02215
Contact: Susan Kosoff

YATES MUSICAL THEATRE FOR CHILDREN
P.O. Box 42
Bloomfield, NJ 07003
(201) 677-0936
Contact: William Yates, Sr.

MIDWESTERN STATES

CLASSICS ON STAGE
P.O. Box 25365
Chicago, IL 60625
(708) 275-6836
Contact: Bob Boburka, Michelle Vacca

DRURY LANE CHILDREN'S THEATRE
2500 W. Drury Lane
Evergreen Park, IL 60805
(708) 422-8000
Contact: John R. Lazzara

DRURY LANE OAKBROOK
Children's Theatre
100 Drury Lane
Oak Brook Terrace, IL 60181
(708) 530-8300
Contact: Anthony DiSantis

FIRST STAGE PRODUCTIONS
929 N. Water St.
Milwaukee, WI 53202
(414) 273-7121
Contact: Rob Goodman

GREAT AMERICAN CHILDREN'S THEATRE CO.
P.O. Box 92123
Milwaukee, WI 53204
(414) 276-4230
Contact: Teri Solomon Mitze

M & W PRODUCTIONS INC.
P.O. Box 93910
Milwaukee, WI 53203-0910
(414) 272-7701
Contact: Michael Wilson

MUSIC THEATRE WORKSHOP
5647 N. Ashland
Chicago, IL 60660
(312) 561-7100
Contact: Meade Palidofsky

OLD LOG CHILDREN'S THEATRE
Box 250
Excelsior, MN 55331
(612) 474-5951
Contact: Don Stolz

SEEM TO BE PLAYERS
P.O. Box 1601
Lawrence, KS 66044
(913) 842-6622
Contact: Ric Averill

WESTERN STATES

A CONTEMPORARY THEATRE
100 W. Roy St.
Seattle, WA 98119
(206) 285-3220
Contact: Philip Schermer

BILINGUAL FOUNDATION OF THE ARTS
421 N. Avenue 19
Los Angeles, CA 90032
(213) 225-4044
Contact: Carmen Zapata

CASA MANANA PLAYHOUSE
P.O. Box 9054
Fort Worth, TX 76107
(817) 332-9313
Contact: Van Kaplan

DENVER CENTER THEATRE COMPANY*
1050 13th St.
Denver, CO 80204
(303) 893-4200
Contact: Kevin Maifield

SEATTLE CHILDREN'S THEATRE
305 Harrison St.
Seattle, WA 98109
(206) 443-0807
Contact: Thomas Pecher

SEATTLE REPERTORY*
155 Mercer St.
Seattle, WA 98109
(206) 443-2210
Contact: Benjamin Moore

SERENDIPITY THEATRE COMPANY*
c/o Coronet Theatre
366 North LaCienega Blvd.
Los Angeles, CA 90048
(213) 652-9199
Contact: Jody Johnston-Davidson

SOUTH COAST REPERTORY
655 Town Center Dr.
P.O. Box 2197
Costa Mesa, CA 92626-1197
(714) 957-2602
Contact: Paula Tomei

THEATRE WEST
3333 Cahuenga Blvd. W.
Los Angeles, CA 90068
(213) 851-4839
Contact: Joe Lucas

Cabaret Rooms

The following is a list of cabaret venues in selected cities across the country. They range from clubs that book up-and-coming performers to those that book only well-known established acts. When contacting the booking agent, be sure to check booking policy (auditions, appointments, open mike nights), tech arrangements, if and how a fee is determined, and whether the club provides publicity.

NEW YORK

THE OAK ROOM AT THE ALGONQUIN HOTEL
59 W. 44th St.
New York, NY 10036
(212) 840-6800
Contact: Arthur Pomposello

B. SMITH'S ROOFTOP CAFE
771 8th Ave.
New York, NY 10036
(212) 247-2222
Contact: Helen Claydon-Way

BIRDLAND
2475 Broadway
New York, NY 10025
(212) 749-2228
Contact: John Valenti
Jazz singers only

THE BITTER END
147 Bleecker St.
New York, NY 10012
(212) 673-7030
Contact: Ken Gorka
Eclectic bookings

THE BLUE NOTE
131 W. 3rd St.
New York, NY 10012
Jazz singers

CAFE CARLYLE
35 E. 76th St.
New York, NY 10021
(212) 744-1600
Contact: René Peyrat or James Sherwin

CLUB AT LA MAMA
74A E. 4th St.
New York, NY 10003
(212) 475-7710
Contact: Meryl Vladimer, (212) 254-6468

DANNY'S SKYLIGHT ROOM AT DANNY'S GRAND SEA PALACE
346 W. 46th St.
New York, NY 10036
(212) 265-8133
Contact: Ken Mallor

DON'T TELL MAMA
343 W. 46th St.
New York, NY 10036
(212) 757-0788
Contact: Sidney Myer
(212) 265-0001

THE DUPLEX
61 Christopher St.
New York, NY 10014
(212) 255-5438 (after 4 PM)
Contact: Amelia David, (212) 989-3015
(10 AM–5 PM)

EIGHTY EIGHT'S
228 W. 10th St.
New York, NY 10014
(212) 924-0088
Contact: Erv Raible

5 & 10 NO EXAGGERATION
77 Greene St.
New York, NY 10012
(212) 925-7414
Contact: Robert Mergler

55 GROVE STREET (UPSTAIRS AT ROSE'S TURN)
55 Grove St.
New York, NY 10014
(212) 366-5438
Contact: Collette Black, (212) 366-9658

THE GREEN ROOM
338 W. 46th St.
New York, NY 10036
(212) 974-8897
Contact: Robert Petito

IRIDIUM
44 W. 63rd St.
New York, NY 10023
(212) 582-2121
Contact: Steve Hall or Ron Sturm
Jazz singers

JUDYS' RESTAURANT & CABARET
49 W. 44th St.
New York, NY 10036
(212) 764-8930
Contact: Richard Hendrickson

KAPTAIN BANANA
101 Greene St.
New York, NY 10012
(212) 343-9000
Contact: Michael or Richard
Revues

MICHAEL'S PUB
211 E. 55th St.
New York, NY 10022
(212) 758-2272
Contact: Gil Wiest, Owner

RAINBOW & STARS
30 Rockefeller Plaza, 65th fl.
New York, NY 10112
(212) 632-4000
Contact: Vivian Antin

THE SUPPER CLUB
240 W. 47th St.
New York, NY 10036
(212) 921-1940

TATOU
151 E. 50th St.
New York, NY 10022
(212) 753-1144
Contact: Allen Middleton

TAVERN ON THE GREEN CHESTNUT ROOM
Central Park at W. 67th St.
New York, NY 10023
(212) 873-3200
Contact: Len Triola
2975 Johnson Pl.
Wantagh, NY 11793
(516) 781-2749

THE TRIAD
158 W. 72nd St.
New York, NY 10023
(212) 595-7400
Contact: Nancy McGraw

WEST BANK CAFE
407 W. 42nd St.
New York, NY 10036
(212) 695-6909
Contact: Rand Foerster or Hank Meiman

WESTBETH THEATRE MUSIC HALL
151 Bank St.
New York, NY 10014
(212) 691-2272
Contact: Arnold Engelman

LOS ANGELES

CATALINA BAR AND GRILL
1640 N. Cahuenga Blvd.
Hollywood, CA 90028
(213) 466-2210
Jazz singers

CINEGRILL
Radisson Hollywood Roosevelt Hotel
7000 Hollywood Blvd.
Hollywood, CA 90028
(213) 466-7000
Contact: J.D. Kessler

GARDENIA
7066 Santa Monica Blvd.
W. Hollywood, CA 90038
(213) 467-7444
Contact: Tom Rolla

JAZZ BAKERY
3233 Helms Ave.
Culver City, CA
(310) 271-9039
Contact: Ruth Price

LARGO PUB
432 N. Fairfax Ave.
Los Angeles, CA
(213) 852-1073

LUNA PARK
665 N. Robertson Blvd.
West Hollywood, CA
(310) 652-0611

LUNARIA RESTAURANT AND JAZZ LOUNGE
10351 Santa Monica Blvd.
Los Angeles, CA 90025
(310) 282-8870
Contact: Bernard Jacoupy

SAN FRANCISCO

THE PLUSH ROOM AT THE YORK HOTEL
940 Sutter St.
San Francisco, CA 94109
(415) 885-6800
Contact: Tracy Walker

CHICAGO

GENTRY
712 N. Rush St.
Chicago, IL 60611
(312) 664-1033
Contact: David Edwards or John Turner

GENTRY ON HALSTED
3320 N. Halsted St.
Chicago, IL
(312) 348-1053

GOLD STAR SARDINE BAR
680 N. Lake Shore Dr.
Chicago, IL 60611
(312) 664-4215
Contact: Bill Allen

TOULOUSE COGNAC BAR
2140 N. Lincoln Park West
Chicago, IL 60614
(312) 665-9071
Contact by mail only: Nancy

YVETTE
1206 N. State Parkway
Chicago, IL 60610
(312) 280-1700
Contact by mail only: Nancy

YVETTE NORTH
604 N. Milwaukee Ave.
Wheeling, IL
(708) 419-0500

YVETTE WINTERGARDEN
311 S. Wacker Dr.
Chicago, IL 60606
(312) 408-1242
Contact by mail only: Nancy

BOSTON

CLUB CABARET AT CLUB CAFE
209 Columbus Ave.
Boston, MA 02116
(617) 536-0966
Contact (send tape, no calls): Frank

DIAMOND JIM'S AT THE LENOX HOTEL
710 Boylston St.
Boston, MA 02116
(617) 536-5300
Contact: Steve Uliss, (617) 421-1438

SCULLERS JAZZ CLUB
Guest Quarters Suite Hotel
400 Soldiers Field Rd.
Boston, MA 02134
(617) 562-4111

REGATTABAR
Charles Hotel, Harvard Square
Cambridge, MA 02138
(617) 876-7777
Contact: Water Music Management
(617) 876-8742
Jazz singers

NEW HOPE, PENNSYLVANIA

ODETTE'S
P.O. Box 127
South River Rd.
New Hope, PA 18938
(215) 862-2432
Contact: Bob Egan, (215) 794-7716

WASHINGTON, D.C.

BLUES ALLEY
Rear of 1073 Wisconsin Ave. N.W.
Washington, DC 20007
(202) 337-4141
Contact: Ralph Camilli

Comedy Clubs

Here are comedy clubs for New York City, Los Angeles, and Chicago and their environs.

NEW YORK CITY

BOSTON COMEDY CLUB
82 W. 3rd St.
New York, NY 10012
(212) 977-1000, Ext. 308
Booker: Risa Barish

CAROLINE'S COMEDY CLUB
1626 Broadway
New York, NY 10019
(212) 757-4100
Booker: Jocelyn Halloran

COMEDY CELLAR—NEW YORK
117 MacDougal St.
New York, NY 10012
(212) 254-3480
Booker: Estee Adoram

COMIC STRIP—NEW YORK
1568 Second Ave.
New York, NY 10021
(212) 861-9386
Booker: Lucien Hold

DANGERFIELD'S
1118 First Ave.
New York, NY 10021
(212) 593-1650
Booker: Linda Rohe

GLADYS' COMEDY ROOM AT HAMBURGER HARRY'S
145 W. 45th St.
New York, NY 10036
(212) 832-1762
Booker: Gladys

GRANDPA'S—STATEN ISLAND
106 New Dorp Plaza
Staten Island, NY 10306
(718) 667-4242
Booker: Top Draw Entertainment
(718) 896-4001

IMPROV AT SHUTTERS
433 W. 34th St.
New York, NY 10001
(212) 279-3446
Booker: Silver Friedman

NEW YORK COMEDY CLUB
241 E. 24th St.
New York, NY 10010
(212) 696-LAFF
Booker: Al Martin

PIPS COMEDY CLUB
2005 Emmons Ave.
Brooklyn, NY 11235
(718) 646-9433
Booker: Seth Schultz

STAND UP NY
236 W. 78th St.
New York, NY 10024
(212) 595-0850
Booker: Cary Hoffman

WEST END COMEDY CLUB
2911 Broadway (113th St.)
New York, NY 10025
(212) 662-8830
Booker: Bob Bleiberg
(212) 861-1564

LONG ISLAND AND UPSTATE NEW YORK

BANANAS—POUGHKEEPSIE
Best Western Hotel (Route 9)
Poughkeepsie, NY 12602
(914) 462-3333
Booker: ComedyWorks (NJ)
(908) 782-6799

BROKERAGE
2797 Merrick Rd.
Bellmore, NY 11710
(516) 785-8655
Booker: Linda Rohe

CHUCKLES COMEDY CLUB
159 Jericho Tpke.
Mineola, NY 11501
(516) 746-2770
Booker: Liz Socci

EAST END COMEDY CLUB
Southampton Inn
91 Hill St.
Southampton, NY 11968
(516) 283-5800
Booker: Top Draw Entertainment
(718) 896-4001

GOVERNOR'S COMEDY SHOP AND RESTAURANT
90A Division Ave.
Levittown, NY 11756
(516) 731-3358
Booker: Andrea Levy

MCGUIRES COMEDY CLUB
1627 Smithtown Ave.
Bohemia, NY 11716
(516) 467-5413
Booker: John R. Ryerson

NEW JERSEY

BANANAS COMEDY CLUB
Holiday Inn
50 Kenny Place
Saddlebrook, NJ 07024
(201) 909-0606
Booker: ComedyWorks (NJ)
(908) 782-6799

CASUAL TIMES
1085 Central Ave.
Clark, NJ 07066
(908) 388-6511
Booker: Top Draw Entertainment
(718) 896-4001

CATCH A RISING STAR—PRINCETON
Hyatt Regency
102 Carnegie Center
Princeton, NJ 08540
(609) 987-1234
Booker: Louis Faranda

COMEDY CABARET—MT. LAUREL
TravelLodge (Rte. 73 & NJ Tpke., Exit 4)
Mount Laurel, NJ 08054
(609) 866-JOKE

MITCHELL'S COMEDY CAFE
5 W. Broad St.
Palmyra, NJ 08065
(609) 829-3161
Booker: Joe Donato

RASCAL'S—AT THE SHORE
1500 Highway 35 South
Ocean Township, NJ 07712
(908) 517-0002
Booker: Top Draw Entertainment
(718) 896-4001

RASCAL'S—WEST ORANGE
425 Pleasant Valley Way
West Orange, NJ 07052
(201) 736-2726
Booker: Top Draw Entertainment
(718) 896-4001

CONNECTICUT

LAST LAUGH AT BROWN THOMSON
942 Main St.
Hartford, CT 06103
(203) 525-1600
Booker: John Schuler

TREEHOUSE COMEDY CLUB—MYSTIC
Best Western Inn (I-95, Exit 90)
Mystic, CT 06355
(203) 536-7126
Booker: Brad Axelrod

TREEHOUSE COMEDY CLUB—NORWALK
22 Isaac St.
Norwalk, CT 06854
(203) 838-2424
Booker: Brad Axelrod

LOS ANGELES

ACME COMEDY THEATRE
135 North La Brea Avenue
Los Angeles, CA 90036
(213) 525-0202

THE COMEDY & MAGIC CLUB
1018 Hermosa Avenue
Hermosa Beach, CA
(310) 372-1193
Booker: Dana Klein

COMEDY EXPRESS
9365 Monte Vista Ave.
Montclair, CA 91763
(909) 624-7867
Booker: Adam Berenson

THE COMEDY STORE
8433 Sunset Blvd.
Los Angeles, CA 90069
(213) 656-6225
Booker: Scott Day

COMEDY LAND
Pampatac Hotel
1717 West St.
Anaheim, CA 92802
(714) 957-2617
Booker: Kelly Jones-Craft

THE GROUNDLINGS
7307 Melrose Avenue
Los Angeles, CA 90046
(213) 934-4747

THE ICE HOUSE
24 N. Mentor Ave.
Pasadena, CA 91106
(818) 577-1894
Booker: Bob Fisher

IGBY'S COMEDY CABARET
11637 West Pico Blvd.
Los Angeles, CA
(310) 477-3553
Booker: Jan Smith

IMPROVISATION—IRVINE
4255 Campus Dr.
Irvine, CA 92715
(714) 854-5455
Booker: Robert Hartman

IMPROVISATION—LOS ANGELES
8162 Melrose Ave.
Hollywood, CA 90046
(213) 651-3625
Booker: Budd Friedman

L.A. CABARET COMEDY CLUB
17271 Ventura Blvd.
Encino, CA 91316
(818) 501-3737
Booker: Ray Bishop

L.A. CONNECTION COMEDY THEATER
13442 Ventura Blvd.
Sherman Oaks, CA 91423
(818) 784-1868
Booker: Kent Skov

LAUGH FACTORY
8001 Sunset Blvd.
W. Hollywood, CA 90046
(213) 656-8860
Booker: Jamie Masada

LONG BEACH COMEDY CLUB
49 S. Pine
Long Beach, CA 90802
(310) 437-6709
Booker: Francine Osborn

UPFRONT COMEDY
123 Broadway Ave.
Santa Monica, CA
(310) 319-3477

CHICAGO AREA

COMEDY WOMB
8030 W. Ogden Ave.
Lyons, IL 60534
(708) 442-0200
Booker: Mark Shufeldt

FUNNY BONE
1504 N. Naper Blvd.
Naperville, IL 60563
(708) 955-0500
Booker: Bert Borth

CHICAGO IMPROV
504 N. Wells
Chicago, IL 60610
(312) 782-6387
Booker: Tom Tenney

ZANIES—CHICAGO
1548 N. Wells St.
Chicago, IL 60610
(312) 337-4027
Booker: Bert Haas

ZANIES—MT. PROSPECT
2200 S. Elmhurst Rd.
Mt. Prospect, IL 60056
(708) 228-6166
Booker: Bert Haas

ZANIES—PHEASANT RUN
Pheasant Run Resort
North Ave., Route 64
St. Charles, IL 60174
(708) 513-1761
Booker: Bert Haas

ZANIES—VERNON HILL
230 Hawthorn Village Commons
Vernon Hill, IL
(708) 549-6030
Booker: Bert Haas

Regional Combined Auditions Nationwide

Remember that dates can change from year to year, so you should write early for information. Also, some auditions move sites from year to year, as noted; others are held in the same city each year.

EAST CENTRAL THEATRE CONFERENCE (ECTC)
Audition Dates: Mid-February (for three days).
Place: Varies within New York, New Jersey, Pennsylvania, Delaware, and Maryland.
Eligibility: Non-Equity and Equity.
Fee: To be determined.
Format: Two minutes for monologue or monologue plus song. Interviews for staff positions; application must be submitted.
Application Deadline: Early January.
For application, send SASE to:
    East Central Theatre Conference Auditions
    Attn: Tom Clark
    Genesee Community College, Batavia, NY 14020
    Phone (716) 343-0055, ext. 6448

ILLINOIS THEATRE ASSOCIATION
Audition Dates: Early March (for three days).
Place: Theatre Building, 1225 W. Belmont, Chicago.
Eligibility: Non-Equity.
Fee: $30, $25 for members.
Format: Three minutes without song, or four minutes with song; accompanist provided; performers and stage managers only.
For application, write to:
    Mr. Wallace Smith, Executive Director
    Illinois Theatre Association
    1225 W. Belmont, Chicago, IL 60657
    Phone (312) 929-7288

INDIANA THEATRE ASSOCIATION
Audition Date: Early February (for one day).
Place: Indianapolis, Indiana.
Eligibility: Member of professional union, or recommendation from professional director.
Fee: Nonrefundable audition fee, to be determined.
Format: Singing or nonsinging, two-minute limit; separate dance auditions. Interviews for tech/design/management.
Application Deadline: Mid-January.
For application, send SASE to:
    Linda Charbonneau
    Indiana Theatre Association
    Butler University Theatre
    4600 Sunset Ave.
    Indianapolis, IN 46208-3443
    Phone (317) 283-9666

LEAGUE OF RESIDENT THEATRES LOTTERY AUDITIONS (LORT)
These are eligible-performer auditions which are held once a year in New York City, Los Angeles, and Chicago. Since there are more applicants than available audition slots, selection is made by lottery, and you may attend only once out of every three successive auditions. There are also interviews for stage managers. Contact Actors' Equity Association for information.

MID-AMERICA THEATRE CONFERENCE AUDITIONS (MATC)

Audition Date: Mid-March (for three days).
Place: Varies within Iowa, Illinois, Kansas, Minnesota, Missouri, North Dakota, Nebraska, South Dakota, Wisconsin.
Eligibility: No residency requirement.
Fee: $30; includes registration fee and access to audition or interview. (After mid-February, fee is $35.)
Format: Two minutes, with or without song; pianist provided. Bring music in correct key. Interviews for technical and design positions. Singing/dancing auditions at end of each day.
Application Deadline: Mid-February. If audition slots are available after cutoff date, later applicants will receive time slots on a first-come, first-served basis.
For application, write to:
  Glenn Q. Pierce
  Mid-America Theatre Conference Auditions
  12528 S. Alcan Circle
  Olathe, KS 66062
  Phone (913) 768-0089

MIDWEST THEATRE AUDITIONS (MWTA)

Audition Date: Mid-February (for three days).
Place: Loretto-Hilton Center, Webster University, St. Louis, Missouri.
Eligibility: No residency requirements. Non-Equity application form, signed by an instructor or director. Dance calls are open to actors who have auditioned previously that day. Equity actors may audition and should request application.
Fee: $25. Bring at least 20 copies of résumé (picture/résumés for callbacks only).
Format: One and a half minutes to present one or two pieces; at least one must be nonmusical. Musical pieces are encouraged; pianist provided. Callbacks same day. Tech/design: portfolio presentation and interview.
Application Deadline: Postmarked by January 1.
For application, write to:
  Peter Sargent, Coordinator
  Midwest Theatre Auditions
  Webster University
  470 E. Lockwood
  St. Louis, MO 63119-3194

NATIONAL DINNER THEATRE ASSOCIATION (NDTA)

Audition Date: Mid-March (for one day).
Place: Varies; usually within Indiana, Kentucky, and Illinois.
Eligibility: Equity and non-Equity companies.
Fee: $25 (or $30 after deadline).
Format: One-minute monologue; 16 bars of song is optional; technicians can send résumé to be made available to producers. Applications are screened.
Application Deadline: Early March.
For application, send SASE to:
  National Dinner Theatre Association Auditions
  c/o David Pritchard
  P.O. Box 726
  Marshall, MI 49068
  Phone (616) 781-7859

NEW ENGLAND THEATRE CONFERENCE (NETC)

Audition Date: Mid-March (for three days).
Place: Boston.
Eligibility: Non-Equity; college students must be 18 or older and have application form signed by instructor or director. (We receive about 1250 applicants and screen to 800.) *Note:* Auditions open to Equity are held in the fall; these are organized by StageSource, 88 Tremont St., #714, Boston, MA 02108. No phone calls accepted.
Fee: $25 for NETC members; $35 nonmember students; $40 nonmember, nonstudent. All fees nonrefundable.
Format: Two audition rooms running concurrently—one for acting only, and one for acting/singing/dancing. Two-minute auditions. Technical and staff interviews also held.
Application Deadline: Postmarked early February; applications available in early December.
For application, send SASE to:
New England Theatre Conference
c/o Northeastern University Dept. of Theatre
360 Huntington Ave.
Boston, MA 02115

NEW JERSEY THEATRE GROUP (NJTG)

The association of the state's 18 Equity theatre companies holds a Job Fair for interns and entry-level technical, administrative, and production staff in April. Equity and non-Equity auditions are in late August and mid-February.
For information, write after January 1 to:
George Ryan, Director of Information Services
New Jersey Theatre Group
P.O. Box 21
Florham Park, NJ 07932
(201) 593-0189

NORTHWEST DRAMA CONFERENCE (NWDC)

Audition Date: Early February (for one day).
Place: Varies, within Idaho, Washington, Oregon, Wyoming, North Dakota, South Dakota.
Fee: $5.
Format: Three minutes, two monologues, plus 16 bars of song; accompanist available. Limited number of slots available.
For application, write to:
Northwest Drama Conference Auditions
Attn: David Krasner
Theatre Arts Dept.
University of Idaho
Moscow, ID 83843
Phone (208) 885-6465; Fax (208) 885-6911

OHIO THEATRE ALLIANCE (OTA)

Audition Date: Mid-February.
Place: Columbus, Ohio.
Eligibility: Non-Equity; must be OTA member and must be pre-registered.
Fee: Audition fee $25, money order or check; contact OTA for current membership rates.
Format: Two minutes; must bring taped accompaniment and player, if singing; callbacks are usually scheduled the same day. Interviews and short portfolio review for tech and management.
Application Deadline: Mid-January.

For application—usually available in late fall—send SASE to:
Ohio Theatre Alliance Auditions
77 S. High St., 2nd fl.
Columbus, OH 43215-6108
Phone (614) 228-1998; Fax (614) 241-5329

OUTDOOR DRAMA AUDITIONS
Audition Date: Mid-March (for one day).
Place: University of North Carolina at Chapel Hill, North Carolina.
Eligibility: Limited to 200 pre-registered applicants who must be at least 18, with previous theatre training or credits. For 15 to 18 companies; a few offer Equity contracts; most casts number about 50.
Fee: $15 nonrefundable application fee.
Format: For actors, one-minute monologue; for singers, one-minute song (accompanist provided); for dancers, choreographer will lead group warm-up and combinations using modern, ballet, and folk styles. Individual interviews for technicians.
For application, send SASE to:
Auditions Director
Institute of Outdoor Drama
CB 3240, NationsBank Plaza
University of North Carolina
Chapel Hill, NC 27599-3240
Phone (919) 962-1328; Fax (919) 962-4212

ROCKY MOUNTAIN THEATRE ASSOCIATION SUMMER THEATRE AUDITIONS
Audition Date: Mid-March (for one day).
Place: Varies within Idaho, Montana, Wyoming, Colorado, and Utah.
Eligibility: Application should include recommendation from teacher or director.
Fee: $15 student membership fee to join RMTA, plus $30 registration fee for "Festivention." Audition fee is $5 student.
Format: Three minutes for two contrasting monologues; may include 16 bars of song; tape deck provided. Interviews for tech/design/staff.
For application, see December issue of *Curtain Call*, or contact:
Daniel Guyette
108 Frasier Bldg.
Theatre Arts Dept., UNC
Greeley, CO 80639
Phone (303) 351-2225

SOUTHEASTERN THEATRE CONFERENCE (SETC)
Audition Date: Early March (for three days); part of SETC Convention. SETC also holds professional auditions in September; application deadline mid-August.
Place: Varies within Alabama, Florida, Georgia, Kentucky, Mississippi, North Carolina, South Carolina, Tennessee, Virginia, West Virginia.
Eligibility: Students must pass fall screening; forms available from college theatre department in early fall. Professionals should write directly to SETC in November/December.
Fee: Students—$15 membership, $15 registration, $10 audition fee; professionals—$40 membership, $35 registration, $10 audition fee.
Format: One and a half minutes for acting and singing; one minute for acting only or singing only. Separate dance auditions. Callbacks are the evening of the same day. Audition briefing at 9 AM the same day. Administrative and tech interviews also held, through Job Contact Service. (This service is available for all nonacting theatre jobs year-round, through monthly *Job Contact Bulletin* and at convention.)
Application Deadline: Early February.

For application, write to:
  Marian Smith
  Southeastern Theatre Conference
  P.O. Box 9868
  Greensboro, NC 27429-0868
  Phone (910) 272-3645

SOUTHWEST THEATRE ASSOCIATION (SWTA)

Audition Date: Mid-February (for one day).
Place: Varies within Arkansas, Louisiana, New Mexico, Oklahoma, Texas.
Eligibility: Union and nonunion.
Fee: Ranges from $15 to $20, depending on membership status in SWTA.
Format: One and a half minutes for acting, plus 16 bars or 30 seconds of a song.
Bring 20 to 25 picture/résumés for callbacks. Bring sheet music. Tapes accepted. For
tech/administration positions, bring portfolio for three-minute interview.
Application Deadline: Postmarked by early February.
For application, write to:
  Molly Risso
  Southwest Theatre Association Auditions
  P.O. Box 4209
  Southeastern State University
  Durant, OK 74701
  Phone (405) 924-0121, ext. 2216 or 2217

STRAWHAT AUDITIONS

Audition Date: West—mid-March (for three days); East—late March (for four days).
Place: West—Los Angeles area; East—Manhattan.
Eligibility: Open to any non-Equity performers, but some screening is done. No
standbys or walk-ins. Staff/design positions open to all by application.
Fee: Performers—$45 for East, $25 for West, $60 for both. Design/tech/staff—$15.
Format: Performers have two minutes to present one monologue and a musical
selection; accompanist provided. Limited number of nonsinging appointments are
also available. Callbacks are posted hourly. Staff/design interviews to be announced.
Application Deadline: Usually two to three weeks before auditions, but appointments
almost always fill up earlier.
Single application form to apply for either West, East, or both. For application, send
business-size SASE to:
  Strawhat
  P.O. Box 1189, Port Chester, NY 10573-8189
  No phone calls accepted.

THEATRE ALLIANCE OF MICHIGAN STATEWIDE PROFESSIONAL THEATRE AUDITIONS

Audition Date: Late February (for two days).
Place: Lansing, Michigan.
Eligibility: Must be at least 18 or in college.
Fee: $25.
Format: Each audition will be limited to two minutes and will include two
contrasting monologues; 16 bars of a song may be added after time limit. Optional
dance auditions. Tech interviews arranged.
Application Deadline: Mid-February.
For application, send SASE to:
  David Pritchard
  Theatre Alliance of Michigan
  Box 726
  Marshall, MI 49068
  Phone (616) 781-7859

THEATRE AUDITIONS IN WISCONSIN

Audition Date: Early to mid-February (one-day workshop, one-day auditions).
Place: Wisconsin Center, Madison, Wisconsin.
Eligibility: Non-Equity, no residency requirements.
Fee: $19.
Format: Actors, two minutes; actor–singers, two and a half minutes. Interviews for tech/design/administration.
Application Deadline: Pre-registration recommended by mid-January.
For application, send SASE to:
    Theatre Auditions in Wisconsin
    Continuing Education in the Arts
    Lowell Hall, Rm.726
    610 Langdon St.
    Madison, WI 53703
    Phone (608) 263-6736

THEATRE BAY AREA GENERAL AUDITIONS (TBA)

Audition Date: February.
Place: San Francisco (for 30 to 40 San Francisco/Bay Area companies).
Eligibility: Priority given to Equity-eligible performers or TBA members.
For information: Dates and all necessary registration information are available only in the October and November issues of *Callboard*. For membership information, write to:
    Theatre Bay Area
    657 Mission St., Suite 402
    San Francisco, CA 94105

UNIFIED PROFESSIONAL THEATRE AUDITIONS

Audition Date: Early February (for two days).
Place: Playhouse on the Square, Memphis, Tennessee.
Eligibility: Must meet at least one of the following criteria: Have a post-graduate degree in theatre (M.A., M.F.A., Ph.D., etc.); be Equity-eligible; have registration signed by a registered UPTA theatre.
Fee: $30, plus 50 copies of photo/résumé sent with registration.
Format: Auditions for acting and singing only, with no separate dance calls (although actors who wish to do so may dance in their audition). One and a half minutes to present a monologue or a monologue and a song.
For application, write to:
    Michael Detroit, Audition Coordinator
    Unified Professional Theatre Auditions
    51 S. Cooper St.
    Memphis, TN 38104
    Phone (901) 725-0776; Fax (901) 272-7530

UNIVERSITY/RESIDENT THEATRE ASSOCIATION (U/RTA) NATIONAL UNIFIED AUDITIONS

U/RTA, a consortium of professional training programs and resident theatre companies, hosts a series of auditions and interviews each year that lead to summer positions with resident companies and to acceptance into graduate programs at member universities, many of which are associated with professional companies. Actors must be nominated by the chair or department head of a college/university theatre program or by the producing director of a professional theatre. Candidates are screened by a panel of evaluators. A final audition is attended by representatives of U/RTA schools, theatres, and guest organizations.
Audition Date: Between late-January and early March.
Place: Held in New York City, Los Angeles, and Chicago.

Master Audition Programs (MAPs): A new set of professional auditions is available to third-year students and recent graduates of U/RTA–member M.F.A. programs. A select group of actors is provided the opportunity to audition before an an invited group of casting directors, agents, and other members of the profession. Contact U/RTA for details.

Application Deadline: Late November or mid-December with late fee.

For information, write to:

University/Resident Theatre Association, Inc.
1560 Broadway, Suite 903
New York, NY 10036
Phone (212) 221-1130

VERMONT ASSOCIATION OF THEATRES & THEATRE ARTISTS (VATTA)

Audition Date: Early March (for one day).

Place: St. Michael's College, Winooski, Vermont.

Eligibility: Equity or Non-Equity; first preference will be given to Vermont residents or students at VT colleges. If space is available, applicants from adjoining areas of New York, New Hampshire, and Massachusetts will be accepted. Not intended for New York City or Boston actors, for most Vermont companies participate in other auditions in those cities.

Fee: Performers—$10 for VATTA and/or Equity members and students; $20 for nonmembers. Design/tech/staff—$5 for VATTA members and students; $10 for nonmembers.

Format: Three minutes for two monologues or one monologue and one song; bring taped accompaniment. Design/tech/staff interviews at the end of the day.

Application Deadline: one week before auditions.

For application, write to:

Vermont Association of Theatres & Theatre Artists Auditions
c/o Greater Burlington Theatre Arts Exchange
P.O. Box 5193
Burlington, VT 05402

Theme Parks and Show Producers

The following is a selected listing, in alphabetical order, of key information for theme parks and theme park show producers. In some cases, the names given below the phone numbers are the people whom performers and technicians should contact; in most cases, they are the entertainment coordinators at the parks. An asterisk (*) designates a parent company.

ACTION PARK
P.O. Box 848
Vernon, NJ 07462
(201) 827-2000
Contact: Personnel Dept.

ALLAN ALBERT PRODUCTIONS
561 Broadway
New York, NY 10012
(212) or (800) 966-8881
Contact: Kathy Carney or Mark Hudson
Around 50 openings each year for both male and female dancers, singers, jugglers, magicians, etc. Allan Albert Productions does the casting for Hersheypark. The shows are mostly musical productions such as a 1950s rock 'n' roll show and a country music show. The company also casts an Italian improvisation show with performers who can sing, a cabaret doo-wop team, a two-man juggling and strolling show, and others.

ASTROWORLD
9001 Kirby Dr.
Houston, TX 77054
(713) 794-3232
Contact: Michael Svatek, Entertainment Dept.
Part of Six Flags Theme Parks Inc.

BUSCH GARDENS ENTERTAINMENT CORP.*
One Busch Gardens Blvd.
P.O. Box 8785
Williamsburg, VA 23187-8785
(800) 253-3302
Parks: Busch Gardens Tampa, Florida; Busch Gardens Williamsburg, Virginia; Cedar Point, Sandusky, Ohio; Cypress Gardens, Winter Haven, Florida; Sea World of California; Sea World of Florida, Orlando; Sea World of Ohio, Aurora; Sea World of Texas, San Antonio; Sesame Place, Langhorne, Pennsylvania.

BUSCH GARDENS TAMPA
P.O. Box 9158
Tampa, FL 33674
(813) 987-5164
Contact: Entertainment Dept.
Professional singers, dancers, musicians, actors, specialty performers, technicians, and support personnel. Comedy show, big band, ice show, the world talent showcase (acrobats, aerialists, jugglers, and comedians), and others.

BUSCH GARDENS WILLIAMSBURG
1 Busch Gardens Blvd.
Williamsburg, VA 23187
(804) 253-3305
Contact: Douglas Minerd, show production manager
In excess of 220 singers (all styles), dancers, actors, musicians, stage managers, technicians, and variety artists. The show package includes popular music, music from films and Broadway, country music, actors in comic street scenes, jazz and tap dance, Italian opera and popular music, German folk music, and dancing and special effects shows.

CEDAR POINT
P.O. Box 5006
Sandusky, OH 44871-8006
(419) 627-2388
Contact: Jay E. Emrich
Part of Busch Gardens Entertainment Corp.
There are over 100 positions available for singers, singer/dancers, musicians, technicians, costumed characters, and costume shop personnel. Dixieland jazz, contemporary country, pop, classic rock 'n' roll, Broadway, and swing.

CYPRESS GARDENS
P.O. Box 1
Cypress Gardens, FL
(813) 324-2111, ext. 233
Contact: Human Resources Dept.
Part of Busch Gardens Entertainment Corp.
Employs 12 singers and dancers.

DISNEYLAND
1313 Harbor Blvd.
P.O. Box 3232
Anaheim, CA 92803
(714) 490-7340 (auditions)
(714) 490-3258 (casting and booking)
Contact: J. Kevin Frawley, talent casting and booking manager

DORNEY PARK/WILDWATER KINGDOM
3830 Dorney Park Rd.
Allentown, PA 18104
(610) 391-7730
Contact: Park Attraction Office
Singers, singer-dancers, musicians, stitchers, technicians/stage managers, and choreographer. Mostly musical revues: country, Motown, rock 'n' roll.

EURO DISNEYLAND
Marne-La-Vallee, France
Inquiries: c/o Walt Disney World Resort (see page 291).
(407) 345-5701

FIESTA TEXAS
P.O. Box 690290
San Antonio, TX 78269-0290
(210) 697-5483
Contact: Entertainment Dept.
450 singers, dancers, musicians, actors, stage managers, and technical personnel. Twelve stage shows and a variety of strolling entertainment and specialty acts. Musical styles range from rock 'n' roll to country to conjunto and tejano. Show bands are also used.

HEARTBEAT PRODUCTIONS
832 So. Cooper St.
Memphis, TN 38104
(901) 278-0138
Contact: Melinda Grable, director of creative services
Corporate/special event productions; musical production shows for parks, casinos, and resorts; costume character touring shows.

HERSHEYPARK
100 West Hersheypark Dr.
Hershey, PA 17033
(717) 534-3177
Contact: Cherie Lingle, entertainment coordinator
See above: Allan Albert Productions

KNOTT'S BERRY FARM
8039 Beach Blvd.
P.O. Box 5002
Buena Park, CA 90620
Job Hotline: (714) 995-6688

OPRYLAND
2802 Opryland Dr.
Nashville, TN 37214
(800) 947-8243
Around 350 openings for singers, dancers, actors, specialty acts, strolling performers, staff conductors, pianists, instrumentalists, stage managers, and technicians every year. All productions include live music.

OSBORNE SHOWS
5118 Goodwin Ave.
Dallas, TX 75206
(214) 631-8414 (audition hotline January thru mid-April)
(214) 824-0128 (year-round)
Casts for Six Flags, Busch Gardens, and Knott's Berry Farm. Openings throughout U.S. and Europe every year. Singers, dancers, actors, musicians, variety acts, and performers with a background in animal training. Musical, magic, audience participation, stunt shows, and animal revues.

PARAMOUNT PARKS*
8731 Red Oak Blvd., Suite 200
Charlotte, NC 28217
(704) 522-9280
Contact: Entertainment Dept.
Parks: Paramount Canada's Wonderland, Vaughan, Ontario, Canada; Paramount's Carowinds, Charlotte, North Carolina; Paramount's Great America, Santa Clara, California; Paramount's Kings Dominion, Doswell, Virginia; Paramount's Kings Island, Cincinnati, Ohio.

PARAMOUNT CANADA'S WONDERLAND
P.O. Box 624
Vaughan, Ontario
Canada, L6A-1F6
(905) 832-7000
Contact: Barbara Granter
Employs singers, dancers, and actors.

PARAMOUNT'S CAROWINDS
P.O. Box 410289
Charlotte, NC 28241-0289
(704) 588-2606
Contact: Rob Sewell, entertainment manager
Employs singers, dancers, actors, and ice skaters.

PARAMOUNT'S GREAT AMERICA
1 Great America Parkway
Santa Clara, CA 95054
(408) 988-1776
Contact: Entertainment Dept.

PARAMOUNT'S KINGS DOMINION
P.O. Box 2000
Doswell, VA 23047-9988
(804) 876-5141
Contact: Paul Haught, manager of attractions

PARAMOUNT'S KINGS ISLAND
6300 Kings Island Dr.
Mason, OH 45040
(513) 573-5800
Contact: Entertainment Dept.

SEA WORLD OF CALIFORNIA
1720 S. Shores Rd.
San Diego, CA 92109
(619) 226-3900, ext. 2552
Contact: Virginia Creamer, Entertainment Dept.
Part of Busch Gardens Entertainment Corp.

SEA WORLD OF FLORIDA
7007 Sea World Dr.
Orlando, FL 32821
(407) 363-2309
Contact: Mike Eaton, manager
Part of Busch Gardens Entertainment Corp. Employs singers and dancers. One show: the Big Splash Bash.

SEA WORLD OF OHIO
1100 Sea World Dr.
Aurora, OH 44202
(216) 562-8101
Contact: Entertainment Dept.
Trainers, skiers, announcers. No song-and-dance shows. All other specialty acts are contracted out.

SEA WORLD OF TEXAS
10500 Sea World Dr.
San Antonio, TX 78251
(210) 523-3312
Contact: Bonnie Bento, show producer
Part of Busch Gardens Entertainment Corp. Street performers, costume characters, character dancers, and street performers for a children's musical show and street performances.

SESAME PLACE
100 Sesame Rd.
P.O. Box L579
Langhorne, PA 19047
(215) 752-7070, ext. 298
Contact: Michael Joyce/Entertainment Dept.
Part of Busch Gardens Entertainment Corp. Musicians, singers, actors, strolling entertainers, dancers, and theatre hosts/escorts. Children's theatre, a Muppet musical show, and the Chromakey show (where kids are "put" into a movie).

SHOW BIZ INTERNATIONAL
5142-B Old Boonville Highway
Evansville, IN 47715
(812) 473-0880
Contact: Maria A. Rivers, senior vice president; Michael Hawk, production assistant
Mostly singers and dancers, but also technicians, magicians, magician's assistants, children's theatre performers, and costume characters. There are over 350 positions available. Musical extravaganza, country–western revues, 1950s rock 'n' roll shows, Broadway revues, magic and illusion shows, Western shoot-outs, and others.

SILVER DOLLAR CITY
HC 1 Box 791
Branson, MO 65616
(417) 338-8084
Singers, dancers, comedic actors, variety artists, and instrumentalists. Six mainstage productions and numerous strolling shows. Performance styles include old time and contemporary country, bluegrass, gospel, Broadway, and Western swing.

SIX FLAGS THEME PARKS INC.*
1168 113th St.
Grand Prairie, TX 75050
(214) 647-8257
Parks: Astroworld, Houston, Texas; Great Adventure, Jackson, New Jersey; Great America, Gurnee, Illinois; Magic Mountain, Valencia, California; Over Georgia, Atlanta; Over Mid-America, Eureka, Missouri; Over Texas, Arlington.

SIX FLAGS GREAT ADVENTURE
P.O. Box 120
Jackson, NJ 08527
(908) 928-2000, ext. 2110
Contact: Michael Korzenok
Dance shows in the streets and in Bugs Bunny Land.

SIX FLAGS GREAT AMERICA
P.O. Box 1776
Gurnee, IL 60031
(708) 249-1776, ext. 4606
Contact: Entertainment Dept.

SIX FLAGS MAGIC MOUNTAIN
Valencia, CA
All parks shows are contracted out. Interested parties should contact:

YLS PRODUCTIONS
P.O. Box 34
Los Alamitos, CA 90720
(310) 430-2890

Or contact:
TOTALLY FUN COMPANY
600 Cleveland St.
Clearwater, FL 34615
(813) 446-8811

For bodysuit and street entertainers:
A. AND R. WALD PRODUCTIONS
P.O. Box 5500
Valencia, CA 91385
(805) 255-4859

SIX FLAGS OVER GEORGIA
P.O. Box 43187
Atlanta, GA 30378
(404) 739-3407
Contact: M.F. Noland Jr. or Torre Stanfill
Singer/dancers, show character performers, stunt performers, and gunfighters. A contemporary country show, a '50s revue, Bugs Bunny's World Games, a Wild West gunfight show, a special Halloween music show, and the Batman stunt show.

SIX FLAGS OVER MID-AMERICA
I-44 & Allenton Rd.
P.O. Box 60
Eureka, MO 63025
(314) 938-5300
Contact: Therese Bargman, Entertainment Dept.

SIX FLAGS OVER TEXAS
P.O. Box 191
Arlington, TX 76010
(817) 640-8900
Contact: Ext. 501
Costume character dancers and singers.

TOKYO DISNEYLAND
Inquiries: c/o Walt Disney World Resort (see below).
(407) 345-5701

UNIVERSAL STUDIOS FLORIDA
1000 Universal Studios Plaza
Orlando, FL 32819-7610
(407) 363-8795
Contact: Entertainment Dept.
Actors, stunt performers, celebrity lookalikes with improvisation skills, singer/dancers. Comedy, stunt, musical, improvisation.

WALT DISNEY WORLD RESORT*
P.O. Box 10000
Lake Buena Vista, FL 32830-1000
Audition Hotline: (407) 345-5701
Dancers, singers, male and female actors with athletic skills, and specialty performers. A variety of musical and non-musical opportunities (including improv) are available at the Magic Kingdom, Epcot Center, Disney-MGM Studios, and Pleasure Island. Performances at the parks themselves include stunt shows and mainstage musicals, among others.

WORLDS OF FUN
4545 Worlds of Fun Ave.
Kansas City, MO 64161
(816) 454-4545, ext. 1350
Singers and dancers. Contemporary country music, and 1960s rock.

Cruise Line Agents and Producers

Many cruise lines hire a booking agent to create an entertainment package for a particular cruise. Some work exclusively with one agent; others use several agents; still others use both booking agents and their own in-house entertainment directors to fill their performance needs. Agents and entertainment directors, in turn, may book revues, acts, or shows produced by an independent production company. Performers interested in cruise work, no matter what their specialty, should introduce themselves to cruise agents and producers. The following list is compiled from information gathered from several established cruise agents, producers, and lines.

ALFORD PRODUCTIONS INC.
P.O. Box 21029
New York, NY 10129-0009
Producer/Director: Larry Alford
Produces song and dance revues for Holland America Line, Commodore Cruise Line (Broadway, popular music, 1930s and '40s revues). Hires strong singers who dance for four-month standard contract. No open calls. Accepts agent submissions, or send picture and résumé. Do not send tapes.

BIG BEAT PRODUCTIONS
1515 University Dr., Suite 108A
Coral Springs, FL 33071
(305) 755-7759
President: Richard Lloyd
Books musical groups, bands, and comedians for Carnival, Norwegian, Sun Line, Discovery, Premier, and Royal Caribbean. Send video or audiotape, picture, and playlist.

BRAMSON ENTERTAINMENT BUREAU
1501 Broadway, Suite 2300
New York, NY 10036
(212) 354-9575
President: James Abramson
Largest booking organization for cruise work. Books comedians, "big name" entertainers, instrumentalists, novelty acts, singers, musicians. Books shows and revues from independent producers. Books for cruise lines such as Cunard, Holland America, Ocean Cruise, Crystal, and Royal Cruise. Accepts videotapes.

GARRY BROWN ASSOCIATES
27 Downs Side
Cheam, Surrey
SM2 7EH England
011-44-181-643-8375
Agent: Garry Brown
Books variety acts, stars, revues, other entertainment for Cunard and other lines. Holds showcases in New York and other major cities seeking talent. Notices placed in Back Stage. *Accepts pictures, tapes, and videos (American, English, European VHS).*

DON CASINO PRODUCTIONS
19511 N.E. 19th Ct.
N. Miami Beach, FL 33179
(305) 935-0137
Casts male and female singers, stand-up comics, novelty acts, novelty instrumentalists, and impressionists. Videos with pictures and résumés are accepted.

FIESTA FANTASTICA
230 S.W. 8th St.
Miami, FL 33130
(305) 854-2221
Producer: Marcelo Palacios; Director of Operations: Joe Israel
Books individual singers and dancers for revues (no variety, specialty, or solo acts) for Holland America, Carnival, and Princess cruise lines. Holds open calls in New York, Los Angeles, Boston, and Chicago. Send pictures, résumés, and videotapes to Casting Department.

GAYLE FORCE ENTERTAINMENT, INC.
11755 Addison St.
Valley Village, CA 91607
(818) 755-0667
Producer: Daniel Heller
Produces revue shows for Holland America. Works with dancers and singers who can dance. Accepts pictures, résumés, videos, and audiotapes.

KENNEDY ENTERTAINMENT
244 S. Academy St.
Mooresville, NC 28115
(704) 662-3501
Producer: Ray Kennedy
Produces revue shows for Cunard, Palm Beach Cruises, and other lines. Works with singer-dancers only on musical revues. Accepts pictures, résumés, and videotapes. Holds seasonal auditions in New York.

ANITA MANN PRODUCTIONS
2500 Santa Monica Blvd.
Santa Monica, CA 90404
(310) 450-7043
Producer: Anita Mann; Vice President: Beverly Jeanne
Produces original revues. Shows for cruise lines, industrials, resorts, and television. Cruise lines include Holland America and Royal Caribbean Cruises. Style of show ranges from Broadway to contemporary. Year-round hiring of strong singers and dancers with major auditions held two to three times a year. Hires novelty acts and technical staff. Send picture, résumé, and videotape to casting department.

HANNA OWEN ENTERTAINMENT AGENCY
22600 Bella Rita Circle
Boca Raton, FL 33433
(305) 462-3750
Owner/President: Hanna Owen
Books for Cunard and other lines. Interested in many types of highly experienced professional performers including opera singers, Broadway or Top-40 singers, novelty acts, and comedians. Accepts pictures, résumés, and recent videotapes. Will not return tapes or material. Submissions from professionals with extensive experience only.

PRODUCTION CENTRAL
2500 W. Olive Ave., Suite 1420
Burbank, CA 91505
(818) 955-7077
President: Allen J. Sviridoff
Produces shows for Holland America Line and others. Send pictures and résumés.

JEAN ANN RYAN PRODUCTIONS
308 S.E. 14th St.
Fort Lauderdale, FL 33316
(305) 523-6399
Producer: Jean Ann Ryan; Vice President: Joanne Maiello
Produces revues and Broadway-style productions for Norwegian Cruise Line. Producing The Will Rogers Follies, S.S. Norway; *Grease,* M.S. Seaward; *Dreamgirls,* M.S. Dreamward; *and* George M!, M.S. Windward. *Also books Las Vegas–style revues and singers for these and four smaller ships. Cabaret and novelty acts booked, as well as illusionists. Hires technical staff. Major audition tours twice each year. Contracts for three to six months. Send picture, résumé, and video/audiotape.*

PETER GREY TERHUNE PRESENTS
P.O. Box 32920
Cape Canaveral, FL 32920
(407) 783-8745
Co-Producers: Peter Grey Terhune and Cathy Abram Terhune
Produces custom revues, shows for cruise lines, industrials, and resorts. Currently producing musical revues for Radisson Seven Seas Cruises, Silversea Cruises, Royal Caribbean Cruise Line, Regency Cruises, and Cunard Line. Shows booked by Bramson Entertainment or independently with cruise lines. Auditions in New York, Los Angeles, Chicago, Nashville, and several colleges and universities in Florida. Send pictures, résumés, and tapes to Jeanine Dwinell.

GREG THOMPSON PRODUCTIONS
921 Elliott Ave. W.
Seattle, WA 98119
(206) 281-0885
President: Greg Thompson
Books and produces musical revues for Celebrity Cruises. Works on a two-show concept: Early show is family-oriented Broadway or Hollywood fare, late show is hotter MTV-style revue. Casts regionally with open calls. Accepts pictures, résumés, audio and video submissions.

CRUISE LINES

Many cruise lines hire entertainment directors to handle bookings for their ships. The responsibilities of these people vary from line to line and from season to season. They may book talent either directly or through agents. Even if you have written to the cruise agents and producers on the preceding list, it might be wise to contact those cruise lines which interest you. The following lines regularly seek and provide entertainment for their patrons.

CARNIVAL CRUISE LINES
3655 NW 87th Ave.
Miami, FL 33178
(305) 599-2600
Hires musicians, sidemen, duos, trios, dancers, magicians, and comedians. Send promotional package including picture, résumé, and demo tape to Entertainment Department.

CELEBRITY CRUISES, INC.
Fantasy Cruises
5200 Blue Lagoon Dr.
Miami, FL 33126
(305) 262-6677
Books a broad spectrum of acts: vocalists, comedians, magicians, jugglers, hypnotists, and ventriloquists. Revues are produced in-house and by Greg Thompson Productions of Seattle and Matrix Entertainment of London. Send picture, résumé, and videotape to Bret Bullock, Director of Entertainment.

COMMODORE CRUISE LINE
800 Douglas Rd., Suite 600
Coral Gables, FL 33134
(305) 529-3000
Send picture, résumé, and a videotape to Pia Lang, Director of Entertainment, for headliners, duos, trios, and island-style bands.

COSTA CRUISE LINES
c/o CSCS
100 South Biscayne Blvd., Suite 700
Miami, FL 33131
(305) 377-4510
Director of Entertainment: Jim D'Amico; Manager of Entertainment: Brian Lunsford
Italian cruise line sailing worldwide hires dancers, choreographers, magicians, novelty acts, and vocalists. Accepts pictures, résumés, and videotapes.

CRYSTAL CRUISES
2121 Avenue of the Stars, Suite 200
Los Angeles, CA 90067
(310) 785-9300
All entertainers are directed to an employment hotline that instructs applicants to submit a videotape to Pete Johnson at the Los Angeles address.

CUNARD LINE
555 Fifth Ave.
New York, NY 10017
Books through Jean Ann Ryan Productions, Garry Brown Associates, Spotlight Entertainment, Hanna Owen Entertainment Agency, and Bramson Entertainment Bureau.

DELTA QUEEN STEAMBOAT CO.
30 Robin Street Wharf
New Orleans, LA 70130-1890
(504) 586-0631
Director of Entertainment: Bill Szymanski; Entertainment Manager: Nancy Gros
Hires performers directly including musicians (especially banjo, ragtime, and piano) and singers who dance (these positions perform staff and managerial duties as well). Contract is usually one year with rotation. Accepts pictures, résumés, and tapes.

HOLLAND AMERICA LINE
300 Elliott Ave. W.
Seattle, WA 98119
(206) 281-3535
Director of Entertainment: Bill Prince
Hires singers, magicians, jugglers, and other specialty acts directly. Videotape or agent submissions only. Books production shows through Anita Mann Productions, Production Central, and Gayle Force Productions in Los Angeles. Contact them for audition information.

MAJESTY CRUISE LINE
Dolphin Cruise Line
901 South America Way
Miami, FL 33132
(305) 358-5122
Entertainment Manager: Vilma Moutsatsou; Production Manager: Jacqui Gibbs
Hires singers, comedians, magicians, jugglers, pianists, duos, and other variety acts directly through Entertainment Manager. In-house producer Jacqui Gibbs

auditions, casts, and develops musical revues around Broadway and Hollywood themes.

NORWEGIAN CRUISE LINE
95 Merrick Way
Coral Gables, FL 33134
(305) 447-9660
Manager of Entertainment: Sue Carper
Jean Ann Ryan Productions functions as in-house production department for musical revues and full-scale Broadway-style shows. Also books outside shows and variety acts. Accepts pictures, résumés, tapes, and agent submissions.

PREMIER CRUISE LINES
400 Challenger Rd.
Cape Canaveral, FL 32920
(407) 783-5061
Entertainment Director: Michael Moore
Casts through independent producers for musical revues. Also books comedians and novelty acts. Promotional material may be forwarded to Entertainment Director.

PRINCESS CRUISES
Entertainment Department
10100 Santa Monica Blvd.
Los Angeles, CA 90067
(310) 553-1770
Director of Entertainment: Rai Caluori
Production shows are generated in-house. Auditions held periodically all over the country. Send videotapes to Fabian Gomez (dancers) or Martin Hall (cabaret and specialty acts).

RADISSON SEVEN SEAS CRUISES
600 Corporate Dr., Suite 410
Ft. Lauderdale, FL 33334
(305) 776-6123
Director of Programming: Jim Cannon
Send publicity pack before calling.

REGENCY CRUISES
260 Madison Ave., 9th fl.
New York, NY 10016
(212) 972-4774
Entertainment Director: Paul McEvoy
Hires production groups, dancers, comedians, and novelty acts. Casting through independent producers, agents, or direct submissions. Entertainers also work as cruise staff.

ROYAL CARIBBEAN CRUISE LINE
1050 Caribbean Way
Miami, FL 33132
(305) 539-6000
Produces revues in-house with casts ranging in size from 10 to 16, featuring singers, dancers, and singer-dancers. Six-month contracts. Annual audition tour goes to New York, Los Angeles, Chicago, Boston, Toronto, London, and several smaller cities. Prefers live audition to videotape. Submit picture and résumé to Mary Ann Delaney, Production Supervisor.

ROYAL CRUISE LINE
95 Merrick Way
Coral Gables, FL 33134
(305) 460-4793
Manager of Entertainment and Cruise Programs: Ms. Morag Veljkovic
Hires variety and cabaret-type acts: comics, ventriloquists, classical artists, jugglers, vocalists, and instrumentalists. Produces production shows, hires production casts. Talent booked directly, as well as through agencies worldwide.

SEABOURN CRUISE LINE
55 Francisco St.
San Francisco, CA 94133
(415) 391-7444
Books only self-contained acts such as cabaret artists, instrumentalists, and comedians. No revues. Send press kit and videotape to Director of Entertainment.

SEAESCAPE CRUISES LTD.
140 S. Federal Hwy., 2nd fl.
Dania, FL 33004
(305) 925-9700
Hires singer-dancers for four different 45-minute revues—two shows per day, seven days per week. Entertainers live on ship with crew. Uses in-house production department. Send pictures, tapes, and/or résumés to the attention of Entertainment Department. Do not call.

SILVERSEA CRUISES
110 E. Broward Blvd.
Ft. Lauderdale, FL 33301
(305) 522-4477
Books all entertainment through Matrix Entertainment in London.

SUN LINE CRUISES
1 Rockefeller Plaza, Suite 315
New York, NY 10020
(212) 397-6400
Entertainment Director: Tina Smith
*Hires singers, dancers, dance groups,
comedians, and magicians for Caribbean
and European cruises.*

WORLD EXPLORER CRUISES
555 Montgomery St., Suite 1400
San Francisco, CA 94111-2544
(415) 393-1565
*Hires classically trained musicians and
singers exclusively. Two-week cruises
feature concerts and lectures on art,
anthropology, botany, and geology of
Pacific Northwest. May–September season.
Contact Ron Valentine, Director of
Operations.*

Presenters' Conferences

Performers who wish to book their own shows can contact the following groups, which organize presenters' conferences. They are not talent agents or talent representatives, and they do not accept headshots or related materials. They can, however, give information about how performers can participate in these events.

THE ASSOCIATION OF PERFORMING ARTS
PRESENTERS
112 16th St., N.W., Suite 400
Washington, DC 20036
(202) 833-2787

MIDWEST ARTS CONFERENCE
c/o Arts Midwest
528 Hennepin Ave., Suite 310
Minneapolis, MN 55403
(612) 341-0755

NATIONAL ASSOCIATION FOR CAMPUS
ACTIVITIES
13 Harbison Way
Columbia, SC 29212-3401
(800) 845-2338

NORTHEAST PERFORMING ARTS
CONFERENCE
c/o New England Presenters
2 Curry Hicks
University of Massachusetts
Amherst, MA 01003-1810
(413) 545-0190

PRODUCERS ASSOCIATION OF CHILDREN'S
THEATRE
c/o Theatreworks/USA
890 Broadway
New York, NY 10003
(No phone calls, please)

SOUTHERN ARTS EXCHANGE
c/o Southern Arts Federation
181 14th St., N.E., Suite 400
Atlanta, GA 30309
(404) 874-7244

WESTERN ALLIANCE OF ARTS
ADMINISTRATORS
44 Page St., Suite 604B
San Francisco, CA 94102
(415) 621-4400

Contributors

Jonathan Abarbanel is a Chicago-based theatre critic and arts business reporter. His work appears regularly in the Dramatists Guild Newsletter and in *TheaterWeek, American Theatre, Variety, Stagebill,* and *Show Music.* In Chicago, he is theatre critic for *North Shore* and *Premiere Chicago* magazines, arts business reporter for *Screen* magazine and *PerformInk,* a theatrical trade paper. He has written special material for CBS and PBS, and sales, training, and corporate image scripts.

Ben Alexander was a copy editor for *Back Stage* from 1991 to 1994. An aspiring playwright, he has been produced Off-Off-Broadway. His works include *The Dance of the Fireflies* and *Phantom Rep.*

Jill Charles is co-author, with photographer Tom Bloom, of *The Actors' Picture/Résumé Book* and is the editor of the annual *Summer Theatre Directory.* She is artistic director of the Dorset Theatre Festival in Vermont, which she co-founded 20 years ago, since which time she estimates that she has looked at about 40,000 picture/résumés.

Maureen Clarke is formerly an associate director of the Riverside Shakespeare Company, in New York City, where she worked for ten years as a teacher, director, verse coach, and casting consultant. She has acted and directed at theatres in New York, Boston, and Denver, and has been writing for *Back Stage* since 1980.

Donna Coe is a former stand-up comic who is currently the comedy columnist for New York's *Daily News* and *Back Stage,* and contributes regularly to various other publications.

Amy Hersh has been staff reporter for *Back Stage* since 1990. Her articles on the performing arts have also appeared in the *Los Angeles Times,* the *Boston Globe, The Christian Science Monitor, New York Newsday, TheaterWeek,* and other publications. Her one-act play, "The Interview," was excerpted in *The Best Men's Stage Monologues of 1993.*

John Hoglund is a contributing cabaret columnist and features writer for *Back Stage,* among other publications. He serves on the board of directors of the Manhattan Association of Cabarets and Clubs and is a member of the Society of Singers. For several years, he worked in Los Angeles as a script doctor on television shows. He has produced many fundraising events for AIDS organizations and other charities. Current projects include a memoir on the life of cabaret legend Sylvia Syms and a biography of Morgana King.

Simi Horwitz is a cultural reporter covering TV, theatre, and books for such publications as the *Washington Post, Variety, Back Stage, TheaterWeek,* and *Opera Monthly,* among others. For the *Washington Post's* "TV Week," she writes news features, profiles, and criticism. For other publications, she covers trends, behind-the-scenes events, and personalities.

Jeffrey Eric Jenkins is a columnist and critic for *Back Stage* and *Back Stage West.* Based in Seattle, he teaches directing at the University of Washington and is serving a three-year appointment as editor of *Athenews.* Over the course of his career, he has directed 28 productions. He holds an M.F.A. degree in Directing from Carnegie-Mellon University.

Michèle LaRue is senior editor at *Back Stage,* with which she has been associated in various capacities for 15 years. Her multifaceted career has also included freelancing as a writer and editor for *Theatre Crafts* (now *TCI*), where she has focused on architecture, costume, and stage design. A member of Actors' Equity since 1976 and of SAG and AFTRA, she has toured extensively, most notably with two one-woman shows. She performs frequently with The East Lynne Company, which specializes in 19th-century American works.

Roberta Lawrence is a New York–based writer, songwriter, and singer. She has written lyrics for jingles, sung for many others, and produced a top-selling crossover jazz record, *Nightwind,* on which she is a featured singer. She has written about music for *Back Stage, Shoot, Musician,* and *ASCAP in Action.* She is currently at work on a novella about the music business.

Esther Tolkoff, an avid museum buff, writes for *Back Stage* and AFTRA publications, as well as for several universities and other organizations. She has contributed to the *New York Times, Seventeen,* and other periodicals. For fifteen years, she was associate editor of *New York Teacher,* where she won several awards. She has performed her own comedy monologue, and has also appeared in independent films and at small theatres in the New York area.

Thomas Walsh is a staff reporter for *Variety* and *Daily Variety* in New York. From 1986 to 1994, he was on the *Back Stage* editorial staff, where his role evolved from part-time proofreader to senior editor, with lots of events in between. He has written for the *New York Times, SportsChannel, Cosmopolitan,* and many others.

Marcia Anne Wood is an actress and singer who has worked in film, television, Off-Broadway, regional, dinner, stock, and children's theatre. A psychoanalyst and former managing editor of *Modern Drama* and of *Psychoanalysis and Psychotherapy,* she is working on a psychoanalytically oriented book for performing artists. She is on the staff of the Institute for the Performing Artist in New York.

Index